N. Brill

Cash's Textbook of Physiotherapy in some Surgical Conditions

other books in the series edited by Joan E. Cash

NEUROLOGY FOR PHYSIOTHERAPISTS

other books in the series edited by Patricia A. Downie

CASH'S TEXTBOOK OF CHEST, HEART AND VASCULAR DISORDERS FOR PHYSIOTHERAPISTS

CASH'S TEXTBOOK OF MEDICAL CONDITIONS FOR PHYSIOTHERAPISTS

by Patricia A. Downie

CANCER REHABILITATION
An Introduction for Physiotherapists and the Allied Professions

CASH'S TEXTBOOK OF PHYSIOTHERAPY IN SOME SURGICAL CONDITIONS

edited by
PATRICIA A. DOWNIE F.C.S.P.

FABER & FABER · London and Boston

First published in 1955
by Faber and Faber Limited
Second impression 1955
Second edition 1958
Third edition 1966
Reprinted 1967
Reprinted with minor revisions 1968
Fourth edition 1971
Fifth edition 1977
Sixth edition 1979

Set, printed and bound in Great Britain by
Fakenham Press Limited,
Fakenham, Norfolk

British Library Cataloguing in Publication Data

Cash, Joan Elizabeth
    Cash's textbook of physiotherapy in some
    surgical conditions. – 6th ed.
    1. Physical therapy
    I. Downie, Patricia A   II. Physiotherapy
    in some surgical conditions
    617'.919   RM700

    ISBN 0–571–04997–4

Contents

LIST OF CONTRIBUTORS   page 13

FOREWORD TO THE FIRST EDITION
by Professor F. A. R. Stammers, C.B.E., T.D.,
B.SC., M.B., CH.M., F.R.C.S.   15

PREFACE   17

1. USING MEDICAL LIBRARIES
by Mr. D. W. C. Stewart, B.A., A.L.A.   19

2. AN INTRODUCTION TO GENERAL SURGICAL CARE
by Miss P. A. Downie, F.C.S.P.   29

3. COMPLICATIONS FOLLOWING SURGERY
by Miss K. M. Thompson, M.C.S.P.   45

4. CARDIAC ARREST AND RESUSCITATION
by Mr. J. R. Pepper, M.A., F.R.C.S.   57

5. GYNAECOLOGICAL CONDITIONS
by Mrs. S. M. Harrison, M.C.S.P.   62

6. HEAD AND NECK SURGERY
revised by Miss P. A. Downie, F.C.S.P.   93

7. PLASTIC SURGERY
by Miss S. Boardman, M.C.S.P.
and Miss P. M. Walker, M.C.S.P.   108

8. AMPUTATIONS
by Miss B. C. Davis, M.C.S.P., H.T., O.N.C.   133

9. INJURIES TO SOFT TISSUES – I   161

10. INJURIES TO SOFT TISSUES – II   183

11. THE PHYSIOTHERAPIST'S APPROACH TO ATHLETIC AND
SPORTS INJURIES   202

12. MULTIPLE INJURIES   206

13. FRACTURES
    by Miss M. K. Patrick, O.B.E., M.C.S.P.   page 210

14. ADVANCED REHABILITATION
    by Miss S. H. McLaren, M.C.S.P.,
    DIP. PHYS. ED. (LOND. AND LIV.)   256

15. CRANIAL SURGERY   271

16. SPINAL SURGERY
    revised by Miss P. A. Dawe, M.A.P.A.   321

    GLOSSARY   357

    LIST OF USEFUL ORGANISATIONS   359

    INDEX   361

Illustrations

PLATES

6/1(a&b)	A patient who has undergone hemi-mandibulectomy	page 100
7/1	Wiring and splinting for jaw fractures	116
7/2(a&b)	Kleinet type splint	119
7/3(a.b.c.)	Rheumatoid hands before and after surgery	123
8/1	Below-knee amputees wearing patellar tendon bearing prostheses	137
8/2	Left below-knee amputation – exercise for unaffected leg	141
8/3	Left below-knee amputee – 'bridging'	141
8/4 8/5 8/6 8/7	Double below-knee amputee practising rolling to sitting with resistance	142
8/8	Weight and pulley work for amputees	144
8/9	Bilateral below-knee amputee practising 'push-ups' for upper limbs	144
8/10	The component parts of the pneumatic pylon (PPAM AID)	148
8/11	Patient walking partial weight-bearing on PPAM AID	149
8/12	Right above-knee amputee on pylon	151
8/13 8/14	Double below-knee amputee on pylons	153 154
8/15	Double above-knee amputee on short rocker pylons	155
8/16	Double above-knee amputee climbing stairs	155
8/17	Patient receiving controlled environment treatment (CET)	156
8/18	Posterior view of above-elbow prosthesis	159
8/19	Anterior view showing strap to operate elbow lock	159

8/20	Close-up of split hook	page 159
13/1	Comminuted fracture of upper tibia and lower femur	211
13/2	Internal fixation of the ulna by a Rush nail	220
13/3	Special caliper used with the A.O. method of treating fractures of the tibia	225
13/4	Impacted fracture of neck of humerus	229
13/5	Monteggia's fracture of radius and ulna	229
13/6(a&b)	Colles' fracture	236
13/7	Bennett's fracture	237
13/8(a.b. c.&d.)	Fractures of the shafts of the tibia and fibula before and after plating	242
13/9	Fracture of lateral malleolus with no displacement of joint mortice	246
13/10	Pott's fracture of both malleoli, with disruption of joint mortice	247

FIGURES

2/1	Cough hold in bed following abdominal surgery	32
2/2	Cough hold sitting in a chair following abdominal surgery	32
2/3	A 'cough-belt'	33
2/4	A patient using a 'cough-belt'	33
2/5	Surgical incisions	35
4/1	Diagram to illustrate the effects of a low cardiac output	59
5/1	The position and relations of the uterus	63
5/2	The ligaments of the cervix	63
5/3	Coronal section of the uterus	64
5/4	The Fallopian tubes	64
5/5	The trigone of the bladder	65
5/6	Lateral view of the pelvic diaphragm	65
5/7	The levator ani muscles	66
5/8	The urethrovesical angles	66
5/9	The superficial muscles of the perineum	68
5/10	Shirodkhar suture	71
5/11	Abdominal incisions used in gynaecological surgery	73
5/12	Cystocele	81
5/13	Urethrocele	81
5/14	Prolapse of the uterus	82

6/1	Lateral view of right facial nerve	page 94
6/2	A strength-duration curve	97
6/3	The nasal sinuses	104
6/4	Cross-fire technique for short wave diathermy to nasal sinuses	105
6/5	Cough hold following thyroidectomy	106
7/1	Skin grafts in relation to layers of the skin	109
7/2	Transposition flap	111
7/3	Abdominal to wrist pedicle	112
7/4	Cross-leg flap	113
7/5	Delto-pectoral flap	114
7/6	Mallet finger	120
7/7	Swan neck deformity of finger	122
7/8	Boutonnière deformity of finger	122
7/9	Surgical treatment of syndactyly	124
7/10	Diagrammatic representation of Thompson's operation	127
7/11	Z-plasty	131
8/1	Bandaging technique for above-knee amputation	145
8/2	Bandaging technique for below-knee amputation	147
9/1	Diagram illustrating reverse scapulo-humeral movement	166
9/2	Diagram illustrating frozen shoulder	167
9/3	Diagram illustrating the significance of pain at certain points of straight leg raising	175
10/1	Posture adopted by a patient with a right-sided nerve irritation	199
13/1	Compression plating	219
14/1	Diagrammatic representation of restoration to health following an accident	258
14/2	Diagram illustrating challenge for patients with painful hands, arms or shoulders	267
14/3	Patient in prone kneeling in preparation for a hip and spine flexion exercise (to mobilise joints following removal of plaster jacket or the equivalent)	267
14/4–14/8	Diagrams illustrating exercises to be avoided	
14/4	Two patients sitting back to back with both arms linked and pulling in opposite directions	268
14/5	Two patients acting as wheelbarrows	268

14/6	Leap-frog	page 269
14/7	Somersaults	269
14/8	Double leg raising	269
15/1	Lateral view of the brain	273
15/2	Sagittal section of the brain	274
15/3	Diagrammatic representation of some of the cortical areas of the brain	274
15/4	The motor homunculus superimposed on the pre-central gyrus	274
15/5	Diagram to show the effects of injury on the visual pathway	277
15/6	Diagrammatic representation of the brain in cross-section	279
15/7	Anterior view of the brain stem and cranial nerves	280
15/8	Right antero-lateral view of the dissected cerebellar hemisphere and peduncles	282
15/9	The circulation of the cerebrospinal fluid	286
15/10	Neck retraction	294
15/11	Extensor (decerebrate) rigidity	294
15/12	Some supratentorial surgical approaches	297
15/13	Surgical approaches to the posterior fossa	298
15/14	Diagrams of atraumatic suction catheters	301
15/15	Common sites for aneurysms	303
15/16(a&b)	Tumour of the right cerebello-pontine angle	313
15/17	Diagram showing the position of the burr hole in stereotaxic surgery for Parkinsonism	316
15/18	Projections of some pain pathways	319
16/1	The meninges	321
16/2	Cross-section of the cervical spinal cord	322
16/3	Spinal cord segments and spinal nerves	323
16/4	Ascending and descending spinal cord tracts	325
16/5	Dermatomes and scleratomes of the upper limb	326
16/6	Dermatomes and scleratomes of the lower limb	327
16/7	Sites and types of spinal tumour	333
16/8	Lumbar intervertebral disc herniations	340
16/9	A shaped foam neck and head support	349
16/10	Various surgical procedures designed to alleviate pain	352

Contributors

MISS S. BOARDMAN, M.C.S.P.
Senior Physiotherapist, Plastic Surgery and Burns Unit
Mount Vernon Hospital, Northwood HA6 2RN

MISS B. C. DAVIS, M.C.S.P., H.T., O.N.C.
Superintendent Physiotherapist, D.H.S.S. Limb Fitting Centre,
Queen Mary's Hospital, Roehampton, London SW15 5PN

MISS P. A. DAWE, M.A.P.A.
Senior Physiotherapist, Department of Surgical Neurology,
Western General Hospital, Edinburgh EH4 2XU

MRS. S. M. HARRISON, M.C.S.P.
Part-time Physiotherapist, The John Radcliffe Hospital,
Oxford OX3 9DU

MISS S. H. MCLAREN, M.C.S.P., DIP. PHYS. ED. (LOND. AND LIV.)
Superintendent Physiotherapist,
The Hermitage Rehabilitation Centre, Chester-le-Street,
Co. Durham DH2 3RF

MISS M. K. PATRICK, O.B.E., M.C.S.P.
District Superintendent Physiotherapist, The General Hospital,
Birmingham B4 6HH

J. R. PEPPER ESQ., M.A., F.R.C.S.
Senior Registrar, Thoracic Unit,
Guy's Hospital, London SE1 9RT

D. W. C. STEWART ESQ., B.A., A.L.A.
Librarian, The Royal Society of Medicine,
London W1M 8AE

MISS K. M. THOMPSON, M.C.S.P.
Formerly Senior Physiotherapist,
Bristol Royal Infirmary, Bristol BS2 8HW

Foreword to First Edition

With the rapid advances that have taken place during the past ten years in anaesthesia, blood transfusion services, chemotherapy, including antibiotics, together with a better understanding of the response of the body to trauma, all surgical procedures have been rendered freer from danger or complication. At the same time, enormous progress has been made by the newer specialities of neurosurgery, plastic surgery and thoracic surgery, the latter more recently embracing several common lesions of the heart. Therapeutically, therefore, surgery has more to offer today than ever before, and physiotherapy has contributed greatly to these exciting developments. It has evolved special pre- and postoperative treatments and exercises, not only for these new procedures, but also for the more orthodox type of operation, and in these latter has minimised the risks of postoperative chest complications and venous thrombosis.

Miss Cash is working in full co-operation with the surgeons at a hospital where all these growing points of surgery are represented and practised, and where, every day, much new knowledge is being gained. It is right and proper, then, that she should record in book form the points of her wide experience and new ideas. Her former book *A Textbook of Medical Conditions for Physiotherapists* dealt mainly with medical ward problems: the present volume is particularly for use in connection with surgical treatment. It is authoritative and right up-to-date, and contains sections on the breast, lungs, heart, abdomen, peripheral vascular disease, kidneys, etc. It will, therefore, fill a much wanted need, and should be as popular as her other book.

F. A. R. STAMMERS

Preface to Sixth Edition

For 25 years this book, like its companion volume on Medical Conditions, has been edited by Joan Cash. Countless numbers of physiotherapists throughout the world have come to be immensely grateful to her for the foresight in first writing the volumes herself and in later years co-ordinating a team of specialists. It is my privilege to continue this tradition and this new edition reflects both the ideas of Joan Cash as well as a number of my own.

I am particularly grateful to Mr. David Stewart, the Librarian of the Royal Society of Medicine, for producing such a succinct and lucid chapter on 'Using Medical Libraries' together with an introduction to the use of references. Today, when research is much talked about, this chapter will, I hope, provide very real help. I am also grateful to Miss S. H. McLaren, M.C.S.P. for her contribution on Advanced Rehabilitation. I accept full responsibility, as editor, for including this, for I am well aware that there are some who regard this particular approach to rehabilitation as unorthodox. I have visited the Hermitage, and partaken in a full day's activities, and I feel that the down to earth philosophy of this centre should be accorded a chapter.

These volumes on physiotherapy must always reflect the whole spectrum of treatment and inevitably this will include the unorthodox as well as the conventional, the researched as well as the unresearched, the simple and the complicated. Yet, always the physiotherapist must remember that she is treating an individual and all her skills need to be adjusted to suit the individual who is seeking her help.

To all the contributors, new and old, I offer my warm thanks for their co-operation; without their help this book would not have been possible. I also thank Audrey Besterman for the line drawings which she has produced with her customary flair from numerous rough sketches! An old Chinese proverb says 'one picture is worth a thousand words'; Audrey Besterman's drawings are certainly worth that!

My final words are directed to the reader: it would be an immense help to know what you would like included in future volumes. Please write and tell me.

P.A.D. 1979

Chapter 1

Using Medical Libraries

by D. W. C. STEWART, B.A., A.L.A.

Medical libraries vary considerably in size and scope of coverage and run from what may be little more than a shelf of books to collections of hundreds of thousands of volumes. All are doing essentially the same job – giving access to some of the considerable body of literature on medical matters which has been building up over many centuries. Medical workers have always been ready to make public their findings though the pattern of publication has changed and continues to change. In 1628 William Harvey (1578–1657) published what some regard as the most important medical book of all time his *De Motu Cordis*, on the circulation of the blood. Harvey's work had been done over a number of years but he did not feel under any pressure to publish any earlier than he did. In contrast, a twentieth century Harvey would first have published a preliminary communication in a letter to the *British Medical Journal* or the *Lancet* and followed it up with perhaps a series of papers in specialised journals. He might then have delivered papers on the subject to various international conferences whose proceedings would be published as monographs or journal supplements emanating from publishers in Prague, London, Amsterdam and Buenos Aires.

In the days of Harvey it was not impossible to be aware of what most other researchers were doing through personal contact but even two hundred years ago this was becoming impossible and more and more reliance had to be placed on the published record of research. Today, medical libraries play a vital role in controlling, through cataloguing and indexing, the output of literature and making it available to potential users.

The average medical library forms part of an institution such as a hospital or research institute and as such will endeavour to identify a readership whose needs it can reasonably try to meet. A teaching hospital library, for example, will be concerned primarily with the needs of medical students, teaching staff, consultants and researchers. It will also cover the needs of other health professionals such as physiotherapists, radiographers and pharmacists and it may also aim to provide for administrative and technical staff not directly concerned with patient care. Provision of nursing literature may also be made but that often depends on whether there is a school of nursing in which case there will probably be a separate nursing library.

It is important to define which is your primary library, that is to say, the one to which you belong and on whose services you have a right to call. It may be the library of a hospital, an authority, a public library system or a professional society. The more libraries to which you can have access the better, as it can be more useful to visit another library if you are working on a subject in which it specialises rather than trying to gather a lot of material by inter-library loan. A visit will also give access to specialised material such as dictionaries and bibliographies which would not normally be made available on loan.

Most libraries produce some kind of printed guide; it may be a lavishly produced booklet or a single duplicated sheet. In addition to digesting this, try to make yourself known to the library staff and get an individual introduction to the library; explain also what you are working on so that the librarian can help you get the most out of the library. Larger libraries such as those of universities have formal introductory procedures for new readers while some have audio-visual presentations on how they work or on the use of some specific types of material such as government publications.

The Catalogue

Make the acquaintance of the catalogue; this is all the more important if it seems daunting in its complexity. It is the key to the library and it is designed both to act as a list of what is held and to provide an alternative approach to the stock from that of the arrangement of books and journals on the shelves. Catalogues are constructed according to fairly elaborate rules to ensure conformity of entry; they deal with how one files a name such as Van Winkle (under 'Van' if he's American, under 'Winkle' if he's Dutch) and how the publications of organisations – as opposed to individuals – should be treated and so on. Unhappily not all libraries use the same rules and large older libraries may have rather old-fashioned styles of entry. Regular use of the catalogue should make the reader familiar with the peculiarities of the system.

Traditional catalogues are on cards filed in cabinets but increasingly common are catalogues on microfilm; they may be on cassettes which can be slipped into a reader and wound on to the appropriate entry or on a series of sheets of microfilm – microfiche – also viewed through a reader. The physical format of the catalogue does not affect the internal arrangement of entries. It is important to know what is in the catalogue and what is not; for example, very few library catalogues aim to list individual articles in periodicals or chapters in books, though a highly specialised library may maintain such an index possibly as a file separate from the catalogue itself.

Most libraries regard the author entry as the 'main entry' so that some catalogues may expect the reader to refer to the author card for the fullest details of the publication in question. While the author of a book is usually an individual the term 'author' is used to cover editors, compilers, sponsoring bodies, government departments and so forth. The name of a publisher is not normally used, so it is rarely any use going to a catalogue knowing that a report was published by the government and expecting to find it under Her Majesty's Stationery Office as it will have its entry under the name of the government department responsible for it. However, a publication such as the *Faber Medical Dictionary* would have an entry under publisher as the publisher's name is an integral part of the title. A good catalogue will try to cover some of the possible headings a reader might approach and there should be a good system of cross references. These consist of '*see*' references which direct from a heading not used, to one which is, such as 'Petrograd *see* Leningrad', and '*see also*' references which refer to a related heading, for example 'Music Therapy *see also* Art Therapy'.

Dictionary Catalogue

A subject approach may be provided by a separate subject catalogue but some libraries inter-file authors and subjects in a dictionary catalogue. Problems can arise here if a word can be used in different senses and a dictionary catalogue distinguishes between, say, 'Brain' as an individual's name (Lord Brain, the distinguished neurologist), the name of something (*Brain*, the neurology journal), the same word as the name of a place and the word as a common noun. A catalogue would file the entries in the order in which I have given them here. Dictionary catalogues should be used in rather the same way as one uses encyclopaedias.

Subject Catalogue

A separate subject catalogue may be arranged by the names of subjects as in a dictionary catalogue or in classified order. A library classification is used mainly for ensuring that books on the same subject are together on the shelves and is based on the principle of analysing subjects into definable groups and assigning to these groups a notation in letters or numbers which places these subjects (and the books or catalogue entries) in correct relationship to each other. Most users of British or American public libraries will have a nodding acquaintance with the widely used Dewey Decimal Classification; this is used in medical libraries but more common is a development of Dewey known as the Universal Decimal Classification (U.D.C.).

UNIVERSAL DECIMAL CLASSIFICATION

In medicine U.D.C. takes as its starting point the discipline, in that its divisions are into anatomy, physiology and pathology to produce filing orders like:

6	Applied Sciences. Medicine. Technology
61	Medicine
611	Anatomy
611.1	Cardiovascular Anatomy
612	Physiology
612.1	Cardiovascular Physiology
616	Pathology
616.1	Cardiovascular Disease

The U.D.C. class 615 covers therapy of all kinds including physiotherapy at 615.8 subdivided into headings such as massage at 615.82. However, the treatment of a disease is classified with material on the disease so that books on physiotherapy will also be filed at other places if they deal with physiotherapy of a specific disorder.

NATIONAL LIBRARY OF MEDICINE CLASSIFICATION

The other commonly used classification is that of the National Library of Medicine which takes the system (cardiovascular etc.) as its basis of arrangement and subdivides by anatomy, physiology, pathology to produce:

WG	Cardiovascular System
WG 200	Heart, general works
WG 201	Cardiovascular Anatomy
WG 202	Cardiovascular Physiology

Physical Therapy is classified at WB 460.

Thus in the one scheme you will find all physiological material together while in the other all cardiological material is in one place. However good a classification may be it is impossible always to keep related material together as many topics have quite complex relationships. Most classifications give librarians some latitude within the rules to suit the needs of the individual library so it is possible to find the same book classified in different ways in two libraries which use the same classification. It is useful to be in the habit of using the catalogue rather than relying on physiotherapy books being on the third shelf down inside the door.

Having found the entry for a book you want in the catalogue it should not be too difficult to find it on the shelves. The information on the catalogue card should include the author, the title and the subtitle, the 'collation' which indicates size, number of pages and other details of physical form, and perhaps an annotation which may provide additional information about the title e.g.:

MORTON, Leslie Thomas, Editor.

Use of Medical Literature. 2nd edition.
London, Butterworth, 1977

x, 462 p

(Information Sources for Research and Development)

In addition the entry will include information such as an accession number which identifies the book for library administrative purposes and a classification number or other indicator of where the book is shelved.

A library may have more than one sequence of books depending perhaps on whether they are earlier than a specific date, available for reference only or of unusual size, so it is important to read the catalogue entry carefully for any indication of this. The libraries of medical schools often have a 'reserve' collection of course reading and standard texts which may be issued for limited periods only.

Periodicals

Medical libraries spend a fairly large proportion of their book grants on periodicals and give this kind of material special treatment. Periodicals may be listed in the catalogue but more often there is a separate list arranged by title which gives an indication of the holdings available. It may also be available as a printed handlist for distribution to readers. In addition the library will maintain a detailed stock record which gives precise details about dates of receipt of issues, what parts have not arrived and so on.

INDEXING PERIODICALS

While the library catalogue lists the book stock in some detail the contents of periodical issues are not normally indexed though special issues of importance may be. Instead, reliance is placed on what are known as 'secondary' publications (usually themselves journals) which index the contents of the 'primary' journals which publish original work. Some secondary publications are designed to keep practitioners and researchers aware of new material appearing while others provide a means of making searches of the literature for information on specific subjects. Occasionally a secondary journal may carry one or two original papers, usually reviews of the literature on some aspect of a subject, while some primary journals may have an abstracting section which draws attention to papers in other periodicals.

The Institute for Scientific Information in the U.S.A. publishes a series of journals called *Current Contents* three of which relate closely to medicine, *Current Contents-Life Sciences*, *Current Contents-Clinical Practice* and *Current Contents-Social and Behavioral Sciences*. There is some overlap between the three. Each issue either details or reproduces the contents pages of the journals it covers and also provides a subject index and a list of authors' addresses. It is a useful means of keeping in touch with what is appearing in journals which your own library may not take and as it is air-freighted from the U.S.A. for rapid distribution in Europe it generally reproduces the contents pages of North American journals before the journals themselves get to this country.

THE INDEX MEDICUS

The *Index Medicus* (or the *Abridged Index Medicus*) is probably the most widely available of all medical indexing sources. It is a monthly index to the contents of some 2 500 medical journals and to a small number of selected congresses, symposia etc., which arranges the papers it indexes according to a carefully compiled list of index terms (Medical Subject Headings or 'MeSH') while also indexing by author. *Index Medicus* has been published almost continuously since 1879 and in its present form it cumulates annually for ease of retrospective searching. It is selective but it covers all aspects of medicine and a good range of journals world-wide though there is a slight bias in favour of U.S. material. Some time spent getting familiar with *Index Medicus* is well worth while.

Index Medicus places physiotherapy in its subject category E2 – PROCEDURES AND TECHNICS – THERAPEUTICS. The main specific heading is PHYSICAL THERAPY; other specific headings of interest to physiotherapists include EXERCISE THERAPY, HYDROTHERAPY, MASSAGE, and ULTRAVIOLET THERAPY. A useful broader heading is REHABILITATION.

Sub-headings are used to assist in arranging entries and include: anatomy, adverse effects, diagnosis, etiology, education, instrumentation, methods, treatment, prevention and so on. An article will be indexed under three or so headings if appropriate and only under the most specific headings available. It is important to check the MeSH list before making a search to ensure that the most appropriate headings are being checked.

EXCERPTA MEDICA

The Excerpta Medica Foundation is the publisher of *Excerpta Medica*, an abstracting journal which appears in 44 sections covering different aspects of medicine from Anatomy to Virology and including a section *Rehabilitation and Physical Medicine*. Papers will be listed in as many sections as are necessary so that an article on the physical training of patients after mitral valve replacement appears in the Rehabilitation and Physical Medicine section as well as in Cardiovascular Diseases and Cardiovascular Surgery. The advantage of *Excerpta Medica* is that it publishes abstracts in English of the papers covered from which the reader may get enough information to make the reading of the original paper unnecessary. Each issue has an index by subject and author while the main part consists of abstracts arranged in subject groups so that an issue can be used as a current awareness source. The headings used in the Rehabilitation and Physical Medicine section include Anatomy, Function Tests, Rehabilitation of Somatic Disorders (subdivided by the site of the disorder), Physiotherapy (subdivided into exercise therapy, massage, electrotherapy etc.), Occupational Therapy, Technical Aids and so on. To assist in retrospective searching an annual index is published.

Only the largest libraries will subscribe to all sections of *Excerpta Medica* but most medical libraries will take enough to cover the main fields of interest of their readers. As the coverage and approach of no two indexing tools is the same there are advantages (though it is time consuming) in making searches in more than one. Index Medicus, Excerpta Medica and the Institute for Scientific Information also offer computerised information services.

Distinguishing References

In using secondary sources it is useful to be able to distinguish between book and periodical references as libraries usually treat them differently. An *Index Medicus* journal reference is presented:

> Modeling procedures in the maintenance of sustained walking in a profoundly retarded girl. Mansdorf IJ. Arch Phys Med Rehabil 58(2): 83–5, Feb 77.

If the article appears in a monograph it looks like this:

> The role of physiotherapy in the overall treatment programme for rheumatoid arthritis. pp 256–9 Gross D.
> In: Wagenhauser FJ, ed. Chronic forms of polyarthritis. Bern, Huber, 1976. WE 344 C559 1975

The last line includes the National Library of Medicine classification number.

An *Excerpta Medica* reference is cited before the abstract and includes the address of the author:

> Early feeding history of children with learning disorders-Menkes J.H. – Dept. Ped., Neurol. Psychiat., UCLA, Los Angeles, Calif. 90210 USA–DEV.MED. CHILDNEUROL. 1977 19/2(169–171) – summ in FREN,GERM

The title of the journal is less clear here but it is *Developmental Medicine and Child Neurology*.

Inter-lending Systems

No library can aim to provide everything its readers could want so libraries co-operate through various inter-lending systems locally, nationally and internationally. A medical library will hold a variety of lists of periodicals held by other libraries and the catalogues of other libraries where these are available. The *British Union Catalogue of Periodicals* lists journals world-wide and indicates which libraries in the British Isles take them. Individual libraries publish their own lists and there are other listings which act as a means of confirming whether a book or journal actually exists. Among the lists is the annual list of current titles taken by the Lending Division of the British Library, the latest edition of which contains about 45 000 periodicals.

The British Library Lending Division (BLLD) collects almost comprehensively in the field of medicine and is the first source on which many medical libraries call if they fail to supply material from their own stock. It aims to provide a rapid service and acts as a referral centre by passing requests it cannot meet to a group of 'back-up' libraries which includes several major university and medical libraries. If required requests will also be sent abroad. The BLLD can only be approached for loans through another library but its reading room at its site near Leeds is open to members of the public.

The Reference Division of the British Library is located at several sites in London and scientific material is housed in the two parts known as the Science Reference Library. Access is available to the general public without formality and a wide range of medical material is held.

Medical library provision in the United Kingdom has improved greatly in the last ten years, particularly outside London, though there is still a wealth of resources in the capital. The *Directory of Medical Libraries in the British Isles* (fourth edition, London, The Library Association, 1977) lists all of the significant libraries and is arranged geographically with supporting indexes; it is an invaluable guide to the resources available in one's area and it also indicates who may use a particular library. The regulations governing access to libraries will vary from place to place and it is a good idea to make enquiries before paying a visit. Every library has its main group of readers to look after first of all and while most are happy to be of help there may be limits to what they can do.

References for Publication

Having found the material which you wish to consult you may then find yourself in the position of writing a paper for publication. There are many books on the writing of scientific papers and publishers will also have their own rules and recommendations on format and presentation. Most medical papers have to supply references to the work of other people which may have been quoted in the text; editors are very hard on the author who produces unsupported statements. Not only must references be provided but they must also be checked for accuracy both in content and presentation. Badly presented or inaccurate references reflect on the general accuracy and diligence of the author and a good paper can be spoiled by inadequate references. Never quote something which you have not read; at the time you read a paper make an accurate and complete note of it avoiding the shorthand like APM&R 3/77 48 which you may be unable to reconstruct accurately when you need to. Note the titles of papers and the last as well as the first page number as some publishers require it. If you have used a variety of libraries in your researches it may help to note where you saw something that took you a while to find as you may want to use it again. Five-by-three inch index cards in a small file are still the best physical means of organising reference lists.

Although I have given examples of how references are quoted in *Index Medicus* and in *Excerpta Medica* this style would not be acceptable to most publishers. The principles of reference citation are laid down in British Standard No. 1629; a leaflet giving examples of medical references has been produced by the former Medical Section of the Library Association. Entitled *Reference Citation Recommendations* it may be obtained gratis from the Association at 7, Ridgmount Street, London WC1E 7AE.

There are two systems for citing references in papers; either by the quoting of the author's name with a superior numeral e.g. Smith[3] or the author's name and the date of the paper e.g. Smith (1976). The second system, generally and inexplicably known as the Harvard system, is now preferred by most journals. In the bibliography references are arranged numerically by the first system and alphabetically by the second system. Some publishers prefer that journal titles be given in full while others recommend abbreviations; a good standard abbreviation list appears in the first issue of *Index Medicus* each year.

When checking the references after typing your paper always check them from the original publication; do not take the short cut of looking them up in the *Index Medicus* for it can make mistakes and it may not give you all the information you need. One of the longest running wrong references appeared off and on in the literature from 1887 to 1938 and was only sorted out when someone took the trouble to read the original paper referred to!

BIBLIOGRAPHY

Morton, L. T. (1972). *How to Use a Medical Library.* 5th edition. William Heinemann Medical Books, London.

Morton, L. T. (Ed.) (1977). *Use of Medical Literature.* 2nd edition. Butterworths, London.

Reference Citation Recommendations (1972). Medical Section, The Library Association, London.

Chapter 2

An Introduction to General Surgical Care

by P. A. DOWNIE, F.C.S.P.

THE TEAM CONCEPT

The total care necessary for patients who undergo any form of surgery involves many people – nowadays called the team. Not everyone will be required for each patient but all are available as and when necessary. The physiotherapist is included in this team and she should be aware of the skills of the others and how they may be utilised to the best advantage of the patient and his family. She must realise that she herself may only have a minor part to play and in many instances no part at all. Some types of surgery will require that the physiotherapist is a very important team member e.g. cardio-thoracic and orthopaedic surgery, while other types of surgery e.g. ear, nose and throat will only require limited physiotherapy. However much she is involved or not in the care of the patient the physiotherapist must always be prepared to co-operate with other members – for example she will need to discuss with the speech therapist what particular breathing exercises are most helpful for a patient who undergoes laryngectomy and subsequently requires to be taught oesophageal speech. Equally she will combine with the occupational therapist to ensure that patients can return home and that the necessary equipment and aids are provided.

In hospital the team will include the following:

1. The medical staff e.g. the anaesthetist, the surgeon and his registrar and houseman, and in cases of malignant disease the radiotherapist and chemotherapist.
2. The nursing staff including nurse specialists such as stoma therapist, mastectomy liaison nurse etc.
3. The occupational therapist, speech therapist, remedial gymnast and physiotherapist.
4. The social worker; the disablement resettlement officer (D.R.O.).

5. The prosthetist will be a vital member of the team where mutilating surgery has been necessary e.g. amputation of a limb or extensive head and face surgery.
6. The dietician.
7. Technicians, radiographers, porters and cleaners.

There should also be links with the community team which will include:

1. The district nurse (community sister).
2. The health visitor.
3. The community physiotherapist.
4. The social services, who usually have an occupational therapist in their team.

At all times the patient, relatives and general practitioner are to be considered as the most important members of the team; the G.P. can often act as the co-ordinator of services and the patient and relatives really determine the extent to which the team are required. The hospital chaplains and parish clergy and ministers should not be overlooked and they should be involved as and when required.

It is not proposed to discuss the individual roles of these team members but it is hoped that each physiotherapist will make it her responsibility to find out what everyone in the team is able to offer and how they can best be used. Participation in ward rounds, in clinics and in case conferences is to be encouraged. Whenever a patient is transferred either to a different hospital or back to the community full details of all treatment as well as an assessment of the patient should be sent to the relevant services.

There has been considerable discussion as to the value of physiotherapy for patients undergoing surgery. Nichols and Howell (1970) undertook controlled trials and the result showed that upper abdominal surgery in particular is likely to inhibit the function of the diaphragm. They concluded that physiotherapy has an accepted part to play in the treatment of established bronchitis by physically aiding the drainage and expulsion of bronchial secretions. They also felt that the problem of postoperative complications was more that of selecting those patients 'at risk', and treating them vigorously *before* surgery, rather than providing unnecessary postoperative treatment in a routine fashion to all surgical patients.

PHYSIOTHERAPY IN GENERAL SURGERY

Patients who undergo surgical procedures may or may not be prescribed physiotherapy. It is probably true to say that no longer does the physiotherapist see routinely every person who appears on a surgical list. Those patients who are referred for pre- and postoperative physiotherapy need to be adequately assessed so that unnecessary treatments are neither carried out nor continued indefinitely. Unless the surgical procedure is an emergency, it is to be hoped that when patients are referred for pre-operative training the physiotherapist will have sufficient time to prepare the patient adequately before the proposed surgery. Patients undergoing extensive abdominal surgery will certainly benefit subjectively and any patient who is known to be either a heavy smoker or who suffers from a chronic chest disorder should receive adequate pre-operative training. In many cases this preparation may be carried out as an out-patient, to save the patient occupying a hospital bed for a week prior to operation.

It is unlikely that patients undergoing minor surgery, endoscopic examination, haemorrhoidectomy, etc. will be ordered physiotherapy *unless* they are known to have a chronic chest condition.

Principles of Physiotherapy for Patients Undergoing Surgery

The general principles involved are:

1. To prevent chest complications, by maintaining lung functions and aiding the clearance of secretions.
2. To prevent thrombosis of the legs by encouraging active leg movements, or if necessary, by performing passive exercises.
3. To maintain muscle power by encouraging simple bed exercises.
4. To help maintain good posture by ensuring that pillows are arranged in a good supportive position.

The approach of the physiotherapist to the patient must be direct, positive and firm. Patients are very quick to sense when someone does not really know what they are doing.

COUGHING

One of the invariable questions will be 'Will I burst my stitches when I cough?' All patients must be reassured about this and shown how they may themselves support their wound when coughing. A sensitive yet firm hand to support the patient's own hands as he holds his wound, will give confidence as well as reassurance. The author has always found that sitting on the bed behind the patient, with the patient able

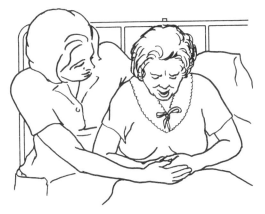

Fig. 2/1 Support from the physiotherapist following abdominal surgery while the patient coughs – in bed

to lean on her shoulder, enables her to use both her hands to support the wound (Fig. 2/1). Sometimes patients are told to bend their knees up as they cough, but this is not always very easy. The head should be flexed as the patient coughs. Patients who undergo surgery are seldom in bed for very long and coughing is very much more easily performed when sitting (Fig. 2/2). Indeed, some patients will find sitting over the side of the bed with their feet supported on the locker, a helpful position in which to cough. Sometimes it helps to give them a 'cough-belt' (Figs. 2/3 and 2/4). These belts are very useful when the patient is a chronic bronchitic with a productive cough as well as being stout. They can be worn loosely and then pulled up tight when they want to cough (Barlow, 1964).

It is not the act of coughing which causes the wound to burst occasionally, although it invariably seems to happen as the patient coughs and he naturally assumes that the coughing was the cause. A

Fig. 2/2 Support from the physiotherapist following abdominal surgery while the patient coughs – sitting in a chair

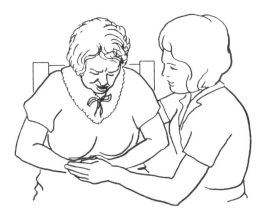

wound breaks down i.e. the sutures give way, almost always because there is an infection or increased serous fluid collection. Just occasionally the suture material may be faulty. If the patient is stout or is known to have a chronic chest disorder, the surgeon may insert some tension sutures as well. These are in addition to the normal suturing of the wound, and are usually threaded through thin rubber tubing so that they can remain in situ without cutting through the skin.

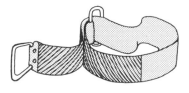

Fig. 2/3 A cough-belt

Fig. 2/4 A patient coughing, with the cough-belt in position

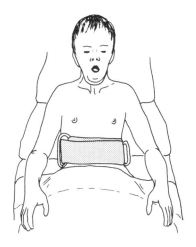

GENERAL POINTS TO BE NOTED BY THE PHYSIOTHERAPIST

Pre-operative

a) Before the patient is seen by the physiotherapist, the notes should be carefully read and any relevant facts noted. For example he may be a heavy smoker, he may have a past history of a leg thrombosis, he may have some disability which could influence his mobility, he may live alone and this could influence how independent he would need to be before being discharged.

b) Introduce yourself to the patient and explain in language which he can understand, exactly what you are going to do and what he will have to do and why all this is necessary.

c) Assess the respiratory expansion of the patient and teach diaphragmatic and lateral costal breathing. It is wise to warn the patient that postoperatively it may be necessary to treat him in side lying and/or with the bed tipped, and he should be shown how to reach this position. If this method has to be used, it is sensible to combine the physiotherapy at a time when the nurses are carrying out nursing procedures so that the patient is not moved unnecessarily.

d) As previously mentioned he should be shown how to hold himself when coughing.

e) Simple foot and leg exercises should be taught and the patient told why they are important. It is not necessary to talk about thrombosis; it is quite simple to explain that the legs will ache if they are kept still after the operation, and that if they are regularly moved this will not happen and they will feel less wobbly when he gets up. The patient should also be told not to sit in bed with his legs crossed at the ankles.

Postoperative

a) The notes must be read and the extent of the operation noted, together with the nursing record of the patient's condition since his return from the operating theatre.

b) The position of drainage tubes, intravenous lines, catheter and type of dressing should be noted.

c) If analgesic drugs have been prescribed, the physiotherapist should arrange that they are given *before* the physiotherapy. Occasionally Entonox (50% nitrous oxide and 50% oxygen) may be used – this has the advantage that the patient can control it and its use can be very effective in pain relief where coughing is essential.

Chapter 3 discusses the application of treatments which the physiotherapist can use pre- and postoperatively. This chapter will now concentrate on some aspects of general surgical procedures and how the physiotherapist may find herself involved. Specialised care following gynaecological, head and neck, cranial and spinal surgery in addition to amputations will be discussed in separate chapters.

SURGICAL PROCEDURES

The actual surgical procedures for different operations will not be described as these can be studied in surgical textbooks. There are, however, certain aspects which are useful for the physiotherapist to have some knowledge of.

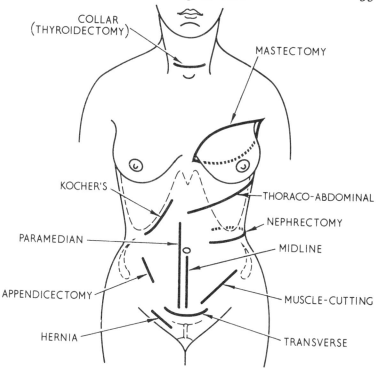

Fig. 2/5 Surgical incisions

Incisions

Figure 2/5 shows some of the basic incisions which are used in surgical procedures. The decision to use which depends on the surgeon as well as the prime requirement of giving adequate access to the diseased area.

CLOSURE OF THE INCISION

The incision may be closed in various ways:

1. Clips are used where an unsightly scar could be distressing to the patient e.g. following thyroidectomy. They are removed 48 to 72 hours postoperatively.
2. Sutures can be absorbable e.g. catgut, non-absorbable e.g. silk, or nylon, invisible intradermal absorbable sutures, or tension sutures (see p. 33).
3. The sutures can be tied as single stitches, as a continuous suture or

as mattress sutures. The advantage of single sutures is that alternate sutures can be removed and if there is any danger of the incision gaping, stitches in the area at risk can remain longer.

4. The size of the suture material will depend on the site at which it is used. Plastic surgery will require very fine material and more numerous stitches, whereas abdominal muscles will require a strong material. Steel wire is used to suture the sternum after the sternum is split in heart surgery, and in some jaw surgery when the mandible is divided and then resutured. If steel wire is used, it is necessary to drill a hole in the bone ends which are to be wired together, through which the wire is threaded.

Drains

Almost all wounds will have some form of drainage left in situ, thus reducing the risk of haematoma formation and subsequent breakdown of wounds.

Drainage tubes can take several forms:

1. A Redivac drain, which is a closed system of drainage using a vacuum principle.
2. Corrugated drains which are either rubber or polythene and drain into the dressing and can be shortened by pulling out gradually before final removal.
3. Intercostal drains which are inserted into the pleural cavity to drain blood and/or air following surgery involving the opening of the chest. They are attached to an underwater bottle/s and this is a form of closed drainage. Where an empyema is being drained the wide bore tubing is sometimes allowed to drain into a dressing (Innocenti, 1979).
4. Internal drains such as a T-tube which is inserted into the common bile duct following an exploration of the common bile duct. These are usually attached to a bottle or bag thus allowing the collection of bile. They are usually in situ for 10 to 12 days.

A caecostomy is sometimes left following colon surgery – this is a drain inserted into the caecum and which allows faecal fluid to escape instead of building up and possibly causing an obstruction. It is usually attached to a bag. It is withdrawn about 10 to 12 days postoperatively. It must *not* be confused with a colostomy. A caecostomy is essentially a safety valve.

Other Tubes

Following surgery, the patient may also have an intravenous infusion – this is to maintain electrolyte balance as well as ensuring both nutrition and hydration. In surgery not affecting the alimentary tract such an infusion will be taken down the morning following surgery.

A nasogastric or Ryle's tube is almost always passed following surgery involving the alimentary tract. This has a dual purpose in that the stomach may be aspirated regularly and, at the appropriate time, feeding may be begun. The physiotherapist should acquaint herself with these essential nursing matters either by discussing them with her nurse colleagues or by reading about them in a good nursing textbook.

A catheter may be passed in the operating theatre and particularly where renal, bladder, rectal or very extensive abdominal surgery has been carried out. It will drain into a bag which hangs from the bed frame. Sometimes the catheter tube may be strapped lightly to the upper thigh and the physiotherapist must ensure that there is sufficient play in the tubing before she starts on too active leg exercises!

SPECIAL POINTS TO BE REMEMBERED BY THE PHYSIOTHERAPIST

Abdominal Surgery

Unless the surgery is specifically for gall bladder disease, inguinal or femoral hernia, or nephrectomy, the incision will be mid-line with extension as necessary to allow for adequate exposure.

After gastrectomy, the patient may develop left pulmonary atelectasis and the physiotherapist needs to emphasise localised breathing to both lower lobes but particularly to the left. The diaphragm will have been handled in the operative procedure and the patient will be reluctant to breathe deeply.

Following cholecystectomy in which a Kocher incision is used, the danger of atelectasis is to the right lower lobe, and so the emphasis must be to the right lower lobe. In addition, if the common bile duct has been explored, there will be a T-tube in situ. This can cause pain and discomfort when the patient breathes deeply. Adequate analgesia must be given *before* the main treatment is given by the physiotherapist and the patient *must* be continually reminded by both nurses and the physiotherapist to breathe deeply.

Adrenalectomy

A bilateral adrenalectomy is most often performed for patients suffering from disseminated cancer and particularly for those with metastatic bone disease. It is also performed for primary tumours of the adrenal glands. The surgical approach is either through the abdomen when the physiotherapy will be as for any abdominal operation, or through bilateral loin incisions i.e. through the bed of the twelfth rib. If the latter approach is used there is always the danger of nicking the pleura with a consequent pneumothorax which may require an intercostal drain to be inserted. Breathing exercises are most important when the loin incision is used.

In addition, if the patient has metastatic bone disease care must be exercised if the deposits affect the ribs. Clapping, shakings and vigorous vibrations must NOT be used; gentle vibrations and resisted bilateral costal breathing should be given. Bed exercises are important but again these must be active and care must be observed if there are deposits in the weight-bearing bones, particularly the femora. Downie (1978a) has described the treatment for these patients.

Breast Surgery

Perhaps no other surgery causes so many reactions. Mastectomy is performed most often for malignant conditions but it should always be remembered that it is also performed for benign lesions e.g. multiple fibromata. The type of surgery varies nowadays from the removal of a lump – 'lumpectomy' – to the full radical mastectomy (Halsted's operation). Probably the most commonly performed operation is the simple or extended simple mastectomy (Patey operation). This latter allows for the removal of the axillary glands with the breast tissue but without the excision of the pectoral muscles.

Whatever surgery is carried out, the physiotherapy allowed will be at the discretion of the surgeon and the physiotherapist MUST ascertain what each particular surgeon will allow by way of movement. If she is unfortunate enough to have little or no contact with the surgeon or if he tells her to 'do what you like', she will be well advised to steer a middle course with regard to arm movements.

Basic guidelines may be summarised as follows:

1. Following lumpectomy, or wedge resection, no treatment should be required.
2. Following local or simple mastectomy without axillary clearance, no treatment should be necessary, but occasionally physiotherapy

may be required to help the patient overcome her fear of movement and thus to encourage a full range of shoulder movements.

3. Following an extended simple mastectomy (Patey), the patient should be encouraged to use her arm for normal daily activities. If stiffness develops, pendular type shoulder exercises are the most useful. In no circumstances must a shoulder be forced.

4. Following radical mastectomy (Halsted), physiotherapy will be aimed at restoration of shoulder movement, particularly elevation and rotation. The pectoralis major and minor muscles will have been excised and pure abduction of the shoulder should not be allowed until all the drains are out and the skin flaps firmly adhered to the chest wall. If abduction is allowed too soon, fluid will collect between the skin flaps and the chest wall and will require repeated aspirations. Apart from causing unnecessary discomfort for the patient, repeated aspirations carry the risk of infection. Pendular type shoulder exercises are the most useful, and all exercises should be active and the shoulder must never be forced.

Some surgeons will bandage the arm to the side for the first week, to prevent abduction and undue movement of the skin flaps. In this case finger, hand and wrist movements should be encouraged, also shoulder shrugging and isometric contractions of the deltoid.

Instruction should also be given in posture correction and how to lift without placing too great strain on the shoulder of the mastectomy side.

In all cases where the physiotherapist is involved in treating mastectomy patients, she must be prepared to enter into the total care of these patients. She should have a knowledge of breast prostheses, of how to adapt brassières and where to purchase suitable swimwear (Downie, 1978b). She should be aware of the emotional problems which can arise following mastectomy (Downie, 1976 and Maguire, 1975), and she should always be ready to listen and to help in any way possible. Co-operation with nurses, social workers, and patient volunteers as well as the doctors is very necessary in this field of care.

LYMPHOEDEMA

In some cases following mastectomy and particularly following radical mastectomy or where the patient has undergone radiotherapy, lymphoedema will occur. Physiotherapy may well be ordered and various methods of treatment are available including massage in elevation, faradism under pressure and the newer compression techniques. There is, as yet, no evidence that any of these has a lasting effect though there is no doubt that all can help to relieve the condition. As well as such specific treatment, the patient should be taught exercises in elevation and how to posture the arm so that drainage may be helped; particularly useful to the patient is to be shown how to position the arm at night in bed, and while sitting watching the television!

Colonic and Rectal Surgery

As with all abdominal surgery physiotherapy will be directed towards the prevention of chest complications but with lower abdominal surgery special attention must also be paid to the prevention of thrombosis. Leg exercises must be taught and supervised thoroughly postoperatively.

Following surgical intervention on the bowel, a paralytic ileus can result leading to great discomfort for the patient with distension of the abdomen. It is important that breathing exercises are encouraged during this period as well as the patient being persuaded to move around in bed as much as possible.

COLOSTOMY

A colostomy is the formation of an artificial anus on the surface of the abdominal wall which can be temporary or permanent. It is sited over the transverse colon or in the lower left quadrant of the abdomen. The lower the siting of the colostomy, the more formed will be the stool. The physiotherapist does not treat the colostomy itself but she should certainly have an understanding of the consequences of such an operation.

When the patient has undergone a combined synchronous abdomino-perineal excision for a carcinoma of the rectum, the colostomy will be permanent.

If a patient is admitted with an acute intestinal obstruction the first stage of relieving the obstruction is often the fashioning of a temporary colostomy. This is followed in about two weeks by an excision and end-to-end anastomosis of the affected colon and about two further weeks later the colostomy will be closed. Sometimes when a resection of the colon is carried out for a carcinoma of the colon, diverticular disease or Crohn's disease, a temporary colostomy may be fashioned so that the anastomosis of the colon can firmly unite before the continuity of the gut is re-established.

When the colostomy is permanent, the aim of rehabilitation must be to ensure that the patient can not only cope with the appliance but does return to a normal life and takes his place fully in society. The Colostomy Welfare Association has done great work in this area; their

volunteers (all of whom have had a colostomy) are all carefully selected
and trained and are willing to visit any patient at the request of the
surgeon or general practitioner. Unlike the Ileostomy Association
they do *not* hold group meetings of colostomists. In recent years
nurses, who have undergone a post-graduate course in stoma care,
have begun to be appointed in the larger hospitals. These are clinical
nurse specialists more commonly referred to as the stoma therapists.
Their role is to advise patients, their families and the nurses in the
understanding of the colostomy and to ensure that the most suitable
appliance is provided for each patient.

The physiotherapist should certainly teach these patients how to lift
correctly and should help to ensure that they get dressed and are able
to walk about not only the hospital and its grounds, but out in the
street as well, before being discharged home.

ILEOSTOMY

Like the colostomy this is an artificial anus on the abdominal wall but
is sited in the right lower quadrant of the abdomen. It is always
permanent and is usually performed following a total colectomy or
pan-procto total colectomy – the latter includes the excision of the
rectum and anus as well as the colon. These very extensive excisions
are performed for patients with ulcerative colitis or extensive Crohn's
disease. These patients are often extremely ill before surgery and will
require a great deal of physiotherapy to help them maintain a good
respiratory function and leg mobility.

As they improve, and in many cases this improvement can be
dramatic, the physiotherapist should teach lifting and generally help
with total rehabilitation prior to discharge.

For these patients the Ileostomy Association organise volunteers to
visit in hospital and after discharge and they have groups all over the
country who meet regularly for social events, holidays, as well as to
discuss new appliances etc.

Genito-Urinary Surgery

NEPHRECTOMY

The removal of a kidney may become necessary when it is diseased as
the result of a malignant tumour; pyonephrosis (gross infection);
tuberculosis; hydronephrosis (dilatation of the renal pelvis due to
obstruction, leading to atrophy of the kidney tissue and impaired
renal function); and occasionally for calculi (renal stones).

The remaining kidney must be healthy before nephrectomy is
undertaken. The incision is usually through the bed of the twelfth rib

but may be higher, through the bed of the tenth rib. Care of the chest is very important and it is not unknown for the pleura to be nicked at operation and for a pneumothorax to occur. An intercostal drain will be inserted and physiotherapy will follow the pattern as for thoracic surgery (Innocenti, 1979).

Whenever a loin incision is used, the physiotherapist should check carefully the posture of the patient, both when lying in bed and when he gets up and starts walking.

PROSTATECTOMY

This operation is usually performed on elderly men, many of whom will have a chronic chest disorder. Chest physiotherapy is therefore very important, and this is an instance where the cough-belt could be used (see p. 32). Prostatectomy is usually performed for benign enlargement of the gland and is carried out through a transverse supra-pubic incision. Carcinoma of the prostate is usually treated by hormonal manipulation but if the condition is causing difficulty of micturition through pressure on the bladder neck, a trans-urethral resection (T.U.R.) of the gland may be undertaken. This is performed endoscopically, and under direct vision the surgeon is able to resect the obtruding tissue.

Early ambulation of these patients is not only desirable but essential; drainage tubes and catheter will need to be secured safely and the elderly gentleman persuaded to walk! Nowadays catheters drain into bags which can be easily carried.

CYSTECTOMY

Surgery for a carcinoma of the bladder will entail removal of the bladder (cystectomy) and the fashioning of an ileal conduit. Not all bladder cancers will need to be treated with radical surgery; radiotherapy is used quite extensively and it is often following such treatment that cystectomy and the formation of an ileal conduit is carried out. An ileal conduit is the formation of an artificial bladder on the abdominal wall, in a manner similar to that of forming a colostomy. In this case a small segment of the ileum is fashioned into a tube and brought out through the abdominal wall, thus forming a stoma. The two ureters are inserted into the ileal conduit and an appliance is attached to the stoma, into which the urine will drain.

Physiotherapy for these patients will include care for the chest, but more especially, teaching them to lift and generally helping them to become active, mobile and capable of being independent before discharge.

An ileal conduit may also be fashioned for patients suffering from chronic incontinence due to certain neurological conditions e.g. children with spina bifida.

GOLD GRAINS INSERTION IN BLADDER

Very occasionally, radio-active gold grains may be inserted for treatment of a circumscribed bladder tumour. If physiotherapy is required the physiotherapist must observe the precautions which are laid down and particularly the time allowed for close treatment of the patient. Radio-active gold has a very short half-life and this time allowance will rapidly increase over five days.

These patients may well be in a poor general state of health and chest physiotherapy is often required. Provided the precautions are observed, there is no danger to the physiotherapist; a portable lead shield may be used to protect the physiotherapist while she encourages the patient to carry out exercises.

Repair of Herniae

A hernia is a weakness in the musculature through which contents of a cavity may prolapse.

HERNIAE OF THE ABDOMINAL WALL

1. A femoral hernia occurs at the femoral ring. It is most common in women.
2. An inguinal hernia occurs at the inguinal canal. It is more common in men. There are two types: *Direct*, which occurs in older people due to associated muscle weakness and increase in abdominal pressure; and *Indirect*, which is congenital and occurs in younger people.
3. An umbilical hernia or para-umbilical hernia occurs either in childhood or at the fifth decade. In adults they are more common in obese patients.
4. An incisional hernia occurs through a previous incision and can be found anywhere.

Repair for these herniae involves excision of the hernial sac where necessary and strengthening of the abdominal wall by means of sutures. Fascia lata may be used like a darn, to repair the groin herniae; this latter procedure is rarely performed now.

Apart from chest physiotherapy as required, hernia patients must be taught to lift correctly. They may also be given abdominal exercises – isometric or inner range exercises but not outer range exercises.

Two other types of hernia are:

1. A hiatus hernia, which is the prolapsing of the stomach through the hiatus of the diaphragm. Repair is usually through a thoracotomy incision and physiotherapy will be as for patients undergoing thoracic surgery (Innocenti, 1979).
2. A strangulated hernia, which is always a serious surgical emergency. The contents of the hernial sac can become trapped if the neck of the sac is very narrow; if the blood supply is impaired, the trapped bowel can become gangrenous. Intestinal obstruction is a not infrequent complication of a strangulated hernia. Physiotherapy is as for abdominal surgery.

REFERENCES

Barlow, D. (1964). 'A Cough-Belt to Prevent and Treat Post-operative Pulmonary Complications'. *Lancet*, 2, 736.
Downie, P. A. (1976). 'Post-mastectomy survey'. *Nursing Mirror*, **142**, 13.
Downie, P. A. (1978a). *Cancer Rehabilitation: an Introduction for Physiotherapists and the Allied Professions*. Faber and Faber.
Downie, P. A. (1978b). *'Rehabilitation'*. Chapter included in *Oncology for Nurses and Health Care Professionals*. Vol. 2 (Ed. Tiffany, R.). George Allen and Unwin.
Innocenti, D. M. (1979). 'Thoracic Surgery'. Chapters included in *Cash's Textbook of Chest, Heart and Vascular Disorders for Physiotherapists*. 2nd edition (Ed. Downie, P. A.). Faber and Faber.
Maguire, (1975). 'The Psychological and Social Consequences of Breast Cancer'. *Nursing Mirror*, **140**, 74.
Nichols, P. J. R. and Howell, B. (1970). 'Routine Pre- and Post-Operative Physiotherapy: A Preliminary Trial'. *Physiotherapy*, **56**, 8.

BIBLIOGRAPHY

Ellison Nash, D. F. (1976). *The Principles and Practice of Surgery for Nurses and Allied Professions*. 6th edition. Edward Arnold.
Taylor, S. and Cotton, L. (1977). *A Short Textbook of Surgery*. 4th edition. English Universities Press.

Chapter 3

Complications Following Surgery

by K. M. THOMPSON, M.C.S.P.

No matter how simple and straightforward an operation, or how physically fit the patient is before he undergoes it, there are always certain risks which cannot be avoided, though preventive measures can lessen their possibility. Some of the complications which may follow surgery are given here in their order of importance to the physiotherapist.

Respiratory Problems

Whenever a general anaesthetic has to be used and opiate anaesthetic agents are administered, the possibility of respiratory problems exists. The anaesthetic may act as an irritant; the cough reflex may be depressed and therefore expectorating secretions is difficult. Thoracic and upper abdominal surgery are most likely to cause respiratory problems.

Thrombosis

Thrombosis of the deep veins of the leg, which may lead to a fatal pulmonary embolism, is always a postoperative danger. The physiotherapist may easily be the person who discovers this during an exercise period, so must always be watchful for the symptoms.

Wound Infections

These are very common due to the prevalence of resistant bacteria. Infections occur even in clean, cold surgery despite the existence in most large hospitals of teams whose task it is to combat infection.

Pressure Sores

Any patient confined to bed must be watched constantly by all who care for him to prevent pressure sores occurring. These may have been precipitated by pressure while on the operating table or they may occur later. Pressure can also be caused from within the tissues, i.e. by the presence of oedema. Vigilance is especially needed where the patient is old, unconscious, immobile or incontinent.

Haemorrhage

Another complication is haemorrhage. This can be primary, occurring within the first 24 hours, or secondary, when it can take place up to three weeks postoperatively.

Muscle Wasting and Impairment of Function

If incisions are very extensive and divide, or in extreme cases damage, muscle or nerve tissue, there can be resultant muscle wasting and impairment of function. This can lead to faulty posture, deformities and, occasionally, stiff joints.

Cardiac Arrest

The ultimate complication is cardiac arrest, and unless immediate action is taken, the symptoms are irreversible. It is therefore vital that it should be recognised at once by everyone who comes in contact with the patient, and that the appropriate action is known and instantly followed.

RESPIRATORY PROBLEMS

Respiratory complications are liable to follow any operation in which general anaesthesia is used. They are most common in thoracic surgery since in those cases the lungs are already involved. After thoracic surgery the highest incidence is probably in abdominal operations, particularly those which require a supra-umbilical incision.

Postoperative respiratory complications are due to retained secretions. Sometimes these secretions are stringy and viscid and therefore difficult to expectorate. Following operation the patient is drowsy, making deep breathing and coughing difficult, and if the incision is thoracic or abdominal, coughing is voluntarily inhibited through fear of pain. Postoperative analgesics make the patient lethargic and the presence of various drips and drains make him relatively immobile and less likely to be able to clear his chest of secretions. Retained secretions may lead to the following problems:

Atelectasis or Postoperative Pulmonary Collapse

This occurs when a plug of mucus becomes lodged in an airway and the air distal to it is absorbed, causing the area to collapse. Collapse of a whole lobe is rare. Segmental collapse is more common and is usually unilateral and basal. Postoperative atelectasis occurs within the first 24 to 48 hours. There is a rise in temperature and respiratory rate followed by a cough with purulent sputum. Patchy atelectasis may be seen on X-ray.

Postoperative Pneumonia

This occurs when the retained secretions become infected and an inflammatory process takes place. It usually presents two to three days postoperatively with a gradual rise in temperature, reduced expansion and X-ray changes. A productive cough follows and purulent sputum may be produced. Broncho-pneumonia frequently occurs in elderly patients following surgery.

Aspiration Pneumonia

Inhalation of stomach contents is the cause of aspiration pneumonia. Inhalation can occur pre-operatively as in elderly patients awaiting surgery for intestinal obstruction. Reflux of gastric contents into the trachea via the oesophagus can also occur during operation when the cough reflex has been abolished by the anaesthetic, or early in the postoperative period. An aspiration pneumonia may be accompanied by severe airways obstruction and pulmonary oedema.

The reduction in depth of each breath, i.e. Vital Capacity (V.C.), which inevitably follows operations on the thorax or abdomen is a further factor in predisposing towards these complications. The diaphragm is responsible for as much as 60 per cent of the normal respiratory movements, but in the first 24 hours after the operation, its movement may be only 20 per cent of the normal. The result of this fact is that the lungs, particularly the bases, are not fully ventilated and the circulation is slowed, with consequent congestion. Not only is the vitality of the lung lowered, but there may be increased filtration of tissue fluid and slight oedema of the lung bases.

Postoperative pulmonary complications delay the patient's recovery; whenever possible they must be prevented and should they occur they need to be treated immediately.

Physiotherapy

The aim of pre- and postoperative physiotherapy is to prevent respiratory complications. However should they occur they must be treated immediately. The main causes of chest complications are a temporarily lowered V.C. and accumulation of secretions due to a decreased cough reflex and diminished respiratory movement. The purpose of physiotherapy is therefore to regain the normal V.C., to stimulate coughing and to encourage the full use of the lungs. In cases where elimination of mucus is difficult, the physiotherapist may assist the patient to remove it, otherwise bronchoscopy may be necessary.

DEEP BREATHING EXERCISES

Deep breathing exercises should be taught pre-operatively while the patient is alert, pain-free and fully co-operative. Emphasis is laid on diaphragmatic and lateral costal expansion with a good, deep inspiration, followed by a relaxed expiration. An understanding by the patient of the value of the correct breathing is essential so that he will co-operate as soon as he recovers from the anaesthetic.

EFFECTIVE COUGHING

The patient should be taught how to cough effectively and with as little pain as possible. This is again best taught pre-operatively. Two points need to be emphasised when teaching coughing. First, strain on the wound will be relieved if the patient supports the operation site with his hands and if he draws his knees up and leans his trunk slightly towards the area of incision. Second, following a good, deep inspiration, a short, sharp expiration produces the easiest and most effective cough.

In order to facilitate the removal of mucus the secretions of the lungs need to be kept moist. Humidification may be achieved in several ways:

a) The simplest method is by Tinct. Benz. Co. (Friars Balsam) inhalations given three times daily. Ideally these inhalations should be given immediately before chest physiotherapy is carried out.

b) Humidifiers which add water, usually warmed, to the oxygen or air which the patient breathes.

c) Where there is a tracheostomy, 1 to 2ml of normal saline may be injected into the trachea.

d) By the use of a nebuliser (e.g. Wright's, Hudson, Bird). In this method a bronchodilator e.g. salbutamol (Ventolin), or a muco-lytic agent can be nebulised for inhalation. Indications for their use are bronchospasm or to thin down thick, sticky sputum.

When in spite of adequate coughing and practise of breathing exercises, mucus does collect and there is danger of collapse, then mechanical assistance will be necessary to remove secretions.

MECHANICAL ASSISTANCE FOR THE REMOVAL OF SECRETIONS

The methods used are percussion, deep breathing exercises with vibrations and postural drainage. Usually there is no reason why a patient should not be posturally drained if it is necessary, but in certain conditions, such as hypertension, hiatus hernia and some aortic surgery, it is contra-indicated. The physiotherapist must be absolutely certain of the patient's condition and where necessary must confirm with the medical officer in charge of the patient whether or not postural drainage is permitted.

If the patient is nursed in the half-lying position, he should be positioned in crook lying or crook side lying for treatment. The foot of the bed may or may not need to be elevated. The breathing exercises, and the movement generally, usually help to relieve the flatulence which so often causes abdominal distension and further hampers breathing!

It must be remembered that practising breathing exercises once a day is useless. To be effective in preventing chest complications, they should be practised for at least five minutes in every hour so that correct breathing becomes a habit. It rests with the physiotherapist to establish a good rapport with the patient and gain his interest, under-standing and co-operation. Frequent short visits are essential until it is clear that the patient is sufficiently enthusiastic to work on his own.

Naso-pharyngeal suction may be necessary in some circumstances where the patient is unable to cough up secretions, despite the assist-ance of physiotherapy, e.g. inability to co-operate, weakness which makes coughing ineffective or sticky sputum which, though the patient is able to cough, he cannot expectorate. In the case of drowsy or unco-operative patients, the catheter may need to be introduced into the trachea in order to stimulate a good cough. Laryngoscopy and/or bronchoscopy may be needed to remove particularly obstinate secretions.

If major chest problems are anticipated e.g. before extensive pulmonary, cardiac or upper abdominal operations or where there is pre-existing lung disease it may be decided to intubate and even ventilate the patient postoperatively for a short while. In this case he will return from theatre with an endotracheal tube in situ. Chest physiotherapy is performed regularly on these patients and secretions removed by suction through the endotracheal tube using a sterile technique. Once the patient is awake and co-operative the endotracheal tube is removed, and since this is often within the first 24 hours, the physiotherapist must persist with frequent treatment to keep the chest clear.

Early mobilisation is an important factor, not only in preventing respiratory complications, but also in the general rehabilitation of the patient. As soon as they are able, patients should be encouraged to move about the bed as much as possible and in the absence of major complications, they usually sit out of bed within the first 24 hours. Drips and drains need not prevent patients from moving from bed to chair and back. Once drains and drips are removed, they should be encouraged to dress and walk about.

DEEP VEIN THROMBOSIS

Thrombosis of the deep veins of the lower limbs may occur in any patient immobilised for any length of time but occurs more frequently in high risk groups e.g. elderly patients, those with a history of previous deep vein thrombosis and those with malignant disease. It can have an insidious onset with no clinical signs or symptoms in the early stages when the main danger is of a fatal pulmonary embolus occurring. A deep vein thrombosis may present with local signs in the lower leg, the calf becoming swollen and tender. Passive ankle dorsiflexion causes pain in the calf muscles (Homan's sign). It may however only show itself when the thrombus becomes suddenly detached and is carried through the right side of the heart to occlude the pulmonary artery, causing a pulmonary embolism.

When a deep vein thrombosis is suspected the patient is treated with anticoagulants and once he is adequately anticoagulated and any calf pain has eased the surgeon usually allows the patient to resume exercising and mobilising, usually with an elastic supporting bandage. He should not stand about, and when sitting he should have the leg elevated.

Physiotherapy

The aim of the physiotherapist is to prevent this complication. Pre-operative instruction will include a programme of active leg exercises and the patient should be encouraged to practise these exercises as well as the deep breathing exercises for at least five minutes in every hour. Postoperatively the leg exercises need to be encouraged and early mobilisation will help to prevent the occurrence of deep vein thrombosis.

If a deep vein thrombosis does develop, the deep breathing exercises should continue but the carrying out of leg exercises will depend on the individual consultant's instructions. Active exercises and mobilisation can usually be continued while the patient is receiving anticoagulant therapy and elastic or blue line bandages may be applied to the whole limb to control swelling and aid venous return.

The physiotherapist should be alert to any pain or tenderness in the calf while treating the patient and must report it to the sister in charge of the ward immediately.

WOUND INFECTIONS

Normally, surgical incisions heal quickly and with little formation of scar tissue and it is perfectly safe for the patient to cough and move around. A wound only breaks down if the suturing material is faulty, if fluid collects under the suture line or the wound becomes infected.

The presence of infection in a previously clean wound is indicated by pain, throbbing and tenderness; the area may become hot, red and oedematous. The sutures tend to cut through the tissues and the wound may gape either along its whole length or in between the sutures.

If the area is already infected, healing is likely to be less satisfactory. Sometimes the very presence of sepsis is an indication for surgery, e.g. a gangrenous appendix, or empyema. Such surgery will involve the use of drainage tubes to permit free drainage of the pus and ensure healing from the base upwards; if tubes remain in for any length of time they can cause irritation of the walls and consequent fibrous tissue formation. In such cases healing becomes difficult when the tube is eventually removed; for this reason tubes are usually shortened and removed as soon as possible, usually between three and seven days, except in the case of an empyema.

Where there is an incision of the abdominal wall, distension can cause bursting either of the whole wound or areas between the sutures; persistent distension is therefore to be avoided.

As a result of any of these factors, scarring may occur in the musculature of the walls of the abdominal or pelvic cavities and consequently there is always the possibility of the contents of the cavity protruding through the weakened area. This condition is known as an incisional hernia.

Physiotherapy

Active exercise is good, as some strain on the wound stimulates the healing process. Excess strain should be avoided. Outer range abdominal exercises or heavy work such as double hip and knee flexion should not be given immediately following abdominal surgery.

If a clean wound becomes infected, cleaning and healing may be stimulated by some form of dry heat. If the infection is superficial, infra-red or radiant heat are satisfactory; if the infection is deep-seated, short wave diathermy should be used. Treatment is best given after the sutures have been cut and the wound allowed to gape so that free drainage is established, and treatment should be given at least twice daily.

The scar may be adherent to underlying tissue and will probably hamper movement, as well as causing discomfort as it pulls on other tissues. In time it may well contract and produce deformity. To prevent this occurring, massage with lanolin may be prescribed after the wound is well healed. Massage should be carried out over the surface of the scar in order to loosen it from the underlying tissue.

Ultrasound therapy is helpful in the treatment of particularly hard scars, such as can occur after surgery for the release of the flexor retinaculum in the carpal tunnel syndrome or after operation for Dupuytren's contracture. Paraffin wax treatment also helps to soften scars and the sooner the treatment can be started, the more successful it will be. Occasionally a scar may be painful, because a superficial nerve becomes entrapped in fibrous tissue. If other treatments fail the fibrous tissue is excised and the nerve freed.

PRESSURE SORES

Patients are mobilised fairly quickly after surgery and pressure sores are unlikely to develop unless the patient is elderly or recovery is delayed or if the patient lies in one position on the operating table for a very long period.

Pressure sores can be divided into superficial and deep sores. Superficial sores begin in the skin and break down leaving a shallow, painful ulcer. Deep sores begin in the subcutaneous tissues, where muscle and fat have less resistance to pressure than skin; destruction may occur in these while the skin covering them shows only erythema. Eventually the skin breaks down and the deeper necrosed tissues are exposed. Both types of sore are due to pressure which occludes the blood vessels and deprives the tissues of nutrition. In a patient with normal sensation this pressure causes discomfort and he alters his position to relieve it, but if there is loss of sensation or he is unconscious or too ill to move, pressure will not be relieved. Other causes may be a) ill-fitting splints; b) friction from rucked sheets; c) persistent soaking of the skin due to incontinence and d) poor skin. The most commonly affected sites are the heels, malleoli, greater trochanters, sacrum and elbows. If a patient is nursed in a propped-up position he tends to slide down and this causes a shearing force on the sacral area, rupturing deeper tissues and small blood vessels and consequently may lead to a deep sacral pressure·sore.

Prevention

Pressure sores should be prevented and this can only be done by regular turning of unconscious or paralysed patients either by manual lifting or by nursing them on turning beds. If the patient is sitting in a chair, he should either be taught to relieve pressure by lifting himself on his arms, or be lifted by a nurse or attendant. Splints must be carefully made and well-finished so that there are no rough areas to cause an abrasion. Sheepskins are frequently used under paralysed or heavy patients to prevent friction and the oil content of a real sheepskin is also beneficial to poor skin. Ripple or water beds, in which the areas of pressure on the patient's body are constantly changed, are another aid to the prevention of sores. They do not however supersede good nursing and regular turning. Physiotherapists can help in this prevention by teaching nurses how to lift and turn patients with minimum effort.

Physiotherapy

When treating a patient the physiotherapist should note any areas of redness or broken skin, and report these to the sister in charge of the ward so that appropriate measures may be taken. If pressure sores occur the physiotherapist may be asked to treat them. If the pressure sore is only superficial, i.e. red and sore, then further erosion may be prevented and healing stimulated by infra-red rays. If the area has broken down, become infected or even necrotic, ultraviolet light may be prescribed. Good team work is essential here as the job will be much easier if the nurse prepares and cleans the area prior to the ultraviolet light being applied and dresses it afterwards. If the pressure area is only reddened with no skin break, an ice cube may be used to massage the area (Marshall, 1971).

HAEMORRHAGE

Haemorrhage may complicate any operation, but is particularly liable when surgery has involved a vascular area, such as the thyroid gland or tonsils. If bleeding is excessive or prolonged, various signs and symptoms will arise; the pulse will be rapid and feeble, blood pressure low, and respirations fast and often of the sighing type. The skin will be cold, clammy and pale. The patient will be restless, feel thirsty and complain of faintness and giddiness. If haemorrhage occurs while the physiotherapist is treating the patient, further help should immediately be summoned and first aid treatment given. If possible the patient should be placed in the lying position and if bleeding is external, digital pressure may be applied above the site of haemorrhage, or directly over the bleeding part.

If sepsis is already suspected, active exercises should be avoided as this could precipitate a secondary haemorrhage particularly between the sixth and fourteenth day.

MUSCLE ATROPHY AND IMBALANCE

The musculature of patients undergoing surgery will vary according to their general health; some patients will be in poor condition such as the elderly patient and those who have been ill for some time, particularly if they are suffering from nutritional disturbances associated with ulcerative colitis or Crohn's disease; others will be in excellent condition but may be affected by the operation.

Muscles may be affected both generally and locally by surgery. Most operations lead to a lessening of general activity and this is as true for a meniscectomy as for a radical pelvic or brain operation. This inactivity can be increased by fear. Reduced muscular activity will lead to a lessened cardiac output, with consequent reduced metabolism.

Locally, muscles in the region of the operation may be affected either through division or through the local nerve supply being damaged. Provided that the muscles are adequately sutured, no lessening of power should result. If the nerve supply is only bruised, full muscle power will return; if however it is divided or excised then there may be residual weakness, e.g. parotidectomy is quite likely to involve damage to the facial nerve and weakness of the facial muscles will result.

Occasionally during operation, stretching of, or pressure on a nerve may occur. If a relaxant drug such as tubocurarine (curare) is used during the operation there is complete absence of tone in the muscles, and consequently no protection for the nerves. If a position is necessary in which pressure on a nerve might occur, there will be a greater tendency for paresis to result and if an Esmarch's rubber bandage is used for a tourniquet in operations on the knee, a drop foot can occur, probably due to ischaemia of the common peroneal nerve. Neurological damage will depend on the extent of the lesion.

In some operations certain positions may be necessary which prevent active use of the muscles, e.g. in operations for recurrent dislocation of the shoulder, where the arm may be fixed in adduction and medial rotation. Muscle power and movement can be inhibited by pain, fear, or as a result of reflex action. As the result of surgery on joints, distension or damage of the capsule can stimulate the nerve endings and reflex inhibition will result.

Whatever the cause, atrophy and hypotonia of muscle will occur in varying degrees following any surgical procedure and the most outstanding effect of this is alteration in posture usually affecting the body as a whole. Atrophy and hypotonia of the spinal muscles will lead to a loss of the erect carriage of the trunk and if the gluteal muscles are also affected an increased pelvic tilt will be followed by spinal deformity. When the patient first gets up and walks, his general posture is likely to be poor; postural flat feet and round shoulders with poking head may be noticeable. If there is unilateral weakness of the trunk muscles then muscle imbalance is particularly noticeable, and may well lead to gross deformity. This is clearly seen following thoracic surgery or where there has been interference with the nerve supply of abdominal muscles. Scoliosis is a likely result and one which can be avoided.

Muscle atrophy can lead to diminished power, with possible serious results, since the muscles are the first line of defence of the joints. Inadequate muscles will result in continuous minor trauma to joint structures with chronic synovitis developing and this is particularly liable to happen following operations on the knee joint unless adequate isometric muscle work is taught.

If the abdominal muscles are affected then their function can be impaired also and not only will posture be disturbed but the intra-abdominal pressure will not be maintained. If intra-abdominal pressure falls, respiration, venous return, defaecation, and support of the abdominal viscera will all be affected. Scarring in abdominal muscles may lead to incisional hernia.

Finally muscle weakness may be a factor leading to stiffness of joints, for if the muscle has insufficient power to move the joint through its full range, then full range is not attained and adaptive contractures can result.

Physiotherapy

Muscle atrophy can be avoided except in the case of nerve involvement. The principle is the practice of active movement, either in the form of active exercises or as static (isometric) work. This should be taught pre-operatively and encouraged for as long as necessary post-operatively. With early mobilisation following surgery, muscle atrophy is rarely seen today.

An important point to be observed is the wearing of shoes rather than slippers; this aids walking and correct posture once the patient is ambulant. The feet are frequently painful after bed rest or varicose vein surgery and exercises for the intrinsic muscles of the foot can be most helpful.

REFERENCE

Marshall, Rosemary S. (1971). 'Cold Therapy in the Treatment of Pressure Sores'. *Physiotherapy*, 57, 8.

BIBLIOGRAPHY

Schonell, M. (1974). *Respiratory Medicine*. Churchill Livingstone.
Sykes, M. K., McNicol, H. W. and Campbell, E. J. M. (1976). *Respiratory Failure*. 2nd edition. Blackwell Scientific Publications.

ACKNOWLEDGEMENTS

The author wishes to thank Mr. R. N. Baird, F.R.C.S. (Ed.), Consultant and Senior Lecturer in the Department of Surgery, Bristol Royal Infirmary; Miss R. Coles, M.C.S.P., Superintendent Physiotherapist, and Miss P. Rundle, M.C.S.P., Senior Physiotherapist, of the Bristol Royal Infirmary, for their help in the preparation of this chapter.

Chapter 4

Cardiac Arrest and Resuscitation

by J. R. PEPPER, M.A., F.R.C.S.

CARDIAC ARREST

This may be defined as a sudden cessation of a functional circulation. It is an emergency which demands prompt recognition. The absence of carotid or femoral pulses is sufficient. There is no need to listen for the heart beat or look for dilated pupils.

Aetiology

The heart arrests either in asystole or in ventricular fibrillation. Asystole is due usually to hypoxia, for whatever reason, or complete heart block. Ventricular fibrillation is commonly the result of an electrolyte imbalance e.g. hypokalaemia.

The common causes of cardiac arrest are:

1. Massive pulmonary embolus which obstructs the circulation and produces myocardial hypoxia.
2. Myocardial infarction which can lead to sudden death probably due to ventricular tachycardia and fibrillation.
3. Pericardial tamponade which restricts filling of the heart.
4. Tension pneumothorax which produces an acute shift of the mediastinum compressing the opposite lung and the heart.
5. Increased vagal tone which can occur during induction of general anaesthesia and may lead to a cardiac arrest when associated with hypoxia and acidosis.

Less common causes include anaphylactic reactions to drugs and air embolism.

RESUSCITATION

Unless the circulation can be rapidly restored, irreversible brain damage will occur within three (3) minutes. The priority therefore is to restore the circulation and ventilate the lungs.

If there is no board under the mattress the patient is transferred to the floor so that effective cardiac massage can be given. External cardiac massage in adults is applied by placing one hand over the other at the lower end of the sternum. The arms should be held straight as this is less tiring for the operator who may have to continue massage for several minutes before further help is available. A rate of massage of 60 per minute is the aim in adults; 80 to 90 per minute in children. In infants and small children the heart lies higher in the thorax so that the massaging hands should be placed over the mid-sternum. Care should be taken to avoid sudden compression of the abdomen as this may cause the liver to rupture.

Initially ventilation is achieved by mouth-to-mouth breathing or a face mask and Ambubag, taking care to maintain an airway. The patient should be intubated with an endotracheal tube swiftly and skilfully; until such skill is available it is safer to continue ventilation by face mask, keeping a close watch on the airway.

While this is going on, medical help will have arrived and an intravenous line and E.C.G. monitor will be set up. If the heart rhythm is ventricular fibrillation, D.C. counter-shock is given starting at 100 Joules (in adults) to restore sinus rhythm. If asystole is present, 1 in 10 000 adrenaline is injected either directly into the right ventricle through the chest wall or into a central venous line to induce ventricular fibrillation which can then be treated by D.C. shock. Sodium bicarbonate is given to correct the acidosis which invariably develops following a cardiac arrest.

The patient who has recently undergone open heart surgery is in a special situation. If after giving adrenaline and continuous external massage for one minute, there is no improvement the chest is re-opened via the recent wound. There are many recorded instances of patients surviving this procedure and leaving hospital in good health.

Once a cardiac output has been restored as shown by the return of the carotid or femoral pulses a search is made for the cause of the arrest and appropriate action taken. An anti-inflammatory steroid, dexamethasone, is generally given as prophylaxis against the development of cerebral oedema. However, the patient may slide into a state of low cardiac output which is insufficient to meet the needs of the vital organs; brain, kidneys and heart.

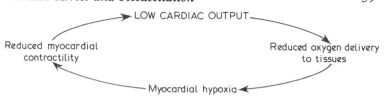

Fig. 4/1 Diagram illustrating the vicious cycle resulting from a low cardiac output

Low Cardiac Output

When such a state exists a vicious cycle develops (see Fig. 4/1).

If this cycle is allowed to continue, cardiac arrest will inevitably recur. On an intensive care unit such a state should be recognised early from the following features:

1. Poor urine output; less than 30ml per hour in an adult.
2. Cool peripheries and if the core and toe temperatures are being measured there will be an increase in the core: toe gradient.
3. Mental confusion deteriorating eventually to unconsciousness.
4. An increasing tendency to acidosis.

Although the causes of low cardiac output are many, the basis of treatment is the same. Initially the filling pressure of the heart is examined by measuring the central venous pressure (right atrial pressure). In some cases it is useful to measure the left atrial pressure as well. Due to the relationship between cardiac output and the filling pressure of the heart as described in Starling's law of the heart, there is a critical range for optimal function of the heart. If the right atrial pressure is below this range which is +5 to +15mmHg, blood, plasma or plasma expanders are given to raise the pressure. By raising the right atrial pressure to the upper limit of this range the heart is placed in the optimal physiological situation. In many instances this simple measure will suffice to restore a normal circulation.

If this is not enough, attention is directed to the state of myocardial contractility. This can be altered by the administration of synthetic catecholamines of which the commonest are isoprenaline and adrenaline. Recently dopamine has come into regular use because of its special beneficial effect on the kidneys. Other drugs in use include salbutamol and noradrenaline. A further drug has appeared recently called dobutamine. All these drugs increase the rate and force of contraction of the myocardium but in practice it is their effect on heart rate which is the limiting factor.

If after applying these measures the patient has not improved an attempt may be made to reduce the peripheral resistance. The aim of this treatment is to reduce the minimum pressure which the left ventricle has to generate in order to open the aortic valve; and thus to reduce the work done by the left ventricle. This is achieved by the administration of peripheral vasodilator drugs which reduce the sympathetic vasoconstrictor drive to arterioles. Hence, whole new vascular beds which were closed are opened up and the capacity of the circulation increases. For this reason the central venous pressure will fall and in order to maintain the heart at its optimal filling pressure, several units of blood or plasma will need to be given. This type of treatment is potentially lethal unless the central venous pressure is maintained. Examples of the drugs which are used include chlorpromazine (Largactil), phentolamine (Rogitine), nitroprusside (Nipride).

In addition the patient may be placed on intermittent positive pressure ventilation (I.P.P.V.), to reduce oxygen requirements by taking over the work of the respiratory muscles and to gain better control of the arterial oxygen tension. The acid base balance is also closely maintained and corrected when necessary.

Until recently no other routine measures were available but there are now various forms of cardiac assist devices of which the intraaortic balloon pump is the only one in regular clinical use.

Intra-Aortic Balloon Counterpulsation

The relationship between the *supply* of oxygen to the myocardium and the *demand* by the energy processes of the myocardium for oxygen becomes critical in low cardiac output states. Drugs which increase the contractility of the myocardium and thus the cardiac output tend to do so at the expense of increased demand by the myocardium for oxygen. Such drugs may increase demand beyond the available supply and thus build up an oxygen debt. Counterpulsation provides a way of improving the ratio between supply and demand.

The concept of counterpulsation is based on the finding that myocardial oxygen consumption is dependent upon the pressure generated by the left ventricle. Counterpulsation does two things: first it increases the diastolic perfusion pressure and second it reduces the pressure against which the left ventricle contracts (a similar effect to that of the peripheral vasodilator drug).

A special balloon catheter is introduced into the descending thoracic aorta via a femoral artery. When the balloon inflates blood is displaced and the diastolic pressure in the aorta is increased. When the balloon deflates the systolic pressure is reduced and the capacity of the aorta for blood increases.

The catheter is attached to an electronically controlled actuator. The R wave of the E.C.G. is the trigger which is picked up by the control unit. The trigger is delayed so that the balloon is inflated during diastole when the aortic valve is closed. Since the majority of coronary blood flow occurs during diastole and is dependent upon diastolic perfusion, the selective elevation of diastolic pressure by the balloon will increase coronary blood flow. Shortly before the onset of left ventricular systole the balloon is deflated. This reduces the systolic pressure against which the left ventricle ejects its blood and so reduces work and hence myocardial oxygen consumption by the left ventricle.

The counterpulsation pump is used in two clinical situations; first in the operating theatre to enable a struggling heart to take on the load of the circulation and so come off cardiopulmonary bypass and second to assist a patient in low cardiac output, either following open heart surgery or as a means of holding a severely ill patient with coronary artery disease for a limited period before emergency coronary artery vein bypass surgery is done.

Chapter 5

Gynaecological Conditions

by S. M. HARRISON, M.C.S.P.

The term gynaecology is derived from the Greek words, *gynae* = a woman and *logos* = a discourse, study or science. Thus gynaecology is the study of the woman as a whole.

It is important to bear in mind that the activity of the genital organs is controlled by the endocrine system, which itself is often influenced by the psyche (mind).

While the symptoms of many diseases are psychosomatic, the mind plays a particularly important role in gynaecological conditions. There is a great deal of fear, anxiety and embarrassment associated with these conditions and their treatment. It is only when we approach the patient with sensitivity and understanding, thinking of each as a complete person, that we can expect our treatments to be effective.

The physiotherapist will meet gynaecological patients in the wards and as outpatients.

Some knowledge of the female pelvis and its contents is essential. The points of special importance for her work are the relationship of one organ to another within the pelvis and the pelvic floor muscles.

ANATOMICAL RELATIONS IN THE PELVIS

The Uterus

The uterus lies in the pelvis with the bladder in front and the rectum behind (Fig. 5/1). It is tilted forward making an angle of 90° to the vagina. Its anterior and posterior surfaces are covered by peritoneum. On each side of the uterus the two layers of peritoneum meet to form the broad ligaments which then attach to the lateral walls of the pelvis. Between the two layers run the round ligaments (round muscles) which eventually enter the deep inguinal ring, pass through the inguinal canal and finally blend with the areolar tissue of the labia majora, thus probably helping to hold the uterus in the anteverted

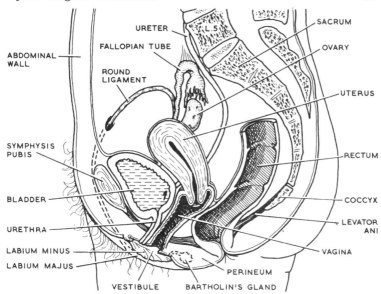

Fig. 5/1 The position and relations of the uterus

Fig. 5/2 The ligaments of the cervix

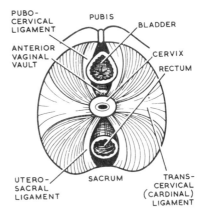

position. The cervix and fornices of the vagina are further supported by the cervical ligaments as shown in Fig. 5/2.

The uterus is a hollow pear-shaped organ whose narrow lower end is termed the cervix. This protrudes into the vagina, a canal which extends downwards and forwards to end in the vestibule i.e. the cleft between the labia minora (Fig. 5/3). The mucous membrane lining the uterus is known as the endometrium.

Opening into the upper angles of the uterus are the right and left

Gynaecological Conditions

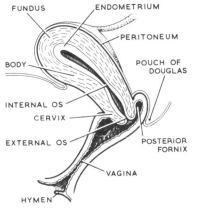

Fig. 5/3 Coronal section of the cervix

Fig. 5/4 The Fallopian tubes

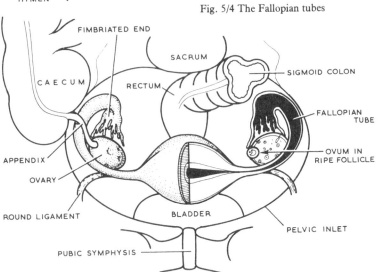

Fallopian (uterine) tubes whose other ends are fimbriated and open into the peritoneal cavity close to the ovaries (Fig. 5/4).

The Bladder

The bladder is a sac capable of considerable distension which acts as a reservoir for urine. It has a flat base which lies parallel to the vagina (Fig. 5/1). The ureters enter the base at an angle and form a triangle with the internal urinary meatus. This triangular area is three or four times as thick as the rest of the bladder and contains thick connective tissue which forms a sheath for each ureteric orifice and becomes the core structure of the urethra, and is called the trigone (Hutch, 1972) (Fig. 5/5).

The involuntary muscle layers in the wall of the bladder are named the detrusor muscle. It is thought that loop-shaped fibres of this muscular layer spiral round the upper two thirds of the urethra

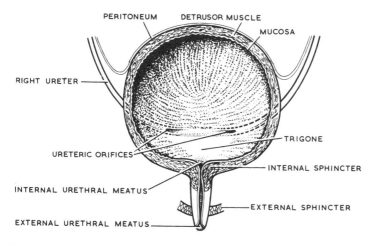

Fig. 5/5 The trigone of the bladder

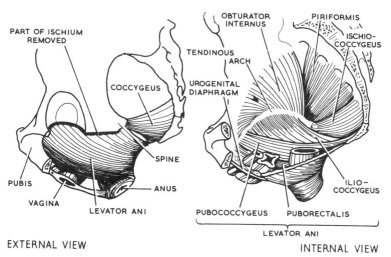

EXTERNAL VIEW

INTERNAL VIEW

Fig. 5/6 Lateral view of the pelvic diaphragm, external and internal, showing urogenital diaphragm

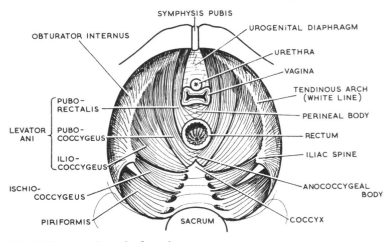

Fig. 5/7 Levator ani muscles from above

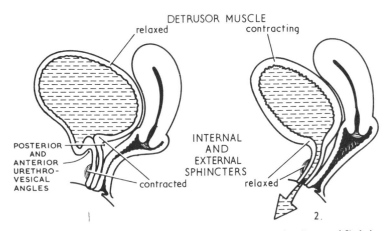

Fig. 5/8 The anterior and posterior urethrovesical angles showing 1) normal 2) their disappearance during micturition

(sometimes called the internal sphincter) and meet the voluntary muscle fibres of the pelvic floor muscles which form an external sphincter round the lower one third of the urethra (Figs. 5/6 and 5/7). The external sphincter makes it possible to stop a stream of urine at will.

It will be seen from Fig. 5/8 that the urethra leaves the flat base of the bladder almost at a right angle, thus forming the anterior and posterior urethrovesical angles. These angles are lost during micturition as funnelling of the bladder base occurs. The posterior angle is frequently missing if the anterior vaginal wall is weakened, allowing the upper part of the bladder base and the urethra to prolapse downwards and backwards. This is often associated with laxity of the pelvic floor muscles and results in stress incontinence (p. 79).

NERVE SUPPLY OF BLADDER

The upper part of the bladder is poorly supplied by autonomic nerve fibres while the area around the trigone is richly innervated (Llewellyn-Jones, 1978). The parasympathetic fibres are derived from S2, S3 and S4 and are motor to the detrusor muscle. The sympathetic fibres mainly derive from L1 and L2 and supply the trigone. In the voiding reflex the sensory stimuli initiated by stretch and tension in the bladder wall are carried to the sacral cord through the afferent fibres of the sacral parasympathetic nerves; the motor branch of this reflex arc is formed by the efferent fibres of these same sacral parasympathetic nerves. Although certain sensory impulses from the bladder (pain and thermal perception) are conveyed by sympathetic fibres, extensive sympathectomy does not alter bladder function. The external sphincter (voluntary) receives its nerve supply from the pudendal nerve (S2, S3, S4).

The Pelvic Floor

All the tissues between the cavity of the pelvis and the surface of the perineum make up the true pelvic floor. It therefore includes peritoneum, fascia, fat and deep and superficial muscles.

SUPERFICIAL MUSCLES

These are individually named as: bulbospongiosus, ischiocavernosus, and superficial transverse perineal muscles. They take origin from the ischium and pubis and are inserted into the central point of the perineum, the perineal body (Fig. 5/9). Anteriorly between the superficial and deep muscle groups there is an extra supporting fascial layer which covers the area between the ischial tuberosities and the symphysis pubis and is called the urogenital diaphragm. The deep transverse perineal muscles are part of the lower border of the urogenital diaphragm and their central point is anchored in the perineal body.

DEEP MUSCLES

These form the most important muscle group and together with the fascia covering their upper and lower surfaces are commonly known as

SUPERFICIAL   DEEPER

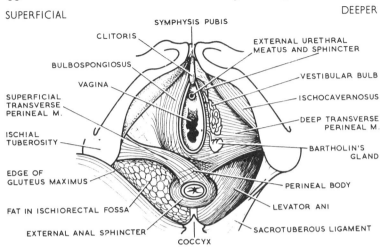

Fig. 5/9 Dissection of the perineum showing the superficial muscles

the pelvic floor muscles, though some authorities use the term 'the pelvic diaphragm' (Fig. 5/6).

The levator ani muscles derive their nerve supply from the third, fourth and fifth sacral nerves. They are sling shaped and arise from the inner surface of the pubis, a thickened line of fascia over the obturator internus muscle and the ischial spine. The fibres pass downwards, backwards and medially to fuse with the fibres of the opposite side in the perineal body, anococcygeal raphe and the coccyx (Figs. 5/6 and 5/7).

As a result of their wide origin the levator ani are sometimes subdivided into muscles naming the point of origin i.e. pubo-coccygeus, ilio-coccygeus, and ischio-coccygeus (Fig. 5/7). The latter two muscles have no connection with the anus, while the pubo-coccygeal portion has some fibres inserted directly into the anal sphincter (pubo-rectalis). Pubo-coccygeus is the important section of the levator ani when stress incontinence and prolapse are being considered.

FUNCTION OF DEEP PELVIC FLOOR MUSCLES

1. Support of the pelvic viscera which is especially important in view of our erect posture.
2. Sphincteric control of the bladder and bowel.
3. Contract reflexly (unless very weak) when the intra-abdominal pressure is raised, e.g. cough or sneeze.

GYNAECOLOGICAL WARD

The range of conditions and operative procedures is large, so the ones most frequently found are listed on the following pages with brief explanatory notes.

Ectopic Pregnancy

This occurs if a fertilised ovum becomes implanted in a site other than the uterine cavity, the Fallopian tubes being the most common extra-uterine site. The tubes will eventually rupture and when this occurs the operation of salpingectomy or salpingo-oophorectomy will be necessary.

Ectopic pregnancy may present as an acute or sub-acute condition. When there is a severe intraperitoneal haemorrhage and the majority of the blood is not removed during the operation, diaphragmatic irritation is often caused by the clotted blood under the diaphragm. Referred pain via C4 and C5 to the supraclavicular area results, and an increase in the incidence of postoperative chest complications is likely.

Pelvic Inflammatory Disease

This is an inflammatory condition of the Fallopian tubes and often of the uterus secondary to bacterial infection. The infection may be primary as in tuberculosis or secondary as in gonorrhoea. Infection may also follow abortion or parturition and occasionally follows such acute inflammatory diseases as appendicitis or diverticulitis.

The disease may present as an acute attack of abdominal peritonitis which is treated by chemotherapy and occasionally by the drainage of any abscesses by the vaginal or abdominal route.

As far as physiotherapists are concerned they are more likely to meet this condition in its chronic form, when they may be requested to give a course of short wave diathermy (see p. 91). The symptoms of this chronic form of the disease are secondary dysmenorrhoea, dyspareunia and a disturbance of the menstrual pattern. Occasionally, under treatment, the condition may be exacerbated. This will be shown by the fact that the patient will be generally unwell and have an increase in her symptoms. Treatment must be stopped until the gynaecologist has been consulted.

It is worth noting that this condition is often abbreviated as P.I.D., and this may lead to confusion with the shortened form of the phrase prolapsed intervertebral disc.

Variations in the Menstrual Cycle

The normal cycle is defined as a blood loss lasting five days every 28 days. The range of this loss may be between one and seven days and the intervals vary between 21 and 35 days, counting from the first day of one period to the first day of the next.

There are a number of descriptive terms applied to abnormalities of the menstrual cycle.

1. Amenorrhoea: the absence of menstruation. This may be primary or secondary.
2. Polymenorrhoea: too frequent periods.
3. Menorrhagia: an increase in the volume of the blood loss occurring at regular intervals. This may be an increase in the volume lost in any given time, or an increase in the duration of the loss, or both at once.
4. Intermenstrual bleeding: bleeding between periods.
5. Postcoital bleeding: bleeding following coitus.

On the whole, a description of the type, frequency and character of the bleeding in simple terms is the easiest way to a clear understanding of a patient's menstrual cycle.

Abdominal Pain due to Nerve Entrapment

In recent years it has been discovered that many women complaining of chronic pain in one or both iliac fossae are suffering from what has been described as the 'nerve entrapment syndrome'. These women are not suffering from gynaecological disease though they may have had gynaecological operations.

This abdominal wall pain has been described as a sharp burning pain in the abdominal wall along the outer border of the rectus sheath. The cutaneous intercostal nerves can be compressed in the posterior wall of the rectus sheath (Mehta, 1973).

Thorough investigations for evidence of serious disease will leave a small group of patients who suffer great discomfort from this condition.

Remission may be spontaneous but frequently symptoms may persist intermittently for a long time.

Diagnosis is confirmed by tensing the abdominal muscles by raising the head and shoulders from a lying position and finding the tender area, about the size of a pea. Coughing also produces the pain.

Infiltration of the tender zone with local anaesthesia relieves the symptoms temporarily and confirms the source of discomfort.

The best results are found to be from injection therapy, using an anaesthetic solution. This produces a differential block with impact on the non-myelinated and small myelinated pain fibres. Operative intervention is seldom necessary.

OPERATIONS USING A VAGINAL ROUTE

DILATATION AND CURETTAGE (D & C)

The cervix is dilated and the uterine cavity is scraped. This is used for diagnostic purposes, removal of polyps, after an incomplete abortion and as a vaginal termination of pregnancy.

SHIRODKAR SUTURE

A non-absorbable suture is placed around the internal os (cervix) (Fig. 5/10), during early pregnancy in women whose defective cervix has

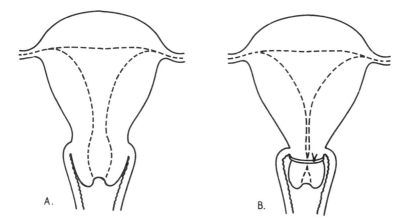

Fig. 5/10 Shirodkhar suture. A. Uterus with an incompetent internal os. B. Non-absorbable suture tied round cervix at level of internal os

dilated prematurely in previous pregnancies, leading to late abortion (18 to 20 weeks). The suture is removed about 14 days before term. Some authorities insert this suture before pregnancy.

CONE BIOPSY

A conical segment is removed from the cervix. It is used as a diagnostic check after cervical smears from a Papanicolaou test have indicated the presence of abnormal cells.

INCISION OF BARTHOLIN'S ABSCESS

An acute infection in the gland of the labium majorum which has to be incised.

EXCISION OF BARTHOLIN'S CYST

An excision of a cyst of the gland at the base of the labium majorum. The cyst is often due to chronic infection.

VULVECTOMY

An excision of the skin in the vulval area for skin disease including malignancy. In the presence of malignant disease it often includes the whole of the vulva and the inguinal glands.

VAGINAL HYSTERECTOMY

The removal of the uterus vaginally for menorrhagia or prolapse.

ANTERIOR COLPORRHAPHY

A repair of the anterior vaginal wall for stress incontinence or prolapse of the bladder (cystocele, p. 80). It is often accompanied by amputation of the cervix. These conditions are observed as bulging or laxity of the anterior vaginal wall.

COLPOPERINEORRAPHY

A repair of the posterior vaginal wall and defective perineum. It may accompany vaginal hysterectomy or anterior repair and amputation of the cervix.

CAUTERY OF CERVIX

This is the treatment of chronic inflammatory conditions of the cervix, symptoms of which are an offensive discharge and dyspareunia.

INSUFFLATION OF THE FALLOPIAN TUBES

This procedure is used to check the patency of the tubes in cases of infertility. Carbon dioxide is blown into the uterus from a pressure apparatus which shows the passage of gas through the tubes on a calibrated drum (kymograph).

OPERATIONS WITH ABDOMINAL INCISIONS

Types of Incision (Fig. 5/11)

Transverse incisions are variations of the Pfannenstiel incision and are commonly known as the 'bikini'. They are relatively bloodless and

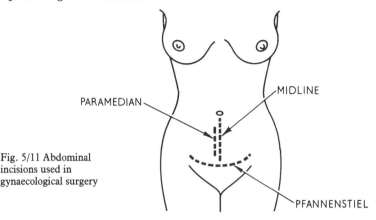

PARAMEDIAN

MIDLINE

Fig. 5/11 Abdominal
incisions used in
gynaecological surgery

PFANNENSTIEL

there is little chance of an incisional hernia. The patient has less postoperative discomfort than with other incisions. The disadvantages lie in its taking slightly longer to perform, and it occasionally gives inadequate exposure for large tumours.

A *mid-line* incision is a longitudinal one in which the linea alba is incised. It can be performed rapidly and is relatively bloodless due to the fibrous tissue being incised. The disadvantages are a definite danger of an incisional hernia developing later, because fibrous tissue heals less efficiently. There is generally more postoperative discomfort.

A *paramedian* incision is made to the right or left of centre and carries a low incidence of incisional hernia. It is slower to perform than a mid-line incision and is likely to produce more bleeding than mid-line or transverse incisions. Postoperative discomfort is similar to that experienced with a mid-line incision.

TOTAL HYSTERECTOMY

The whole uterus is removed. Occasionally the cervix is left in situ, thus becoming a subtotal hysterectomy.

HYSTEROTOMY

A termination of pregnancy by removing the fetus and products of conception through an incision in the uterus.

WERTHEIM'S HYSTERECTOMY

The removal of the whole uterus, tubes and ovaries, upper half of the vagina, broad ligaments and the lymph nodes around the iliac vessels and the lateral pelvic walls. It is performed for carcinoma of the cervix and occasionally for carcinoma of the uterus.

MYOMECTOMY

The removal of fibroids from the uterus. It can also be done vaginally if the fibroid is being extruded as a polyp.

VENTROSUSPENSION

A correction of the position of the uterus from the retroverted to the anteverted position by shortening the round ligaments or by drawing them through the peritoneum and rectus muscles and suturing them to each other in front of the rectus muscles.

OVARIAN CYSTECTOMY

A removal of an ovarian cyst with conservation of a remnant of the ovary.

OOPHORECTOMY

The removal of one or both ovaries.

SALPINGECTOMY

The removal of one or both Fallopian tubes for disease, or removal of a portion of both as a form of sterilisation.

SALPINGO-OOPHORECTOMY

A removal of a Fallopian tube and an ovary. It can be bilateral. It is sometimes associated with hysterectomy.

BIOPSY OR WEDGE RESECTION OF THE OVARY

A diagnostic biopsy operation on the ovary for endocrine problems.

FALLOPIAN PLASTIC OPERATIONS

Restoration of patency to a blocked Fallopian tube in an attempt to cure infertility.

PELVIC EXENTERATION

A radical operation for pelvic malignant disease which entails removal of the uterus, rectum or bladder or both with transplantation of ureters and colostomy.

POSTERIOR COLPOTOMY

An aspiration or drainage of the pouch of Douglas through the posterior fornix.

LAPAROSCOPY

A means of visualising the abdominal contents after the induction of a pneumoperitoneum without making a large abdominal incision. Operative procedures can be carried out by this method, e.g. ovarian biopsy and sterilisation using diathermy.

PRESACRAL NEURECTOMY

This is done for primary spasmodic dysmenorrhoea. The fibres of the presacral nerve lying in front of the first part of the sacrum are divided.

Operations for Stress Incontinence

VAGINAL

See anterior colporrhaphy (p. 72).

ABDOMINAL

These are a series of abdominal or combined abdominal and vaginal operations, the principle of which is the construction of some form of sling to reform the posterior vesico-urethral angle of the bladder (Fig. 5/8). Such operations are named after their originators, e.g. Aldridge, Millin, Marshall-Marchetti-Krantz, and others. These may be accomplished by the insertion of artificial substances, natural transplanted tissues, or the use of contiguous tissues (vaginal). These materials are anchored either to the periosteum and ligaments of the bony pubis or the sheath of the rectus abdominis.

PHYSIOTHERAPY

Most patients in the ward will be having an operation, so the work of the physiotherapist will be similar to that on other surgical wards but with certain additions and some differences in technique.

Deep Vein Thrombosis

Patients who have had a pelvic operation appear to be particularly susceptible to deep vein thrombosis, therefore special precautions should be taken:

1. If Tubigrip or an elastic bandage has not been applied prior to operation or in the theatre, the physiotherapist may be asked to apply this when the patient returns to the ward.

2. The foot of the bed can be elevated and a bed cradle used to facilitate frequent foot and leg movements.
3. Extra emphasis should be placed on deep breathing, practised frequently, to improve venous return.

COUGHING FOLLOWING THE PFANNENSTIEL APPROACH

Due to the frequency of the use of the Pfannenstiel incision the author has found that the best way to assist the patient with postoperative breathing and coughing is as shown in Figure 2/1, p. 32.

The instructions are:

1. Blow out slowly and continuously until the lungs feel empty.
2. Shut the mouth and draw air up through the nose slowly, feeling the chest expanding. When the chest feels comfortably full start blowing out again.
3. After emptying and filling the lungs three or four times, a sharp command 'cough now' is given, while firm pressure from the patient's and physiotherapist's hands is given over the incision. If the patient has sutures in her vagina or perineum she should apply firm pressure over her sanitary pad when she coughs. This will lessen the bulging of the abdomen or perineum and greatly increase the patient's comfort and confidence.

Graduated Exercises

A scheme of graduated exercises in the form of a duplicated list is very useful. Each patient can be given a list at the time she is taught pre-operative breathing. A brief explanation about the list given at this time shows the patient that the breathing exercises are part of a programme of continuous care which aims to reduce the effects of the anaesthetic and the operation and speed her restoration to normality.

As well as the three exercises already mentioned above the following should be included: strengthening exercises for the abdominal and back muscles; and correct lifting methods.

PELVIC TILTING

This encourages the viscera to move away from the incised abdominal wall, so increasing the patient's comfort. It should be taught in the crook-lying, lying, sitting and standing positions to encourage an upright posture.

PELVIC FLOOR EXERCISES

These are vital because the pelvic floor needs re-education due to the condition or as a result of the surgery. The starting date must be agreed by consultation with the surgeon.

Infra-Red Radiation and Short Wave Diathermy

Heat can be very effective in speeding the healing of infected and slow-healing wounds or haematomas. The dilatation of the capillaries and arterioles in the superficial tissues allows more blood to flow to the tissues, thus aiding the reaction to and clearing of the infection because more white blood cells are present. The increased metabolism in the heated area results in an increased demand for oxygen and nutrients and the output of waste products.

Care should be taken to ensure that an adequate area of skin around the incision is exposed to the heat, as thermal sensation in the proximity of a wound is frequently impaired. The presence of metal in the form of metal clips or buttons anchoring a continuous suture is a contra-indication to any form of heat treatment.

Physiotherapists working in an obstetric or gynaecological department will find themselves in a very emotional atmosphere. This emotion may reveal itself in a coarseness and vulgarity which they may find distasteful and unbecoming to women. At the opposite extreme they will find a reticence and embarrassment that makes it difficult to achieve any satisfactory contact with the patient.

There are, however, certain repetitive phenomena which physiotherapists will meet in both specialities. These are emotional in origin and tend to occur about the third and the ninth day after delivery or a major operation.

After parturition the 'let down' and relief accompanied by discomfort in the perineum and breasts often cause depression on the third day. On the eighth or ninth day, particularly in primigravidae, the realisation of the responsibility that they have now assumed weighs heavily upon them.

The same thing applies, though the reasons are somewhat different, after major gynaecological operations. The second and third post-operative days are often the most uncomfortable. At this time some patients start to show concern about the effect of the operation on their femininity. This is particularly true of a hysterectomy. On the ninth or tenth day, just prior to her discharge, the patient becomes worried about her ability to reassume her role as a complete woman and mother.

GYNAECOLOGY IN THE OUTPATIENT DEPARTMENT

Since there are many gynaecological conditions where physiotherapy is not indicated, the role of the gynaecologist is to select those patients who will benefit from the particular skills of a physiotherapist.

As some of these skills are only acquired as a result of post-registration training, it is accepted that some stages of the treatments which follow cannot be undertaken by a student. However, a student can learn much by observing an experienced physiotherapist treating a patient and assisting where appropriate.

Treatments are likely to fall into two categories:

1. Restoration of function by re-education of the pelvic floor muscles.
2. Short wave diathermy.

Symptoms of Weak Pelvic Floor Muscles

The pelvic floor muscles have many functions so a wide range of symptoms can be expected to show if the muscles are weak. The most important of these are listed below, together with the patient's descriptions of the symptoms. A patient may present with one or many of these symptoms:

1. Stress incontinence: leaking of urine when coughing, sneezing, laughing or on exertion.
2. Cystocele, urethrocele, rectocele: a bulgy lump just inside the vagina.
3. Vaginal laxity: lack of satisfaction during coitus and inability to retain a contraceptive diaphragm or tampon.
4. Uterine prolapse: heaviness in the vagina or something coming down.
5. Frequency: passing urine very often.
6. Obesity: symptoms get worse as weight increases.

Each of these symptoms will be discussed individually before any treatment is described.

Incontinence

This can be divided into four types and all are non-neurogenic, i.e. they do not originate in the nervous system. They are: complete incontinence; overflow incontinence with retention; urge incontinence; and stress incontinence.

Stress incontinence is the most relevant to this text but brief notes about the other types are also included.

COMPLETE INCONTINENCE

This is due to the development of a fistula which allows urine to leak into the surrounding tissues. The rate of this flow is dependent on the size of the fistula.

The most common sites of a fistula are: (*i*) between bladder and vagina (vesicovaginal); (*ii*) between ureter and vagina (ureterovaginal); (*iii*) between urethra and vagina (urethrovaginal).

The causes of a fistula may be congenital or acquired. Examples of the latter include childbirth, surgery, radiotherapy, or a new growth.

Treatment is surgical.

OVERFLOW INCONTINENCE

Overflow incontinence with retention of urine is generally caused by an obstruction to the outflow of urine. This causes the bladder to fill and overflow, giving passage to small amounts of urine at frequent intervals. The causes of overflow incontinence with retention may be a mass in the pelvis such as a retroverted gravid uterus, a fibroid or an ovarian cyst; or it may be caused by trauma to the bladder or its nerve supply during a pelvic operation or childbirth, which results in the mechanism of the micturition reflex being damaged. Impaction of faeces in the elderly is very common as an additional cause and is often overlooked.

Treatment varies with the cause. Physiotherapy is not indicated.

URGE INCONTINENCE

Urge incontinence occurs when the desire to micturate overwhelms the voluntary capacity to control bladder function, and spontaneous emptying of the bladder occurs at any time.

This is an inflammatory condition which can be acute or chronic. Infected residual urine causes irritation of the base of the bladder (the trigone) giving a basal trigonitis. This causes the micturition reflex to be released earlier than usual

Treatment is by antibiotics or surgery.

Stress Incontinence

This may be defined as the accidental voiding of varying amounts of urine down the urethra when the intra-abdominal pressure is raised as in a cough, sneeze, or during physical exertion. The number of activities which induce leakage vary with the severity of the condition.

This is the most interesting type of incontinence to the physiotherapist because the choice of treatments lies between physiotherapy and surgery. Well directed physiotherapy can so often make surgery unnecessary. Women with stress incontinence are always distressed and embarrassed by their condition. However the word 'stress' does not indicate an anxiety state but describes a sudden increase in intraabdominal pressure resulting in the involuntary passage of urine.

CAUSES OF STRESS INCONTINENCE

1. Weakness of the deep pelvic floor muscles.
2. Loss of elasticity of the connective tissue of the pelvic floor due to overstretch.
3. Atrophy of the urethral musculature leading to a decrease in urethral turgor.

The withdrawal of hormones in menopausal women makes them particularly prone to the second two conditions. The administration of oestrogen or a combination of oestrogen and androgenic hormones often relieves the condition. The loss of urethral turgor causes a loss of resistance to the passage of urine in the urethra and can be an important factor in incontinence.

Weakness of the pelvic floor muscles is almost always due to the effects of childbearing, where postnatal exercises have been omitted or ineffectively taught.

Cystocele and Urethrocele

The anterior vaginal wall may prolapse independently of any uterine descent. When the upper part is involved the bladder herniates backwards due to its connection to the vagina via the pubocervical fascia (Fig. 5/12). A lump is formed which the patient can feel and if the condition is severe the bladder is incompletely emptied. The residual urine easily becomes infected and frequency and dysuria are then additional symptoms.

If the lower part of the anterior vaginal wall prolapses, the urethra is displaced backwards and a urethrocele develops (Fig. 5/13).

Causes. Prolapse may be caused by prolonged pressure by the presenting part in the second stage of labour or too rapid expulsion of the fetus. Damage to the urogenital diaphragm precipitates a urethrocele.

Prolapse of the posterior vaginal wall produces a rectocele.

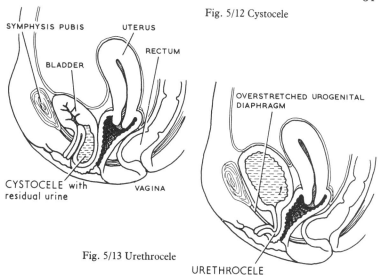

Fig. 5/12 Cystocele

Fig. 5/13 Urethrocele

Vaginal Laxity

The muscles of the pelvic floor play an important part during sexual intercourse. Muscular insufficiency can lead to sexual problems; also difficulty in retaining a contraceptive diaphragm or tampon in the vagina.

Prolapse of the Uterus

The word prolapse means 'to slip out of place'. When the uterus prolapses, the upper vagina which is attached to the uterus is drawn downwards as well.

Three degrees of uterine prolapse are recognised (Fig. 5/14):

CAUSES

Deficiency in the uterine supports predisposes to prolapse. Three main reasons for the supports to become weaker are:

Congenital;

Overstretching during childbirth, especially if the patient bears down before she is fully dilated. A prolonged second stage with a large baby will also damage the uterine supports, as will too much pressure on the fundus of the uterus when attempting to deliver the placenta;

Withdrawal of hormones at the menopause.

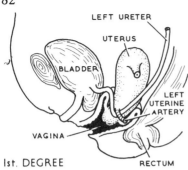

LEFT URETER
UTERUS
BLADDER
LEFT UTERINE ARTERY
VAGINA
RECTUM
1st. DEGREE

Fig. 5/14 Degrees of uterovaginal prolapse

First degree. Here the uterus descends inside the vagina to, or almost to, the introitus

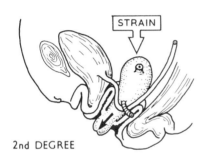

STRAIN
2nd DEGREE

Second degree. Here the cervix projects beyond the vulva when the patient strains

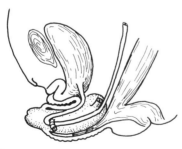

3rd DEGREE
COMPLETE PROCIDENTIA

Third degree. In third degree prolapse or complete procidentia, the whole uterus lies outside the vagina and most of the vagina is inside out. The cervix may become ulcerated and the acute angulation of the urethra causes difficulty in the initiation of micturition. Hydronephrosis can occasionally be present. It is interesting to note how quickly these severe changes can resolve when the prolapse is reduced. A period of bed rest and vaginal packing generally precedes operative treatment for procidentia

Frequency

The word frequency should only be used to denote a repeated desire to pass urine even when the bladder is empty. This occurs with urge incontinence, but can frequently be met in patients with stress incontinence where their fear of leaking urine is linked subconsciously with a desire to keep their bladder empty – so the repeated attempts to pass urine become a habit. This could be called 'self-induced frequency', and can be regulated by bladder training (see stress incontinence, p. 85).

Obesity

If the patient is overweight she has a lot of extra fat around and in between her pelvic organs. This puts considerable extra weight and strain on her pelvic floor, especially if she has a persistent cough.

It should be noted that local vaginal infections, such as trichomonas, will be treated by the gynaecologist, as will involutional vaginitis which is particularly found in menopausal women. The latter responds readily to the administration of oestrogen.

Once a physiotherapist has a full understanding of the symptoms she may find in a patient, she can start considering the treatment.

RESTORATION OF FUNCTION BY RE-EDUCATION OF PELVIC FLOOR MUSCLES

A therapist specialising in obstetrics and gynaecology should undertake this treatment. Initially patients are seen individually. Quiet, privacy and time (about 40 minutes) are required.

Method

1. History.
2. Explanation.
3. Assessment of pelvic floor muscles and initial teaching.
4. Routine of exercises.

HISTORY

The following points should be covered.

a) Parity.
b) Type of delivery. Episiotomy and stitches are not important, since an episiotomy performed to enable a quicker delivery of the baby is

good obstetric practice. It is relevant to enquire about the length of the first and second stages of labour. A persistènt anterior lip of the cervix or prolonged pushing are likely to produce extra stretching and weakening of ligaments and muscles of the pelvic floor. A fast second stage can be equally traumatic.

Forceps extraction does not generally produce added trauma, though a high rotation may do so.

c) What weight were her babies? Was polyhydramnios present?
d) Did she do postnatal exercises? Was exercise for the pelvic floor included?
e) Menstrual cycle.
f) Contraception method.
g) Dyspareunia? Sexual satisfaction?
h) Micturition habits. Frequency? Urgency? Nocturia? Stress Incontinence? What activity makes her leak urine? Does she have to change her pants often during the day? Does the leaking prevent social activity? Does she wear a pad?
i) Bowel habits?
j) Weight? Large or small frame; shoe size is a useful guide.
k) Any conditions which make her cough or sneeze frequently? Smoking?
l) Anything else relevant?

EXPLANATION

This should include simple details about the anatomy of the pelvis, with a diagram. Relate the patient's symptoms to her weak pelvic floor and need for re-education.

ASSESSMENT OF THE PELVIC FLOOR MUSCLES AND INITIAL INSTRUCTION

This is an essential part of the treatment. The muscles are not visible so the therapist must use a digital check to assess their contraction. *Method:* The patient either lies on her left side with knees comfortably drawn up, or she is in crook lying with knees slightly apart. The therapist washes her hands, puts on disposable gloves and with thumb and index finger of her left hand separates the labia and notes if there are signs of vaginal irritation. She asks the patient to cough, and notices any bulging at the introitus, also any leakage of urine. She then introduces the index and middle finger (or middle only) of the right hand slowly, keeping in mind the direction of the vagina and locates the fornices and cervix and checks the state of the vaginal walls. Great care must be taken during this procedure especially if the woman is nulliparous.

The therapist withdraws her fingers until the distal two phalanges are palpating the posterior vaginal wall. Say to the patient 'Squeeze my fingers as much as you can'; the strength of the pelvic floor muscles will be evident by the resulting sensation if you remember that strong muscles will nip the fingers very firmly. It is frequently helpful at this point to ask the patient to 'Squeeze your back passage and your birth canal' as this may improve the strength of the contraction. The patient must be told to be aware of the squeezing and lifting sensation in her vagina (and back passage) as she performs the exercise as this is her only proof that the correct muscles are working.

When the therapist is satisfied that the patient is able to do this and can feel that the muscles are working, she withdraws her fingers. The patient repeats the contraction, checking the sensation in her vagina and relating this to her home practice. She should also learn to do the contractions while in sitting and standing positions as these will be the most convenient for her everyday life.

A vaginal pressure gauge or perineometer, as made by the American gynaecologist A. H. Kegel (1949) is a useful teaching aid and can also show improvement in the strength of the muscles as the pressure is shown to rise on the gauge.

Finally, explain to the patient that a definite routine must be followed if the treatment is to be effective.

ROUTINE FOR EXERCISES

The patient should commence a routine of hourly contractions of the pelvic floor muscles; 'Four contractions every hour on the hour', each contraction to be held for four seconds. The ring of a cake timer or alarm clock can be useful as a stimulus until the brain becomes used to the regime. Discussion will ensure that a schedule is worked out to suit the patient's everyday activities.

Reminders can be given to the patient to contract or brace her pelvic floor whenever she coughs, sneezes or lifts heavy objects – this will prevent the sudden increase of intra-abdominal pressure overstretching the pelvic floor. Stopping and starting the flow of urine while micturating, exercises the muscles and provides an indication of strengthening if the stream is stopped more completely.

Obesity: If the patient is overweight she should reduce her intake of food or be referred to a dietician.

Persistent coughing and sneezing: Chest or allergy clinics may be of assistance. Smoking must be reduced if that is the cause of the coughing.

Follow-up appointments: Patients return for assessment at three or four week intervals. Those with less severe symptoms will be ready for discharge after about three months (see results below).

Group Therapy

When several patients living near the hospital require treatment weekly exercise sessions as a group can be very beneficial. Patients gain much from contact with others who have similar problems and an element of competition enters for the overweight patients during the weekly 'weigh-in'. The 'pelvic floor group' meets once a week for about 20 minutes. Very little equipment is required; any moderate-sized room is suitable.

EXERCISES

Pelvic floor contractions are practised in all the variations of lying, sitting and standing, making the positions relate to the patient's daily life. To prevent fatigue of the pelvic floor muscles, strengthening and mobilising exercises for the abdominal and back muscles are interspersed. Posture correction is also taught.

As the pelvic floor muscles increase in strength the contractions can be made more difficult to sustain by practising them while skipping, running or jumping. Coughing, sneezing and lifting with the pelvic floor contracted must also be taught. Duplicated reminder lists of exercises will aid the patient's memory as great emphasis is laid on home practice. The overweight patients are weighed each week and their weight is recorded.

Results – A Group of 212 Patients with Stress Incontinence Treated by Muscular Re-education 1970 – 1976

1.	Success (no further stress incontinence)	199	93%
	Failure	13	7%
		212	

2.	Failures – Causes	
	Severe cough	3
	Gross obesity	1
	Inappropriate selection in gynaecological clinic (too much utero-vaginal prolapse)	9
		13

3. Duration of successful treatments

3–5 months	154	77%
6–9 months	45	23%
	199	

4. Pre- or postmenopausal

Pre-menopausal	154	72%
Postmenopausal	58	28%
	212	

5. Previous failed repairs for stress incontinence (S.I.), then treated by muscular re-education – 16 out of 212

One previous repair for S.I.	11
Two previous repairs for S.I.	2
Three previous repairs for S.I.	3
	16 all successful

6. Obesity in group of 212

* Normal weight	133	59%
5kg overweight	79	41%

* Standard tables height/weight

POINTS OF INTEREST FROM RESULTS

1. Initial diagnosis of stress incontinence was made clinically – cystometry was not used.
2. In all but 16 cases (previous repairs) muscular re-education was the first treatment of choice.
3. Stress incontinence which persists through one or more operations to remove it can frequently be cured by muscular re-education of the pelvic floor muscles.

Faradism

The author does not use vaginal faradism as part of the programme. If, however, a patient has such gross weakness of her pelvic floor muscles that she can get no sensation of muscular contraction, then vaginal faradism may be used as a sensory stimulus for about six treatments.

METHOD

Scott electrodes (Scott, Green and Couldrey, 1969) can be used or individual vaginal electrodes can be made for each patient. A 12.5cm (5in) length of malleable zinc is rolled round a pencil to give it shape. When the pencil is withdrawn all edges are turned in about one eighth of an inch and the long sides pressed together until they just meet. A lead can then be attached to one end either through a hole in the electrode or a metal clip, to make connection to the faradic source.

With the patient in crook lying a large 15×22.5cm (6×9in) indifferent electrode and wet lint pad is placed under the sacrum. The patient can insert the vaginal electrode herself. If unwilling to do so the therapist will find it easy if she remembers that the vagina angles downwards and backwards in crook lying.

The intensity should be increased until the patient is feeling a strong contraction of her pelvic floor muscles, within the limits of comfort. She should be encouraged to try to contract the muscles actively with the surges a few times in each treatment.

FARADISM UNDER GENERAL ANAESTHESIA

Some authorities have used several maximal faradic stimuli to the perineal body of an anaesthetised patient, and claim this aids the strengthening of the pelvic floor muscles; others have not been able to show this when repeated.

Electronic stimulators for the pelvic floor muscles, either as implants or vaginal/rectal electrodes connected to batteries worn round the waist are the subject of experiment with indefinite results at present. It would seem that these techniques require further liaison between clinician and therapist (Brown, 1977).

SHORT WAVE DIATHERMY

The resolution of some gynaecological conditions can be accelerated by the application of deep heat.

The short wave diathermic current is of high frequency and alternating, and does not stimulate motor or sensory nerves. It is ideal for heating tissues as deeply placed in the pelvis as the female reproductive organs.

Physiological Effects

Short wave diathermy produces heat in the tissues; the resulting rise in temperature accelerates metabolism and causes an increased blood flow to the area.

Uses

The increased blood flow through the area together with increased flow of oxygen and nutrients and the removal of waste products make the resolution of inflammation the main use of short wave diathermy in gynaecological conditions. Pain produced by an inflammatory process will also be relieved as the inflammation resolves.

Method

The two most useful methods of arranging the electrodes are cross-fire and contra-planar.

CROSS-FIRE

The tissues in the pelvis are very vascular and therefore have a very high dielectric constant. The cross-sectional area of the pelvis is larger than that of the electrodes. These two facts combine to make the superficial tissues receive more heat than the deep ones.

To prevent this overheating of the superficial tissues, the field can be passed through the pelvis in two directions. This involves moving the electrodes to a position at right angles to their previous position halfway through the treatment.

In this way half the treatment could be given antero-posteriorly through the pelvis with the patient in the lying position, and the second half with the patient in the side-lying position with legs curled up and the electrodes over the pelvic outlet and the lumbo-sacral area of the spine.

To limit the spreading of the field and encourage deep heating the electrodes should be widely spaced from each other, and air (which has a low dielectric constant) used as a spacer between skin and electrode where possible (Scott, 1975).

CONTRA-PLANAR

In conditions which produce vaginal discomfort it is useful to have the distribution of the field uneven, and thus get a concentration of heat over the electrode nearer the skin.

The patient sits low in a deck chair (cotton or linen canvas only) with her thighs apart, with a large flat electrode under her perineum, (with a suitable amount of felt spacers or towelling between her and the electrode). The other electrode can be placed over the abdomen making sure that the skin/electrode spacing is greater than in the other electrode.

Alternatively the perineal electrode could be of the condenser type and be placed under the chair close to the canvas. If the abdomen is heavily scarred the directing electrode could be placed behind the lumbo-sacral region.

A course of 12 treatments each lasting 20 minutes is satisfactory. At least two treatments should be given per week.

Precautions Especially Relevant in the Treatment of Gynaecological Patients by Short Wave Diathermy

CLOTHING

The patient should remove all her garments from her waist down to her feet. The skin of the abdomen, buttocks and thighs can be adequately inspected for scars or other blemishes.

SKIN SENSATION

Every area that is to be treated should be tested for sensation to heat and cold, paying particular attention to any scarred area which may show altered reactions.

MOISTURE

Great care should be taken to see that the perineum and inner aspects of the thighs are dry, as moisture will cause a concentration of the field. If the patient is obese a dry Turkish towel could be placed between her thighs.

INTRA-UTERINE DEVICES

These contraceptive devices have been found to lose their shape when subjected to short wave diathermy. Metal devices like the 'Copper 7' concentrate the field.

It is the author's opinion that short wave diathermy is *contraindicated* for a patient fitted with an intra-uterine device.

MENSTRUATION

It has been the practice not to treat a patient who is menstruating. The author has found it unnecessary to suspend treatment at this time unless the patient has very heavy periods or secondary dysmenorrhoea.

The sanitary protection should be removed before treatment, whether it is pad or tampon, and the perineum thoroughly dried. The patient can sit on a paper towel if she feels she may soil the towelling.

A clean pad or tampon can be replaced after treatment.

The presence of pacemakers, hearing aids or items of replacement surgery should be checked for in the usual way.

Conditions Treated by Short Wave Diathermy

PELVIC INFLAMMATORY DISEASE

Details of this condition are given on p. 69. Short wave diathermy is used in the treatment of the chronic phase of this disease.

CHRONIC CATARRHAL ENDOCERVICITIS

Symptoms of this condition are deep tenderness in the transcervical and uterosacral ligaments, dragging backache, dyspareunia and vaginal discharge.

The cervix of the patient is cauterised under a general anaesthetic. If after three to six weeks there is residual tenderness of the ligaments and dyspareunia, short wave diathermy will aid resolution.

DISCOMFORT IN THE VAGINA OR INTROITUS

This symptom may be found at the postnatal examination. Short wave diathermy can hasten the patient's return to normal.

INFERTILITY

Some authorities use short wave diathermy to promote changes in the cervical mucus appearing to result in better penetration of the uterus by the spermatozoa.

The role of the physiotherapist does not only lie in the treatment of the patient's symptoms as mentioned in this chapter.

Prophylaxis must be her aim. Her knowledge of the musculoskeletal changes in pregnancy, labour and the puerperium must be used to minimise the effects of these processes on women.

Patient care starts during antenatal classes and should include instruction to the pupil midwives and district midwives who have no obstetric physiotherapist working with them.

Constant attention should be given to postnatal exercise schemes to ensure they contain the right exercises and are taught effectively. Patients in the postnatal ward who have a history of stress incontinence should have the ability to contract their pelvic floor muscles checked in the physiotherapy outpatient department after their postnatal examination. Further teaching and checking should continue for three to six months and if problems occur the gynaecologist should be consulted.

It is by this combination of prophylaxis and active treatment that the physiotherapist can contribute so much in the alleviation of some of the problems of modern women of all age-groups.

REFERENCES

Brown, A. D. G. (1977). 'Postmenopausal urinary problems'. *Clinics in Obstetrics and Gynaecology*, **4**, 1.
Hutch, J. A. (1972). *Anatomy and Physiology of the Bladder, Trigone and Urethra*. Appleton-Century-Crofts.
Kegel, A. H. (1940). 'The Physiologic Treatment of Poor Tone and Function of the Genital Muscles and of Urinary Stress Incontinence'. *Western Journal of Surgery, Obstetrics and Gynaecology*, **11**, 527.
Llewellyn-Jones, D. (1978). *Fundamentals of Obstetrics and Gynaecology*. Vol. 2 Gynaecology. 2nd edition. Faber and Faber.
Mehta, M. (1973). *Intractable Pain*. W. B. Saunders.
Scott, B. O., Green, V. and Couldrey, B. M. (1969). 'Pelvic Faradism, Investigation of Methods'. *Physiotherapy*, **55**, 8, 302.
Scott, P. M. (Ed.) (1975). *Clayton's Electrotherapy and Actinotherapy*. 7th edition. Baillière Tindall.

BIBLIOGRAPHY

Garrey, M. M., Govan, A. D. T., Hodge, C. H. and Callander, R. (1974). *Gynaecology Illustrated*. 2nd edition. Churchill Livingstone.
Jeffcoate, Sir N. (1975). *Principles of Gynaecology*. 4th edition. Butterworths.
Kegel, A. H. and Powell, T. O. (1950). 'The Physiologic Treatment of Urinary Stress Incontinence'. *Journal of Urology*, **63**, 5, 808.
Llewellyn-Jones, D. (1977). *Fundamentals of Obstetrics and Gynaecology*. Vol. 1 Obstetrics. 2nd edition. Faber and Faber.
Mandelstam, D. (1977). *Incontinence – A Guide to the Understanding and Management of a very common complaint*. William Heinemann Medical Books.
Mandelstam, D. (1978). 'The pelvic floor'. *Physiotherapy*, **64**, 8, 236.
Noble, Elizabeth (1978). *Essential Exercises for the Childbearing Year*. John Murray.
Phillipp, E. E., Barnes, J. and Newton, M. (Eds.) (1977). *Scientific Foundations of Obstetrics and Gynaecology*. 2nd edition. William Heinemann Medical Books.

ACKNOWLEDGEMENTS

The author expresses her gratitude to Mr. J. A. Carron Brown, Consultant Obstetrician and Gynaecologist to the United Norwich Hospitals, who has helped her with this chapter, giving his time most generously. Thanks are also due to many colleagues in the Department of Obstetrics and Gynaecology at the Norfolk and Norwich Hospital, to Mrs. D. Mandelstam M.C.S.P., of the Edgware General Hospital and The Disabled Living Foundation, and Mrs. P. Yudkin, Medical Statistician at the John Radcliffe Hospital, Oxford.

Chapter 6

Head and Neck Surgery

revised by P. A. DOWNIE, F.C.S.P.

Rather than discussing ear, nose and throat conditions as in previous editions, this chapter will consider those disorders of the head and neck which the physiotherapist may encounter from time to time. The anatomy and physiology of the head and neck and its contents, can be studied in any standard textbook and it is not proposed to describe this except where it is necessary to explain the disorder and its consequent treatment.

BLOCK DISSECTION OF CERVICAL LYMPH GLANDS

A block dissection of the cervical lymph glands is frequently carried out when there is malignant disease in the head and neck region. Sometimes it is performed as a procedure in itself but it may well be part of a more radical procedure involving either removal of the larynx, a hemi-mandibulectomy, or glossectomy. It may be bilateral or it may involve only one side. The spinal accessory nerve is almost always divided or excised in the process of dissection; this is because of its anatomical position and also because quite often it is involved in the disease process.

Physiotherapy

The most important requirement for these patients is the teaching of shoulder shrugging exercises before operation and then ensuring that they are carried out postoperatively. The physiotherapist may be asked to treat the chest as well, though this is not required routinely. If however the patient is a known smoker or chronic bronchitic, and many of them are, and if the surgery is more extensive than a straightforward block dissection, chest physiotherapy may be required.

Shoulder exercises however are the main requirement together with encouragement to move the neck. If exercises are not taught, encouraged and supervised, the trapezii will atrophy and a frozen shoulder will quickly follow. All this is preventable (Downie, 1975).

FACIAL PALSY

Facial palsy is one of the complications of disease of the middle and inner ear. The facial nerve can be compressed or damaged in any part of its course, but as a complication of aural disease it is in its intratemporal course that it will be affected. During this part of the course the nerve, in the narrow bony facial canal, runs from the internal auditory meatus laterally above the labyrinth for a short distance. It makes a right-angled turn back (the genu) then runs down and back in the

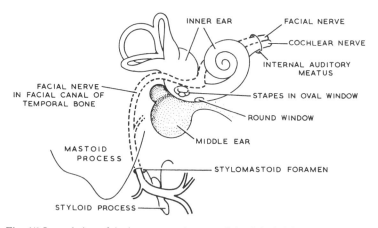

Fig. 6/1 Lateral view of the intratemporal course of the right facial nerve

medial wall of the tympanic cavity (Fig. 6/1) and finally passes vertically down in the posterior wall of the cavity surrounded by mastoid air cells. The bony wall of the canal is very thin and it may actually be deficient at one or more points.

Due to its position the canal and nerve may readily be involved in ear diseases and in surgery, the nerve becoming inflamed, compressed or injured.

Acute infections of the middle ear can involve the sheath of the nerve, especially if an infected mastoid air cell lies just above the nerve in the absence of the bony wall of the canal.

Erosion of the bony wall of the canal is liable to occur in chronic suppurative otitis media, either by infection or a cholesteatoma.

In surgery the nerve may be damaged during the operation or by the displacement of fragments of bone. It may be compressed by haemorrhage or oedema.

In addition to involvement in diseases of the ear the nerve may also be damaged in this part of its course in fractures of the temporal bone. Idiopathic facial palsy (Bell's palsy) can also occur. The cause is unknown and there is no apparent disease of the ear. Groves (1971) postulates the theory that vasospasm results in swelling and ischaemia and consequently compression of the nerve. Such ischaemia could be the result of exposure to draughts and cold.

Types of Lesion

The lesion may be a neurapraxia due either to compression by blood or exudate, or caused by bruising. Alternatively, there may be degeneration of the nerve if compression is not relieved or the nerve is damaged during surgery. A combination of both types of lesion is possible.

TREATMENT

A very careful assessment has to be made before treatment can be decided upon, in order to estimate the type and level of the lesion. Such assessment includes a test of motor function, nerve conductivity tests and strength-duration measurements, electromyography, and lacrimation, hearing and taste tests. Treatment is then decided upon according to the above tests and the speed of onset and progression of the paralysis.

Facial paralysis developing during acute middle ear infections will usually recover completely without special treatment when the primary condition is dealt with.

Should the paralysis occur in chronic suppurative otitis media, exploration is usually considered essential. The facial canal is opened and if there is fibrosis and degeneration, the sheath of the nerve is incised, fibrous tissue removed and a nerve graft is carried out. Any cutaneous nerve may be used. Recovery is likely to be slow – some months – and may not be complete.

The onset of facial palsy immediately after aural surgery is likely to indicate that the nerve has been damaged. The surgeon will explore at once and carry out a decompression or graft according to what he finds.

A delayed paralysis following surgery will indicate either too tight packing in the ear, slight contusion of the nerve or, if the paralysis is increasing, bleeding into the facial canal. This will require either removal of the packing or exploration of the facial canal.

Idiopathic facial palsy rarely requires treatment. Many patients recover within two to three weeks without treatment. Some patients recover very slowly, those in whom some nerve fibres have degenerated. A few never gain full recovery and in these there has been total degeneration. Some surgeons treat the patient with adrenocorticotrophic hormone (A.C.T.H.) and claim excellent results, others have tried decompression but as yet there is no certain proof that this is effective. Usually treatment is medical and includes reassurance of the patient, care of the eye, exercises for the facial muscles and support for the paralysed muscles.

In all cases general care of the patient as described above for idiopathic facial palsy is essential and physiotherapy is usually ordered.

Physiotherapy

Physiotherapy is usually ordered whatever the type of lesion, since there will be a short or long period before full recovery of the facial muscles. In some cases complete recovery may not occur.

The measures which may be taken include: nerve conductivity tests; strength-duration curves; movement using proprioceptive neuromuscular facilitation (P.N.F.) techniques; infra-red therapy; occasionally ice therapy; occasionally electrical stimulation.

NERVE CONDUCTIVITY TESTS

When facial palsy appears immediately after surgery, a nerve conductivity test may be requested at an early stage, from three to ten days. If the nerve has been completely severed there will be immediate failure in conductivity and no muscle response, whereas if there is a muscle twitch the nerve cannot have been severed.

The usual method of carrying out the test is to have the patient in the lying position. A small button electrode is placed at the exit of the nerve from the stylomastoid foramen and the indifferent electrode on the neck. A pulse of one milli-second is used. The intensity of current needed to obtain a minimal visible contraction on the normal side is compared with that needed on the affected side.

STRENGTH-DURATION CURVES

These are carried out, when necessary, to determine the type of nerve lesion and the patient's progress (Fig. 6/2).

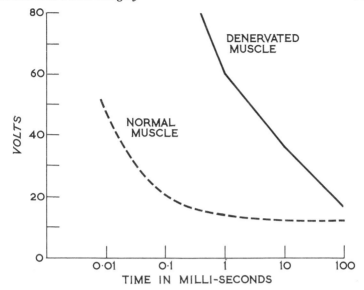

Fig. 6/2 A strength-duration curve

MOVEMENTS

While there is no ability to contract the muscles the physiotherapist may do the movement for the patient, who is asked to try to 'feel' it and to attempt to hold it. As power begins to return the patient tries to join in and P.N.F. techniques may be used. A spatula can be placed inside the cheek and the patient is asked to pull the cheek in as it is pressed out by the spatula.

INFRA-RED AND ICE THERAPY

The small, delicate facial muscles waste quickly, and can become fibrotic and contracted if recovery is delayed. Stimulation of the circulation and nutrition is therefore valuable, consequently gentle heat is often given before movement. Ice could be used but it has the disadvantage of causing rupture of tiny superficial veins, which is not desirable on the face.

ELECTRICAL STIMULATION

This is rarely used today but occasionally if a patient cannot get the 'idea' of the movement, when paralysis has been present for some time, electrical stimulation can be used until he has acquired the 'feel' and knows what to try to do.

In some patients as the nerve recovers, associated movements tend to occur, for example, as the patient closes the eye the corner of the mouth shoots up. It may be difficult to prevent this but if the patient is shown what is happening he can be encouraged to make an effort to control it.

The physiotherapist will encourage the patient to take care of the eye, stressing that he should not go out without covering it. If trouble does occur she must report it at once.

HYPOPHYSECTOMY

This is the surgical removal of the pituitary gland (hypophysis cerebri). It is frequently performed on patients who have multiple bone metastases resulting from a primary carcinoma of breast, prostate or occasionally thyroid. It is known that some of these tumours are hormone dependent and although bilateral oophorectomy and/or adrenalectomy are more frequently performed, some units prefer the operation of hypophysectomy.

The results of this operation can be quite dramatic particularly in the relief of pain if that has been the predominant feature.

Hypophysectomy may be carried out by a neurosurgeon, or an E.N.T. specialist. If surgical removal is considered undesirable, ablation of the gland may be achieved by the implantation of yttrium rods in the pituitary fossa. This latter will be carried out under radiographic control by a radiotherapist. Surgical removal of the gland or radiation ablation is normally carried out using a trans-sphenoidal approach and under general anaesthesia. Two other approaches may occasionally be used, the trans-frontal or trans-ethmoidal.

Following surgery the patient will require replacement drug therapy for the rest of life; this will include steroids, thyroid extract and occasionally pitressin.

Physiotherapy

Breathing exercises should be taught pre-operatively and it should be carefully explained to the patient that as he will be nursed in a recumbent position postoperatively, these exercises are very important. He must also be told to avoid blowing his nose, and to reduce coughing to a minimum so that a cerebrospinal fluid leak is avoided.

If the metastatic bone disease has affected the vertebral column it is not uncommon to find that these patients are in a spinal jacket and in which case breathing exercises are even more vital.

Bed exercises should be taught and encouraged and mobilisation and general rehabilitation will need to be assessed and graded according to the patient's condition and capabilities.

JAW SURGERY

Increasingly, the physiotherapist is being more involved in the treatment of patients who undergo jaw surgery for malignant disease. Maxillo-facial fractures are dealt with in Chapter 7, likewise the plastic surgical repair following extensive tissue excision for malignant disease. This short section will confine itself to hemi-mandibulectomy, maxillectomy and partial glossectomy.

Many cancers involving the jaw are considered curable but often the surgical excision has to be radical. For both these reasons rehabilitation is important.

Hemi-Mandibulectomy

Breathing exercises should be taught pre-operatively and jaw movements as well as neck movements should be checked. Following a simple hemi-mandibulectomy, the postoperative physiotherapy will be straightforward. Once the drains are removed the patient should be encouraged to open and close his mouth; these movements should be carried out in front of a mirror so that the mouth is opened symmetrically. Provided the excision does not include the mandibular symphysis there should be no problem and function should be rapidly restored (Plates 6/1a and 6/1b).

If the symphysis is excised there is nearly always a tendency to drooling, which makes eating and drinking both messy and difficult. Intensive exercises to the lips with finger assistance or resistance may help in the retraining. A prosthesis is almost always inserted either at the initial excision or as a secondary procedure.

Social rehabilitation, i.e. enabling the patient to take his place in society once more, is almost the most important aspect. This can mean seeing that he is able to mix with people, go into shops etc.; the physiotherapist should be prepared to help in this.

Following maxillectomy and glossectomy, breathing exercises should be encouraged. If general classes are held·all these patients should be encouraged to partake and extra head and neck exercises should be incorporated for them. If a block dissection of the cervical lymph glands is carried out at the same time the special requirements discussed on p. 93 should be noted.

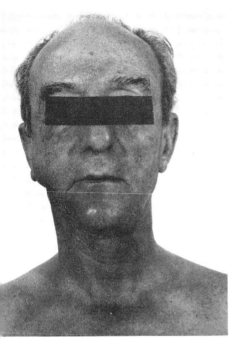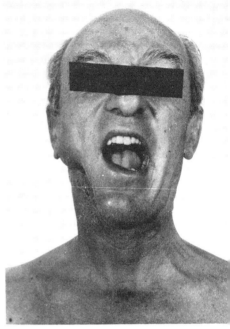

Plate 6/1a&b A patient who has undergone right hemi-mandibulectomy and block dissection of lymph glands. b) Shows the range of movement

CARCINOMA OF THE LARYNX

Cancer of the larynx accounts for one per cent of all cancers diagnosed and the incidence is higher in men than in women. Smoking and an excess intake of alcohol are said to be contributory causes.

Primary treatment for the disease will either be by radiotherapy or cytotoxic drugs thus allowing the voice to be preserved. Many of these patients are elderly and the physiotherapist may be asked to treat the chest of some of those undergoing radiotherapy. Very occasionally the larynx becomes extremely oedematous during radiotherapy and an emergency tracheostomy may need to be performed. These patients will certainly need treatment. If postural drainage is felt to be necessary to aid the adequate clearance of sputum, this is usually possible but the physiotherapist should first ask the prescribing doctor.

If the recurrent laryngeal nerve is involved, patients will have difficulty in coughing, and will require much encouragement. If radiotherapy and/or cytotoxic drugs fail to control the disease then surgery will be carried out.

Laryngectomy

The entire larynx will be removed and if necessary a bilateral or unilateral block dissection of the cervical lymph nodes – this will be dependent on the extent of the disease.

Physiotherapy

Pre-operative breathing exercises should be taught and the physiotherapist should consult with her speech therapist colleague to learn how she can help in the preparing of the breathing control which will be required for the teaching of oesophageal speech. The patient will have had the operative procedure explained by the doctors and will know that he will have a permanent tracheostomy. The physiotherapist should be prepared to reassure the patient that this 'hole in the neck' will in no way affect his daily activities.

Postoperatively, breathing exercises and vibrations and shakings are usually all that is required: it is more effective if the physiotherapist combines with a nurse who will suck the secretions out, while the chest is vibrated. Postural drainage is *not* advocated for the first three to four days, because it is very uncomfortable for the patient. If necessary he can be put down on his side either flat or with two pillows.

These patients are up very quickly and unless they were in poor condition pre-operatively or had to undergo very extensive surgery, they should not present problems. Shoulder joint and girdle movements should be encouraged and likewise neck movements, once the drains are out. Later, these patients should be encouraged to dress and be taken out and about in the hospital grounds and the street, prior to discharge.

MÉNIÈRE'S DISEASE

This is a disease first described by Prosper Ménière in 1861, in which there is an increase in the quantity of endolymph in the labyrinths. It is characterised by sudden attacks of vertigo, nausea and vomiting, tinnitus and deafness. The attack may last less than an hour, several hours or longer and there may be premonitory signs such as a dull ache in the ear or there may be no warning. Some patients have a history of tinnitus and increasing deafness in one or both ears, but otherwise the ears are normal.

The actual cause is unknown though many theories exist. One fairly widely accepted theory is that there is spasm of the blood vessels supplying the labyrinth, resulting in ischaemia. This theory is reinforced by the fact that vasodilator drugs and cervical sympathectomy appear to bring about an improvement in the condition. It is also found that attacks are sometimes precipitated by stress and anxiety and exposure to cold. The attacks are slightly more common in men than women and first occur before the age of 50.

Once an attack has occurred the patient tends to become tense and depressed. This is partly due to the tinnitus and partly because the patient is frightened of how this condition may affect his everyday life. An attack may be so severe that the patient may fall and be quite unable to walk and such an attack might be serious in his work or, for example, when driving a car. The vertigo may not be as severe or prolonged as this and after one or two attacks the condition may never occur again. Attacks can usually be controlled by conservative treatment.

Medical Treatment

This is directed towards the reduction of the hypertension of endolymph, relief of fear and depression, and control of symptoms. During a severe attack the patient should lie flat in bed with the head supported by pillows. The nausea is controlled by drugs such as Stemetil (prochlorperazine maleate), and sedatives; tranquillisers will relieve anxiety. Between attacks salt and water restriction and vaso-dilator drugs such as nicotinic acid and Priscol (tolazoline hydro-chloride) are often valuable.

If this treatment does not prove effective, conservative surgical treatment or radical surgery in the form of total destruction of the labyrinth may prove necessary.

Surgical Treatment

This may be conservative, in the form of surgical sympathectomy, decompression of the labyrinth or selective destruction of the labyrinth by placing the tip of an ultrasound applicator on one end of the lateral semicircular canal.

Ménière's disease may also be treated by total destruction of a labyrinth by withdrawing the membranous lateral semicircular duct through an opening in the bony capsule or by removing the utricle through the oval window.

These operations are followed by vertigo, particularly severe after total destruction, but usually lessening gradually over a period of several weeks. When there has been selective destruction the patient is warned that he may suffer from mild attacks of vertigo for about three months. During this time vertigo is controlled by drugs but physio-therapy is often helpful.

Physiotherapy

Occasionally vertigo persists and physiotherapy may then be ordered. The giddiness is aggravated by any change of position and is particularly bad on sudden movements of the head or eyes. For this reason the patient tends to hold the head and eyes still and to move the trunk slowly and carefully. The neck and shoulder muscles therefore become tense and often remain so, long after the giddiness has permanently disappeared.

The object of physical treatment is to gain relaxation of tense muscles and to overcome the fear of giddiness, until it completely ceases and the patient is capable of carrying out normal activities with normal self-confidence. If these aims are not achieved, the tenseness continues and activities are limited through fear of the unpleasant sensation of vertigo.

The exact routine of exercise varies. It is common to begin with eye movements, first slowly, then quickly, and then a combination of both. The use of long and short focus is also valuable. Provided that the head is supported, head bending forward and rotation may also be given. Head backward bending is often avoided as it seems to produce more vertigo. On the next day, the same movements may be practised in the long-sitting position and head rolling and head extension may be added, performed first with the eyes open and then with eyes closed. These movements should also be performed slowly at first and then quickly, and then changing rapidly from one speed to another. Shoulder movements to gain relaxation are now added and slow trunk movements. The patient can then join a class of other patients, so that the spirit of competition may enter into the treatment. Exercises in sitting, stressing trunk and head flexion and extension, are given, and standing, trying to gain steady balance, is added. Progression is made daily by adding exercises in standing and by using changes of posture, first with the eyes open and then closed. Ball throwing makes a useful exercise to obtain balance and co-ordination. Ball work may be developed in standing and walking so that moving about freely is encouraged. Later balance walking, walking round objects and passing other people should all be used.

Patients vary in their progress and exercises must be chosen accordingly. The mental make-up of the patient has a great deal to do with the rate of recovery. The treatment should be pressed to the limit of tolerance of the individual, and encouragement given in order to restore confidence. The patient has to learn that a movement which makes him a little giddy has no untoward effects, and the next day that same movement may well fail to produce giddiness.

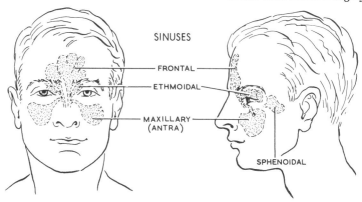

Fig. 6/3 The nasal sinuses

NASAL SINUSITIS

This is an inflammation of the mucous membrane lining the nasal sinuses (Fig. 6/3). It may be acute or chronic. The maxillary sinus is most often affected.

Acute Sinusitis

Acute sinusitis is most often caused by the virus of the common cold. It also results from chronic dental infection, trauma or infected tonsils and/or adenoids. Infection is especially likely to occur if there is partial obstruction of the opening from the nose to the sinus, such as may be present when there is a deflected nasal septum, enlarged adenoids or an allergic state of the nose causing swelling of the nasal mucous membrane. Sinusitis is also often associated with chest infections.

The inflammation is characterised by swelling and exudate with increased secretion of mucus. If the organism is virulent, the patient's resistance low or the exudate cannot drain adequately, due to blockage of the opening, the exudate may become purulent. Symptoms are general and local. There is a slight rise in temperature, a feeling of general malaise and headache. Pain is usually present, sometimes with tenderness on pressure. If the maxillary sinus is affected pain is felt in the cheek in the region of the upper teeth; in frontal sinusitis it is just under the upper margin of the orbital cavity; in ethmoidal sinusitis at the upper part of the side of the nose.

Nasal discharge is mucoid at first in most patients, but after a few days may become purulent. Once adequate drainage is established, relief of pain may be expected and within a few days the condition may be cleared and discharge ceases.

Chronic Sinusitis

Chronic sinusitis often develops insidiously following either an acute attack which fails to resolve completely, or repeated colds or tooth infection. Permanent changes take place in the lining membrane of the sinus and sometimes in the bony walls. The mucous membrane becomes thickened and fibrotic, cilia disappear, mucous glands hypertrophy and a thick sticky mucus is difficult to move. The secretions therefore stagnate and become infected.

Constant absorption of toxins and swallowing of infected material upsets the general health and causes chronic gastritis so that the patient is likely to complain of headache, tiredness and digestive disturbances.

Local symptoms are mucopurulent nasal discharge and pain in the face, worse in the morning since secretions have accumulated during the night. A postnasal drip is often very worrying to the patient.

Physiotherapy

If physiotherapy is ordered it will probably take the form of short wave diathermy. Chronic sinusitis can respond quite dramatically to short wave diathermy which should be applied using the cross-fire technique (Fig. 6/4). Very mild doses of short wave diathermy of short duration should be given so that the circulation and vitality of the mucous membrane is stimulated without increasing tissue metabolism and the activity of micro-organisms. If there is an increase in symptoms, particularly pain, treatment MUST be stopped. Very occasionally, short wave diathermy is prescribed for acute sinusitis; in this case it must be given with even greater care.

Fig. 6/4 Diagram showing cross-fire technique for short wave diathermy to the nasal sinuses

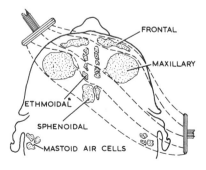

THYROIDECTOMY

Surgery of the thyroid gland can take the form of a partial, hemi- or total thyroidectomy. Total thyroidectomy is rare, except in the case of malignant disease when it may be combined with a bilateral block dissection of the cervical lymph nodes.

More often a partial or hemi-thyroidectomy is performed and is carried out through a collar incision (p. 35). Pre- and postoperative chest physiotherapy may or may not be given. If it is, particular attention should be paid to the upper lobes of the lung, for it is these that are most likely to develop atelectasis. Because of the close proximity of the recurrent laryngeal nerve to the thyroid gland, it may be bruised at operation thus making coughing more difficult, as well as giving the patient a degree of hoarseness of speech. Many patients are very frightened about coughing and one method of support is shown in Figure 6/5. Clips are normally used to close the incision and will be

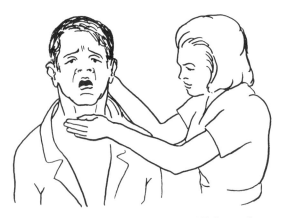

Fig. 6/5 Method of support for a patient while he coughs following thyroidectomy. One hand on the occiput, and the other over the incision

removed very quickly – probably half on the first postoperative day and the remainder on the third day. Following thyroidectomy, patients are rapidly mobilised and can be discharged on the sixth postoperative day, unless after-treatment is required e.g. radiotherapy or chemotherapy in the case of malignant disease.

Occasionally, a patient presents with a retro-sternal thyroid and if this necessitates the splitting of the upper part of the sternum, then the physiotherapy care will be a modification of that which is given for a thoracotomy. Again, emphasis will be on the upper lobes of the lungs.

With any surgery in the neck region, patients are apprehensive about moving their heads. The physiotherapist should encourage head and neck movement and see that a correct posture is rapidly regained. The positioning of pillows is important and the physiotherapist can teach the nurse the best way to give maximum comfort and a good head position by the judicious placing of them.

REFERENCES

Downie, P. A. (1975). 'The rehabilitation of patients following head and neck surgery'. *Journal of Laryngology and Otology* **LXXXIX**, 12.
Groves, J. (1971). 'Facial paralysis'. Chapter included in Vol. 2 *Scott-Browne's Diseases of the Ear, Nose and Throat*. 3rd edition (Jt. Eds. Ballantyne, J. and Groves, J.). Butterworths.

BIBLIOGRAPHY

Downie, Patricia A. (1978). *Cancer Rehabilitation: an Introduction for Physiotherapists and the Allied Professions*. Chapter 8. Faber and Faber.
Stell, P. M. and Maran, A. G. D. (1978). *Head and Neck Surgery*. 2nd edition. William Heinemann Medical Books Ltd.

Chapter 7

Plastic Surgery

by S. BOARDMAN, M.C.S.P. and P. M. WALKER, M.C.S.P.

The term plastic surgery was used by the Germans at the beginning of this century to describe surgery concerned with 'moulding of tissues.'

The first recorded reconstructive surgery was performed in India 600 years B.C. where amputation of the nose was a common punishment, and forehead skin was used to construct a new nose. Tagliococci, an Italian surgeon, reconstructed noses using an arm flap in the 16th century. The recorded use of free skin graft dates from the 19th century when new techniques were described by Jacques Reverdin, Ollier and Thiersch in Paris, and Wolfe in Glasgow. The challenge of mutilating injuries during the First World War stimulated the development of plastic surgery and it became a speciality in its own right. The pioneer in the U.K. was Sir Harold Gilles. During the Second World War, surgeons such as Gilles, Kilner, MacIndoe and Mowlem laid the foundation of the speciality as it is now known.

THE SKIN AND ITS FUNCTION

It should be remembered that skin is not just a collection of epithelial cells, but a composite organ of epidermis and dermis (Fig. 7/1). The epidermis is stratified and is made up of five layers of cells, the deepest of these, the stratum germinatum, being the cell producing layer.

The dermis is made up of two layers. In the upper layer lie the capillary loops, the smallest lymphatics and nerve endings, including touch corpuscles, while the deeper layer consists largely of fibrous tissue with an interlacing of elastic fibres, and this rests directly on subcutaneous tissue. This latter consists of bundles of connective tissue interspersed with fat cells. The glandular parts of some of the several glands and deep hair follicles lie in this area. This subcutane-

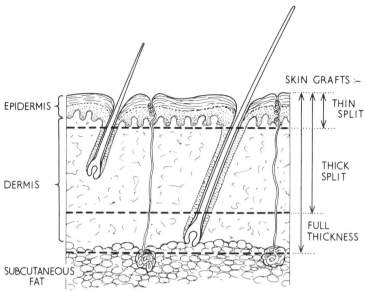

SKIN GRAFTS :–

EPIDERMIS

DERMIS

SUBCUTANEOUS FAT

THIN SPLIT

THICK SPLIT

FULL THICKNESS

Fig. 7/1 The layers of the skin showing from where the various types of free skin grafts are taken

ous layer serves to support blood vessels, lymphatics and nerves and protects underlying structures.

The skin is the largest organ of the body, representing about 16 per cent of the total weight of the normal adult. It has many functions, but the two most important when considering skin loss, are protection against invasion by bacteria, and prevention of fluid and protein loss from the body.

If primary healing does not take place, surgery may be required to provide skin cover.

There are two methods of skin transfer:

1. Free skin grafts, which are without a blood supply for up to 48 hours after transfer.
2. Skin flaps, which are joined to the body by a functioning arterial and venous flow.

Free Skin Grafts

These may be split skin or full thickness.

SPLIT SKIN

These can vary from the very thin to three-quarter skin thickness. They are cut with a knife or dermatome. Such grafts are used in the grafting of burns. After cutting, they are spread on Tulle Gras for ease of handling and applied to the raw areas.

The donor sites heal within 10 to 12 days. The grafted area may be nursed exposed or with dressings, according to the wishes of the surgeon. The recipient area must always have a good blood supply and be free from necrotic tissue and infection, (particularly haemolytic streptococcus).

For the first 48 hours, a split skin graft survives on the exudate from the underlying granulating tissue. By 48 hours, capillaries will have grown into the graft and vascularised it. Haematoma or tangential movement of the graft will prevent vascularisation and the graft will fail.

Following skin grafts, exercises may be commenced at about five to seven days. Joints not directly involved in grafting may be moved, but movements of these must not cause friction on newly applied skin. Once the grafts are well established, the application of a bland cream to soften scars is desirable, e.g. lanoline or hydrous ointment may be used. This should be *gently* kneaded in; heavy-handedness must be avoided otherwise blistering occurs.

Split skin grafts often contract considerably, and may have to be replaced or released at a later stage, more split skin or full thickness grafts being added, or skin flaps used.

FULL THICKNESS GRAFTS

Wolfe Grafts: These are small full thickness grafts of skin excluding fat, usually taken from the post-auricular or supraclavicular area to repair facial defects, such as eyelids. The donor site will not regenerate and must itself be closed by a split skin graft or direct suture. Full thickness skin graft contracts less than a split skin graft and so is the graft of choice for releasing contracture of the eyelids which can lead to corneal ulceration.

Skin Flaps and Pedicles

These consist of skin and subcutaneous tissue.

They take their own blood supply, and can be used to graft over areas where the blood supply is poor, or non-existent, as over cortical bone, cartilage, joint and bare tendon. Flaps do not contract so can be used to prevent or correct deformities. In order to maintain the viability of the flap, transfer of skin can sometimes only be done in stages. In some flaps, there is a 'random' supply of blood vessels. Other flaps are designed to include at least one sizeable artery or vein; the latter type can be much longer. Examples of these arterial or axial pattern flaps are the forehead and delto-pectoral flaps.

The principal types of flaps are:

1. Transposition flaps.
2. Pedicle flaps.
3. Direct flaps.
4. Free flaps – due to the advent of microsurgery.

TRANSPOSITION FLAPS

These are used to replace defects by transposing skin and subcutaneous tissues from an adjacent site, the donor site being covered by a split skin graft or sutured directly (Fig. 7/2). They are often employed

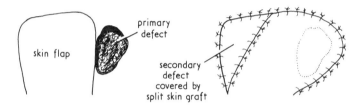

Fig. 7/2 Transposition (rotation) flap used to cover a defect

in the grafting of pressure sores, and in themselves demand little treatment from the physiotherapist.

PEDICLE FLAPS

Pedicle flaps raised and sometimes tubed are used most often for the replacement of traumatic defects of the face and neck, although in this day and age they are less commonly used. From a physiotherapy point of view the acromio-thoracic and abdominal pedicles are important ones to mention. Pedicles may be raised from the upper chest wall, the lower end being swung into position to repair the nose or chin defect, and held in place for three weeks. This will necessitate a mild side flexion and rotation of the neck. They may also be raised from the abdomen and transposed either to the face and neck or a limb via an intermediary (Fig. 7/3), e.g. a pedicle raised on the abdomen can be attached to a wrist and after three weeks it is detached from its base and carried by the wrist to the lower leg as replacement skin.

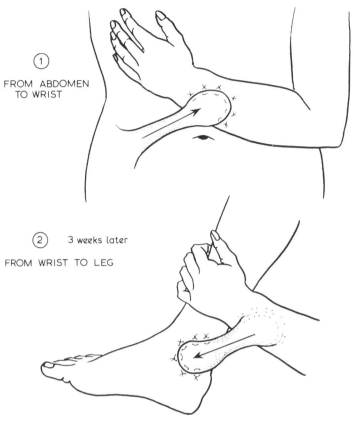

① FROM ABDOMEN TO WRIST

② 3 weeks later
FROM WRIST TO LEG

Fig. 7/3 1) The abdominal pedicle is raised and attached to the wrist. 2) The abdominal pedicle end is detached and re-attached to the ankle area

DIRECT FLAP

These are open, their undersurface remaining raw throughout their attachment period.

CROSS-LEG FLAPS

The cross-leg flap is perhaps one of the most common in use, one leg being the donor for the other. A flap is raised; one end is attached to the recipient site, and the other remains attached to the donor site (Fig. 7/4). The donor site itself is then resurfaced with a split skin graft. The position is maintained for three weeks, during which time the physiotherapist supervises joint care and muscle function. Some of these repairs entail acrobatic positions and often lead to discomfort in the joint involved, and muscle spasm. Such tension and consequent pain may be relieved by the application of heat or ice and massage to the muscles and joints involved. Extreme care must be taken to prevent damage to the flap by heat, for the circulation is reduced and burning and destruction may ensue. It must be remembered that the area is anaesthetic and the patient may be unable to give adequate warning of excess heat. Deep kneading can relieve spasm and discomfort in a matter of a few days. Exercises too are given in the form of static muscle contractions and movements of joints wherever possible.

Other examples of direct flaps are: abdominal, delto-pectoral and groin flaps.

FREE FLAPS

This is a flap which is completely detached from the donor site and transposed directly to the recipient area. Using a microscope, the blood vessels are dissected out (at least one large artery and vein) and anastomosed with vessels in the recipient area.

This method of transferring a flap is of infinite value, and more of these will obviously be used in the future as there is no hindrance to movements, the donor and recipient sites being unattached.

Pedicle and direct flaps are both means of 'making good' one area, by robbing another. They can be transposed from one limb to another via an intermediary, e.g. a flap or pedicle raised on the abdomen can be attached to the wrist, and after three weeks it is detached from its base and carried by the wrist to the lower leg as replacement skin. Incidentally, ununited fractures are often encouraged to heal when the compound site is given good skin cover.

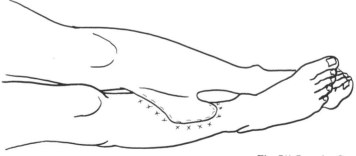

Fig. 7/4 Cross-leg flap

THE USE OF PLASTIC SURGERY

Conditions seen in the Plastic Surgery Unit may, for simplicity, be divided into those requiring:

1. Head and neck surgery.
2. Hand surgery.
3. Trunk and limb surgery.
4. Cosmetic surgery.

HEAD AND NECK SURGERY

This entails radical surgery dealing with such conditions as carcinoma of the jaw, tongue, bony and skin structures of the face.

Having undertaken radical excision of the malignant area, it will be necessary to perform reconstructive surgery, which could include raising of pedicles, delto-pectoral or forehead flaps to replace the soft tissues (Fig. 7/5).

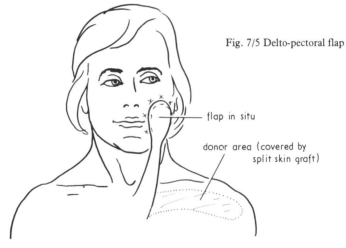

Fig. 7/5 Delto-pectoral flap

flap in situ

donor area (covered by split skin graft)

When bony structures such as the mandible and maxilla are excised, reconstruction may be carried out by the use of bone grafts or artificial prostheses.

PHYSIOTHERAPY

Pre-operative physiotherapy may include an explanation of the procedures to be undertaken, including the possible necessity of tracheostomy, difficulty in speech, eating and general discomfort. Breathing exercises must be taught. They are usually carried out in the half-lying position as grafts may be applied at the time of surgery, and the least amount of movement during the first few days is desirable to prevent skin loss. Leg exercises are taught for the prevention of thrombosis.

Postoperatively on return from theatre, the patient may have a tracheostomy and is nursed in a half-lying position – flaps or pedicles may have been used for the soft tissue reconstruction and bone grafts for bony reconstruction. Breathing exercises to clear the chest are carried out, maintaining the half-lying position. Patients with tracheostomies receive regular suction. Leg exercises must also be performed.

Special attention is paid to pedicles and flaps to prevent:

a) kinking, and b) torsion. Either of these could cut off the blood supply and lead to necrosis.

If, however, the patient develops a chest condition, treatment for this must take preference over the reconstructive surgery in which case the patient may be tipped, turned and moved for postural drainage.

It should be noted that radical head and neck surgery can lead to psychological problems and patients need constant reassurance and aid with communication which may include speech therapy. Ultimately, they will need help to adjust to society at large.

Facial Fractures

These are admitted to a plastic surgery unit as they are often accompanied by severe lacerations as a result of patients going through a windscreen. Other factors causing these injuries include direct blows, e.g. punches.

The most common fracture sites are:

1. Mandible.
2. Maxilla.
3. Zygoma.
4. Nose.

N.B. The first aid treatment in dealing with facial fractures must be noted.

Patients should *never* be laid on their backs, because the tongue can fall back and obstruct the airways.

FIXATION

A mandible is fixed by interdental wiring or cap splints. The maxilla

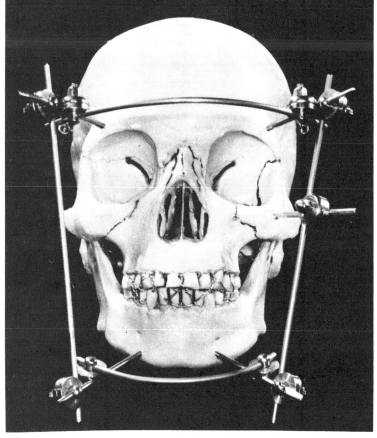

Plate 7/1 Interdental wiring and external splintage following fracture of both maxilla and zygoma

and zygoma are usually fixed by interdental wiring and external splintage (Plate 7/1).

The nose is immobilised by either: a) plaster of Paris splint, b) two small metal plates on either side of the bridge or c) Orthoplast.

Fractures involving the zygoma may lead to trismus i.e. difficulty in opening the mouth.

PHYSIOTHERAPY

Most of these patients present as emergencies. When first seen wiring and splintage may be present and the nose may also be packed.

Breathing exercises are carried out because the patient may have a considerable amount of blood in the mouth and back of the throat which could lead to chest complications. As the teeth are wired together, difficulty may be experienced in expectorating. Suction is carried out via the gap in the interdental wiring. Packing of the nose will exclude nasal suction.

After the splintage is removed, if trismus is still present, short wave diathermy to the temporo-mandibular joint is given, using low dosages.

Jaw osteotomies are performed for abnormal bite and/or cosmetic reasons and are treated as a fractured jaw.

Cleft Lip and Palate

Any combination of cleft lip and palate may be present:

a) Unilateral cleft lip.
b) Bilateral cleft lip.
c) Unilateral lip and palate.
d) Bilateral lip and palate.
e) Palate only.

First, the cleft lip is repaired at about three months. If it is bilateral the second side is repaired six weeks after the first side.

At nine to twelve months the palate is repaired, i.e. before the child commences speech.

Just before the child starts school, revision of scars and any nasal deformity are undertaken.

PHYSIOTHERAPY

Chest physiotherapy may be necessary as some children become undernourished, due to feeding difficulties, and therefore are more prone to chest infections. This will include postural drainage, turning and vibrations, both pre- and postoperatively.

Facial Palsy

This may be congenital or acquired, causing great distress to the patient. The face symmetry may be improved with surgery. The most common operation is the fascial sling. Fascia may be taken from the tensor fascia lata and attached to the zygomatic arch and the zygomaticus muscle, thereby hitching up the sagging muscles.

HANDS

Hand surgery and rehabilitation must aim towards producing maximum function, cosmetic appearance being of secondary importance.

One of the major problems following hand surgery is stiffness. Some causes of stiffness are: a) oedema, b) pain, c) immobilisation, or d) scar tissue.

The more the above problems are reduced to a minimum, the more chance the patient has of regaining good function.

Crush Injuries of Hands

Following crush injury there is gross swelling, due to the presence of excess tissue fluid and also excessive bleeding. The patient is taken to theatre and the tissue is decompressed by the evacuation of blood and fluid. Dead tissue should be excised to prevent infection occurring.

Fractures are reduced and if unstable are fixed with Kirschner wire. Nerves and blood vessels are repaired and skin loss made good by split skin grafts or full thickness flaps. *The hand is elevated to minimise oedema.*

PHYSIOTHERAPY

Immediately after the operation physiotherapy is commenced and shoulder and elbow exercises are carried out.

It may be possible to carry out hand movements in the early stage, if a skin graft has not been applied; should it be applied movements are deferred for five days. From the commencement of treatment, joint range should be measured at frequent intervals.

Oedema is controlled by massage, exercises in elevation and a pressure bandage.

At the earliest opportunity, active exercises are commenced to each individual joint and the hand as a whole, as well as accessory movements.

When the incision has healed and skin grafts settled, a bland cream is massaged into the scars to soften them. At a later stage, if the scars have become adherent, ultrasound may be used.

It must be remembered that gross hand deformities may also cause psychological problems, with which the patient may need some help. If these deformities prevent him from returning to his former work, a hand assessment should be carried out and a meeting with the disablement rehabilitation officer (D.R.O.) should be arranged in order to find the patient more suitable work.

Tendon Repairs

PRIMARY REPAIR

This is the surgery of choice, i.e. where possible, suturing the two ends together soon after the injury has occurred.

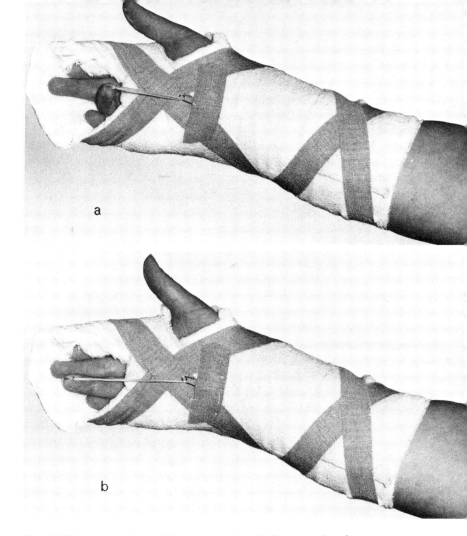

Plate 7/2 Kleinet-type splint. a) The resting position. b) Extension of the finger

After the repair, the patient is treated in a Kleinet-type splint (Plates 7/2a and b). This splint allows for active movement in all the joints, including those affected by the tendon repair.

Flexor tendons: Extension of the finger is allowed within the limits of the splint. Following this, the patient relaxes the finger and the elastic band will return to its former position of flexion, thereby offering resistance to the antagonists and giving reflex relaxation of the agonists.

Extensor tendons: The finger is held in maximum extension to prevent the tendons becoming slack as the patient begins to mobilise the finger.

In both cases, the splint is removed after three weeks.

PHYSIOTHERAPY

Immediately postoperatively, the patient is instructed to exercise within the Kleinet splint, actively extending the finger and allowing the elastic band to flex it.

After three weeks the plaster of Paris is removed and gentle active exercises are commenced. Massage with a bland cream may be given to the scar.

At five weeks, gentle resisted exercises are started; passive stretching may be required at six to eight weeks as the tendons often become adherent within the flexor sheath and thus there may be difficulty in extending the finger. At eight weeks a dynamic splint to aid extension may be applied.

SECONDARY REPAIR

Flexor tendon graft: If the surgeon is unable to carry out a primary suture, a tendon graft will almost certainly be necessary.

A silastic rod may be inserted for about six weeks in order to keep the flexor sheaths open while the patient regains full passive movement, which may be lost due to inactivity since the time of accident. The graft is then inserted. This is usually taken from palmaris longus or extensor digitorum brevis tendon.

Kleinet splinting is again used and the splint removed after three weeks when active physiotherapy is commenced.

Following tendon grafts and repairs, the aim must be to regain full range movements and it must be impressed upon the patient the need to exercise frequently when at home. It will require maximum effort and co-operation on his part to obtain a good result.

Mallet Finger

This is a common injury in which the extensor tendon is avulsed from its attachment at the base of the distal phalanx (Fig. 7/6).

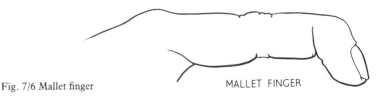

Fig. 7/6 Mallet finger

MALLET FINGER

TREATMENT

The finger is splinted for six weeks with the distal interphalangeal joint hyperextended.

Following this, gentle mobilisation commences, with instruction given on the wearing of the splints during activities likely to cause recurrences of the injury.

Dupuytren's Contracture

This is a condition affecting the palmar aponeurosis in which thickening, fibrosis and contracture occur.

TREATMENT

Surgery is performed removing the affected tissue and skin may be transposed from the dorsum of the finger to repair the defect or a skin graft used. Some surgeons leave the wound of the palm open and encourage early movement.

Physiotherapy commences immediately postoperatively, to prevent stiffness of those joints not involved in surgery.

Recently, mobilisation of the affected joints has been commenced at two to five days, the hand being placed in a polythene bag or silicone oil.

Once healing has occurred, massage and ultrasonics may be given to soften the scars.

Rheumatoid Arthritis

Prophylactic Synovectomies

These may be performed with the hope of preventing further damage. The hypertrophic synovium is removed and active exercises are commenced after five to ten days in order to regain function.

Common deformities seen in rheumatoid arthritis are:

1. Ulnar deviation.
2. Subluxation of the metacarpal phalangeal joints.
3. Swan neck deformity (Fig. 7/7).
4. Boutonnière deformity (Fig. 7/8).

A replacement arthroplasty may be used to correct deformities of the metacarpal phalangeal joints. This is performed using silastic joints, e.g. Swanson's.

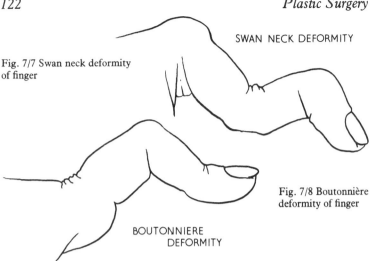

SWAN NECK DEFORMITY

Fig. 7/7 Swan neck deformity
of finger

Fig. 7/8 Boutonnière
deformity of finger

BOUTONNIERE
DEFORMITY

PHYSIOTHERAPY

Immediately postoperatively, the patient is mobilised within the
retraining splint. Gentle passive movements may also be given to these
new joints. After three weeks, when supervised by the physiotherapist, the splint may be removed for treatment, although the
patient is encouraged to wear the splint for about three months (Plates
7/3 a.b.c.).

Correction of Deformities

Deformities involving the interphalangeal joints, such as Boutonnière
and swan neck, are corrected by Harrison pegs. These are small,
angled, polypropylene pegs inserted into the medullary cavity of
phalanges and which, in effect, arthrodese the joint in a functional and
stable position.

TREATMENT

This being a form of arthrodesis, mobilisation of the affected joint
must *not* be undertaken. As the patient has been immobilised in
plaster of Paris, it may be necessary to mobilise the other joints.

Plate 7/3 (*opposite*) a) Rheumatoid arthritis of the hands. b) Following surgery, the
patient wears a retraining splint. c) The hand, with the splint removed

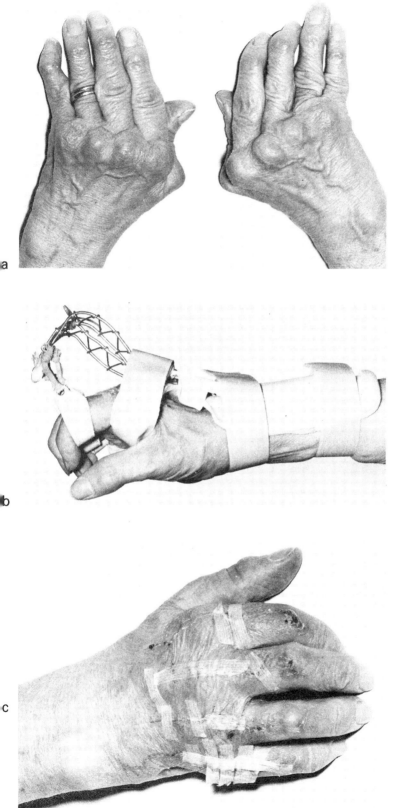

Ulnar Styloidectomy

This is performed either because of pain, or to prevent rupture of the extensor tendons. Little physiotherapy is required.

Syndactyly

This is the condition where two or more digits are joined by a skin web. Occasionally bony continuity may be present.

TREATMENT

The fingers are separated surgically and a skin graft may be inserted (Fig. 7/9). Once the skin grafts have settled, physiotherapy in the form of active movements is commenced.

Pollicisation

This is an operation devised to replace the thumb using another digit. This is transferred with intact vessels and nerves, and implanted on to the thumb metacarpal.

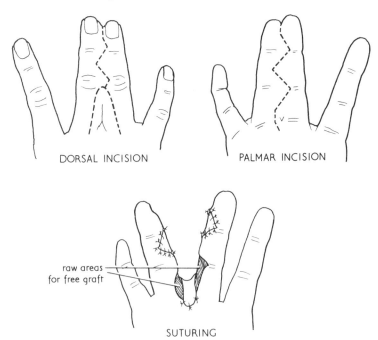

DORSAL INCISION   PALMAR INCISION

raw areas
for free graft

SUTURING

Fig. 7/9 Surgical treatment of syndactyly

PHYSIOTHERAPY

This is commenced when the plaster is removed, i.e. when bony union has occurred. It must be noted that the new joint and skin sensation of the thumb continues to be that of the transposed digit, therefore re-education should be directed with this in mind.

TRUNK AND LOWER LIMB

Pressure Sores

If pressure sores fail to heal, it may be necessary to excise the sore and any underlying necrotic tissue including bone, and cover it with skin. This is usually performed by the use of a transposition flap and most commonly to the sacrum, ischial tuberosity and/or greater trochanters.

Transposition or rotation flap: This is a rectangle or square of skin and subcutaneous tissue which is rotated around a pivot into an immediately adjacent defect. The donor area is covered by a split skin graft to cover this defect (Fig. 7/2).

The patient if possible is nursed on a low air loss bed, the flap being exposed and free from pressure.

PHYSIOTHERAPY

Breathing exercises to prevent chest infections are given and wherever possible active movements to all joints. Care must be taken to ensure that there is no stress on the flap which would endanger the circulation. It must be remembered that many of these patients have neurological conditions, such as paraplegia and multiple sclerosis. It is, therefore, most important to carry out passive movements in order to prevent contractures. Total rehabilitation must be planned to suit their condition.

When the flap is stable and circulation satisfactory, this is at approximately three weeks, the patient is allowed up for short periods. The length of time is gradually increased as the circulation in the flap continues to improve. A careful watch must be kept and if the flap shows signs of breaking down, the patient must be returned to bed and the pressure removed.

Malignant Melanoma

This is a malignant, pigmented tumour which often presents as a dark mole which grows rapidly and later becomes irritant and occasionally bleeds. Wide excision and skin graft is the treatment of choice.

Approximately 7cm either side and 10cm towards the nearest lymph nodes is removed and a split skin graft used to cover the defect. Block dissection of the nearest lymph nodes may also be undertaken.

PHYSIOTHERAPY

As this condition can affect any part of the body, physiotherapy is given accordingly.

Lower limb: The grafted area is immobilised and if a block dissection of the groin nodes has been performed, the patient is nursed with the hip in flexion. Movements are given to the distal joints to maintain circulation, prevent thrombosis and stiffness in the limb. Movements are given to the other limb.

After two weeks, gentle mobilisation to the hip joint is commenced followed by walking at about three weeks. A double thickness layer of Tubigrip is applied for ambulation, and it may be necessary to wear this for many months. Swelling may occur because of interference with the lymphatic drainage.

Upper limb: If this condition occurs in the upper limb, and a block dissection of the neck glands has been performed, it is essential to give postoperative breathing exercises. The patient's chest condition must always be noted and, if necessary, treated.

Lymphoedema

This may be congenital or acquired. Oedema is due to a blockage of lymphatic vessels. Acquired lymphoedema often follows surgery where excision of lymph glands has been undertaken; in the tropics, filariasis can be a cause.

TREATMENT

1. *Thompson Operation – or buried dermal flap:* In this operation fat and lymphoedematous tissue is excised, usually from groin to ankle or wrist to axilla around half the circumference of the limb. One of the resulting two flaps is de-epithelialised and then sutured between the muscle bellies (**Fig. 7/10**). This establishes a communication between the usually patent deep system of lymphatics which subsequently drains the more superficial layers. The remaining flap is sutured over the de-epithelialised area and a pressure dressing applied. The patient is nursed in bed with the leg elevated for 10 days or until the wound has healed.

PHYSIOTHERAPY

Chest physiotherapy and ankle exercises to prevent thrombosis are

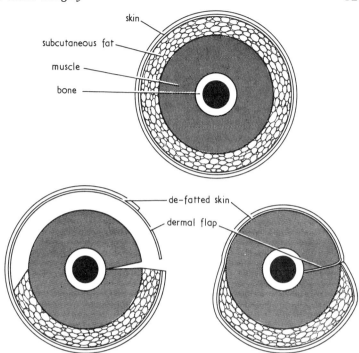

Fig. 7/10 Diagram showing the Thompson operation for lymphoedema

carried out. At 10 days, if the wound has healed, a Bisgaard bandage or a layer of Tubigrip is applied and the patient swings the leg over the side of the bed. At 10 to 12 days, weight-bearing commences followed by walking re-education, as the patient has often been in bed for two to three weeks and the wound is extensive.

2. *Charles Operation*: In this operation the skin and lymphoedematous tissue is excised down to deep fascia, from knee to ankle, the skin being separated and used to cover the defect.

PHYSIOTHERAPY

The leg is immobilised until the skin graft has become established. After seven days, gentle active movements are commenced and weight-bearing allowed at 10 to 12 days with a double layer of Tubigrip being worn for support.

Ulcers and Lacerations with Skin Necrosis

These conditions usually occur in older patients and those patients with impairment of blood supply or who through the use of drugs and radiotherapy develop paper thin or fibrotic skin.

Ulcers

The patient is admitted for bed rest, elevation of the leg and cleaning of the ulcer. Once clean and healthy looking, a split skin graft is applied to close the defect.

PHYSIOTHERAPY

Pre-operatively, maintenance exercises to increase circulation, prevent thrombosis, decrease oedema and prevent joint stiffness are carried out.

Postoperatively the patient will continue the maintenance exercises, but care must be taken not to disturb the skin grafts. At 10 days the patient swings the leg over the side of the bed and walking may commence at 12 to 14 days, wearing a double layer of Tubigrip for support.

Lacerations

Skin necrosis may be caused by lacerations and failure to heal after suturing. The laceration may be jagged and surrounding tissue necrotic. In this case a skin graft is used to cover the defect.

PHYSIOTHERAPY

Postoperatively physiotherapy is carried out as for ulcers.

Compound Fractures

The fractures most commonly seen on a plastic surgery unit are compound fractures of the tibia and fibula, where skin loss is evident. A fracture will not unite if there is inadequate skin cover, and if infection occurs serious problems such as osteomyelitis may ensue.

The aim of treatment is to provide skin cover as soon as possible, by the use of a skin graft. The quality of skin must then be improved so as to prevent further breakdown and consequently, frequent hospital admissions. A free flap is applied but if this is impossible a cross-leg flap or tube pedicle will be used.

The patient must be nursed in either an above-knee plaster with a window over the site of skin loss or in traction with a Steinmann's pin through the calcaneum.

PHYSIOTHERAPY

Maintenance exercises are carried out as for orthopaedic patients; sandbags, springs, etc. being used to maintain the strength of the good leg and arms.

Breathing exercises are carried out if necessary, but as the majority of these patients are young men, chest complications are rare. If however patients present with multiple injuries, e.g. fractured ribs, sternum, mandible etc., breathing exercises then become a necessity.

As soon as skin cover has been achieved, patients are often referred back to the orthopaedic surgeon and therefore the final rehabilitation is carried out from the orthopaedic ward.

COSMETIC SURGERY

Rhinoplasty

This is a plastic operation to improve the appearance or function of the nose. It is undertaken for congenital or post-traumatic deformities and is often a two stage operation consisting of:

1. Sub-mucal resection.
2. In-fracture, i.e. the nasal bones are separated from the maxilla, thus allowing them to be mobilised and the correct position attained.

Immobilisation is carried out by the use of plaster of Paris.

Face Lifting

This is to eliminate wrinkles; an incision being made in front of the ears, the skin undermined and pulled tight. This may also be accompanied by eyelid reductions etc.

Dermabrasion

This is used to flatten irregularities of the skin such as are caused by acne etc. Sandpaper or wire brushes are used to perform the operation.

Port Wine Stains

These are congenital birth marks. They may be excised and skin grafted.

Abdominal Lipectomy

This is performed to remove excess fatty tissue from the abdomen. It is also known as an apronectomy.

Mammaplasty

This is carried out to reduce or augment breast tissue.

Mammary hypoplasia: This is lack of breast tissue which may be congenital or acquired. Augmentation is achieved by the insertion of a silicone prosthesis.

Mammary hyperplasia: This is an increase in breast tissue which is again congenital or acquired and surgery may be carried out to remove this excess tissue.

Bat or Prominent Ears

The operation is usually performed on school children who are often teased about the condition. This is corrected by the excision of some post-auricular skin and alteration of the cartilaginous tissue of the ears if necessary.

PHYSIOTHERAPY

Little physiotherapy is carried out for any of the above conditions unless the patient has an underlying chest condition. In the case of mammaplasty, breathing exercises may be required as tight strapping around the chest impedes lung expansion.

OTHER CONDITIONS

Hypospadias

This is a congenital deformity whereby the urethra opens on to the undersurface of the penis or perineum. The aim of surgery is to move the opening forward to the tip of the penis. This is done by:

1. Releasing the chordae.
2. Creating a gutter through which the urethra may pass and inserting a temporary catheter.
3. Skin grafting around the catheter.

As this is mostly performed on young children, little or no physiotherapy is needed.

Scar Revision

Disfiguring scars, i.e. those following trauma must be allowed to settle before further surgery is contemplated. The most simple procedure is to excise and resuture.

Z-PLASTY

This is an operation whereby the course of the scar is altered i.e. to try to allow the scar to blend in with the surrounding tissue by, wherever

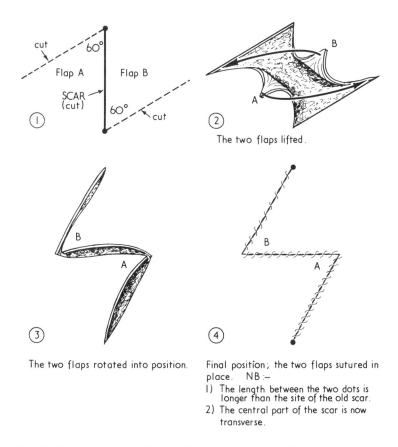

The two flaps lifted.

The two flaps rotated into position.

Final position; the two flaps sutured in place. NB :—
1) The length between the two dots is longer than the site of the old scar.
2) The central part of the scar is now transverse.

Fig. 7/11 Diagrams to show a Z-plasty. (Cut one out for yourself on paper)

possible, lying in the same direction as the skin lines (Fig. 7/11). Larger scars may be excised and replaced by skin grafts or flaps.

In this chapter, we have only mentioned conditions and operations commonly seen in a Plastic Surgery Unit; naturally surgeons have their own interests, muscle grafts are performed for facial palsy, excision arthroplasties and arthrodesis of finger joints by use of pegs, and many new procedures are being tried and improved upon. Although physiotherapy techniques differ slightly, the primary aim throughout is to rehabilitate the patient to full function wherever possible.

BIBLIOGRAPHY

Calman, K. C. (Ed.) (1976). *Recent Advances in Plastic Surgery*. Vol. 1. Churchill Livingstone.

Grabb, W. C. and Smith, J. W. (1973). *Plastic Surgery: A Concise Guide to Clinical Practice*, 2nd edition. Little, Brown and Co., Boston.

Laing, J. E. and Harvey, Joyce (1972). *Management and Nursing of Burns*. 2nd edition. English Universities Press.

Lister, G. (1977). *The Hand: Diagnosis and Indications*. Churchill Livingstone.

Macallan, E. S. and Jackson, I. T. (1971). *Plastic Surgery and Burns Treatment*. William Heinemann Medical Books.

McGregor, I. A. (1975). *Fundamental Techniques of Plastic Surgery and their Surgical Applications*. 6th edition. Churchill Livingstone.

Muir, I. F. K. and Barclay, T. L. (1974). *Burns and their Treatment*. 2nd edition. Lloyd-Luke (Medical Books) Ltd.

O'Brien, B. (1977). *Microvascular Reconstructive Surgery*. Churchill Livingstone.

ACKNOWLEDGEMENT

The authors thank Mr. Brian Morgan, F.R.C.S., Consultant Plastic Surgeon at University College Hospital, London and at the Plastic Surgery Unit, Mount Vernon Hospital, Northwood, for his help and encouragement in the preparation of this chapter. They also thank Dr. A. R. Bell, M.B., Ch.B., Clinical Assistant, Department of Physical Medicine, Mount Vernon Hospital, Northwood for her help.

Chapter 8

Amputations

by B. C. DAVIS, M.C.S.P., H.T., O.N.C.

Amputation of a limb performed for vascular disorders when other treatment has proved ineffective, or amputation as a result of trauma, malignancy or deformity should be accepted as a positive form of treatment, relieving the patient of a painful, useless, dangerous and often infected extremity.

After amputation has been performed, the patient can be rehabilitated to a fully independent life, return to work, and in time become as active as he was prior to amputation, depending upon his general condition.

The amputee needs time and help to overcome the psychological shock resulting from the loss of a limb. He realises that he is different from other people and, more important, that this difference will be apparent. He will be uncertain of his future and will need encouragement from all members of the rehabilitation team: the surgeon, nursing staff, physiotherapists, occupational therapists, social workers, the medical officer at the Limb Fitting Centre, prosthetist and the patient's general practitioner. All these people must work in close co-operation with one another.

Rehabilitation is one continual process from the time the surgeon decides to amputate, until such time that the patient is independent with his definitive prosthesis. This may take six weeks, although the patient is unlikely to remain in hospital for the whole of this period.

Amputations of upper and lower limbs involve differences in cause, age-group and rehabilitation, and so will be considered separately. The ratio of lower limb to upper limb amputees is of the order of 20 to 1.

LOWER LIMB AMPUTATIONS

This is the larger group of amputees and these patients are seen in greater numbers by physiotherapists.

Indications for Amputation

The causes of lower limb amputation together with the approximate percentage of cases are as follows:

Peripheral vascular disease and diabetes	73
Trauma	12
Malignancy	6
Congenital deformities	2
Other	7

It is seen that peripheral vascular disease and diabetic gangrene, both diseases associated with the elderly, account for the majority of lower limb amputations, and accordingly in any one year 70 per cent of new lower limb amputees are over the age of 60. These patients often have many of the other problems associated with the elderly: cardiac involvement, low exercise tolerance, arteriosclerosis of the cerebral vessels causing possible hemiplegia and diminished mental ability, poor respiratory function, reduced visual acuity, poor healing, osteoarthrosis and neuropathy.

Traumatic amputations more commonly affect the younger age-groups and are mostly necessitated by road traffic accidents and industrial injuries.

Malignant disease is also a reason for amputation in patients in the younger age-groups.

Amputations for congenital deformity and limb length discrepancies are usually performed on children and young adults. This is best delayed until the patient is old enough to decide for himself that he wishes to have the operation performed.

The Limb Fitting Service

Before discussing the treatment of the amputee, it is important to understand something of the prosthetic service available to the patient. This obviously varies in different countries, but in the United Kingdom a uniform and comprehensive service is offered to all amputees.

There are 28 Limb Fitting Centres throughout England, Wales and Northern Ireland which are administered directly by the Department of Health and Social Security. There are also five centres in Scotland for which the Scottish Home and Health Department is responsible. The patient is referred to his nearest centre by the surgeon at the hospital at which he had his amputation. There he is seen by a Medical Officer who will be responsible for his limb fitting programme and prosthetic rehabilitation. The patient is examined, assessed and usually measured for his temporary prosthesis on his first visit.

The patient remains under the care of the Artificial Limb Fitting Service all his life, for he will continually require repairs and replacement of his artificial limb. He will also be supplied with sufficient woollen or cotton stump socks, bandages, walking aids and other appliances as he requires them.

Should the patient move to another part of the country he is transferred to his nearest Regional Limb Fitting Centre.

All artificial limbs are made by independent manufacturers under contract to the Department of Health and Social Security.

Surgery and Levels of Amputation

Whatever the pathology predisposing to amputation, there are many factors which will influence the surgeon in his selection of level of amputation. As well as the pathology, the surgeon will also consider factors such as surgical techniques, viability of tissue, prostheses and not least important the patient's particular needs, taking into account his occupation, importance of good cosmesis, age and sex.

HINDQUARTER AMPUTATION

This amputation is performed almost solely for malignancy as a life-saving procedure and here, obviously, the pathological factors are of prime importance. The surgeon has no choice but to remove the entire limb and part of the ilium, pubis, ischium and sacrum on that side, leaving peritoneum, muscle and fascia to cover and support the internal organs.

HIP DISARTICULATION

This procedure is commonly performed in cases of malignancy; it may also be necessary following extensive trauma but is seldom done for vascular insufficiency. The limb is disarticulated at the hip joint and the bony pelvis is left intact, thus producing a good weight-bearing platform.

MID-THIGH AMPUTATION

This is the amputation which is perhaps most commonly seen in the elderly group of patients. In the patient with vascular disease, an above-knee amputation is one in which primary healing occurs more readily than the through-knee or below-knee amputation. However, compared with these other levels, the above-knee amputee will have more difficulty in learning to control his prosthesis and in achieving a good gait and, in the case of the elderly patient, the attainment of total independence will be more of a problem. Proprioception from the knee joint will be lost and the patient must bear weight on the prosthesis at the ischial tuberosity. Hip flexion contractures occur very easily unless care is taken to prevent them, the shorter stumps tending to become flexed and abducted (due particularly to the strong pull of tensor fascia lata). The longer above-knee stumps by contrast tend to become flexed and adducted (there will be more of the adductor group intact and these muscles have a mechanical advantage over the pull of the short tensor fascia lata).

The surgeon makes the above-knee stump as long as possible, but must leave 4½–5 inches (11·5–12·5cm) between the end of the stump and the knee axis in order to leave space for the knee control mechanisms to be put into the prosthesis. If, however, there is a hip flexion contracture, a long stump is a disadvantage as the end of the long stump magnifies the contracture and the prosthesis will be very bulky to accommodate this.

Many surgeons use the myoplastic technique or a myodesis in which muscle groups are sutured together over the bone end or attached to the bone at physiological tension. The muscles therefore retain their contractile property, circulation to the stump is improved, and the stump will be more powerful in the control of a prosthesis.

AMPUTATION AT KNEE JOINT LEVEL

This includes disarticulation of the knee and the Gritti-Stokes amputation. In the former, the tibia together with the fibula is disarticulated at the knee joint. The patella is retained and the patellar tendon is sutured to the anterior cruciate ligament, the hamstrings are sutured to the posterior cruciate ligament and so act as hip extensors. A strong powerful stump results with no muscle imbalance, and full end bearing is possible on the broad expanse of the femoral condyles. Most of the proprioception of the knee joint is retained.

In the Gritti-Stokes technique, the femur is sectioned transversely through the condyles and the condyles are trimmed down medially and laterally. The articular surface of the patella is shaved off and the patella positioned at the distal end of the femur. Bony union should occur and weight is taken on the patella.

Full end bearing is possible on the knee disarticulation, but due to the relatively smaller weight-bearing surface in the Gritti-Stokes amputation, this is often not possible and a certain amount of weight must be taken through the ischial tuberosity. However, the Gritti-Stokes amputation necessitates smaller skin flaps with better vascular nutrition and therefore primary healing is more certain.

BELOW-KNEE AMPUTATION

If at all possible, the surgeon will elect to perform a below-knee amputation. The great advantage is that the normal knee joint with its proprioception is retained and therefore balance and a good gait pattern will be more easily attained, particularly if the patient is able to wear a patellar tendon bearing prosthesis which leaves the knee function unrestricted (Plate 8/1). The optimum level is $5\frac{1}{2}$ inches (14cm)

Plate 8/1 Two patients with below-knee amputations wearing patellar tendon bearing prostheses. Note that control of the prosthesis depends entirely upon the hip and knee joints and muscles, particularly the quadriceps and hamstrings

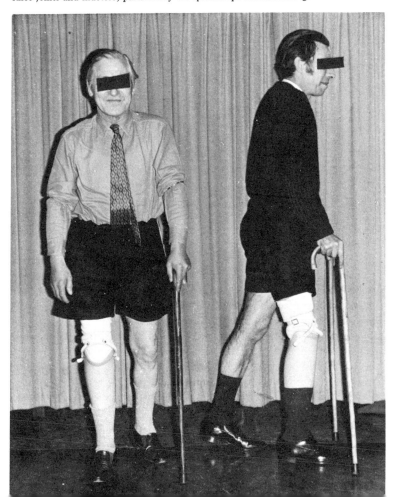

below the tibial plateau, although a patient with a slightly shorter
stump would still achieve good function with a prosthesis.

The fibula is sectioned slightly more proximally than the tibia, and
the end of the tibia is bevelled to avoid a prominent bone end.
Frequently a myoplastic technique is used, resulting in the advantages
previously described.

SYMES AMPUTATION

This involves disarticulation at the ankle joint and removal of the
medial and lateral malleoli to the level of the articular surface of the
tibia. This amputation is not done in vascular conditions, as a higher
level will always be necessary due to insufficient blood supply. Good
end bearing is possible, the heel pad being sutured into position over
the distal end of the tibia and fibula.

FOOT AMPUTATIONS

Trans- and midtarsal amputations result in relatively little locomotor
difficulty, the main problem being that of the provision of satisfactory
footwear.

PHYSIOTHERAPY

The physiotherapist's role in the rehabilitation of the amputee can be
considered in three stages: pre-operative, postoperative (pre-
prosthetic), and prosthetic.

Again it must be emphasised that rehabilitation is one continual
process, the final goal for the patient being independence on his
definitive prosthesis and a return to normal activities, within the
limitations of his age and condition.

Pre-Operative Stage

Treatment at this stage is of course most applicable to the patient with
vascular disease, and in these cases a pre-operative exercise programme is very valuable. Many of these patients have been at home or
in hospital confined to bed or to a chair because of a lesion of the foot,
gangrene or ischaemic pain. If the patient has been walking at all he
will only have been hobbling from one room to another, the joints of
the affected leg will be held in a position of flexion (the reflex response
to pain) and his general condition will be poor.

The physiotherapist should assess the patient's physical abilities
and also take into account his mental attitude and home conditions.
On the basis of this assessment she will commence and progress the

physical treatment programme, at all times with reference to the surgeon, nursing staff and other members of the rehabilitation team.

During the pre-operative stage, the patient begins to adapt to his changing circumstances, learns to know the staff who are concerned with his rehabilitation, and perhaps meets other amputees who are progressing towards independence. At this stage the therapists and social worker should be finding out about the patient's home situation, if possible meeting close relatives and involving them in the patient's programme of rehabilitation. The psychological aspect is very important and the physiotherapist can do much to help and motivate the patient at this stage.

Depending upon the time available and the general condition of the patient, the following should be included in the treatment programme:

1. Strengthening exercises for the upper trunk and upper limbs to facilitate crutch walking, transfers and for moving up and down the bed.
2. Strengthening and mobilising exercises for the lower trunk, necessary for all activities, rolling, sitting up, walking.
3. Strengthening exercises for the unaffected leg for crutch walking, standing, transferring.
4. Exercises for the affected leg to increase the range of movement and improve stability of those joints which will remain after amputation.
5. Crutch walking, if possible, non-weight-bearing with the affected leg.
6. Maximal independence including ability to move about the bed using the unaffected leg, rolling, prone lying.
7. It is important to teach wheelchair activities even though it is hoped that the patient will ultimately achieve independence on a prosthesis. A few weeks will elapse before he receives this and in the meantime he should be encouraged to be as independent as possible. Many of the elderly patients do not manage with any degree of safety on crutches.

Postoperative Stage

The aims of treatment at this stage are:

1. Prevention of joint contractures.
2. To strengthen and coordinate the muscles controlling the stump.
3. To strengthen and mobilise the unaffected leg.
4. To strengthen and mobilise the trunk.

5. To teach the patient to regain independence in functional activities.
6. To control oedema of the stump.
7. Early ambulation.

Physiotherapy will be commenced the day following operation. It should always be remembered that most of the patients undergoing amputation for vascular reasons have been heavy smokers for many years, therefore chest complications are not uncommon. Routine postoperative breathing exercises should be commenced on the first day.

PREVENTION OF CONTRACTURES

Attention should be given to the position of the patient in bed. The stump should lie parallel to the unaffected leg with the joints extended. There should be no pillow under the stump and there should be fracture boards beneath the mattress. Both physiotherapists and nursing staff should keep a check on the patient's position. The patient should understand its importance and be encouraged to maintain it.

A routine of prone lying, with all joints in as much extension as possible, is commenced as soon as the patient can tolerate it, usually on the third postoperative day, ideally for 15 to 20 minutes, three times daily. If the patient is unable to lie prone because of cardiac or respiratory problems, he should lie supine for as long as he can tolerate it, again two or three times a day.

STRENGTHENING OF THE STUMP

Isometric work for the muscles of the stump is started three days after operation. As the wound heals, manually resisted isotonic work can be given and gradually progressed. It is inadvisable, particularly when the myoplastic technique has been used, to give strong resisted work until about 14 days after surgery, as there will be much suture material in the wound and care must be taken not to pull on this.

The physiotherapist must at all times watch for any muscle imbalance and pay particular attention to the weaker groups, which will most likely be the extensors of the hip and knee and possibly the hip adductors, in fact, those muscles necessary to oppose a potential contracture (p. 136). Stability of all joints of the stump will be essential in the effective control of a prosthesis.

STRENGTHENING AND MOBILISING THE UNAFFECTED LEG

Strong isometric 'holds' with the hip and knee in extension (Plate 8/2)

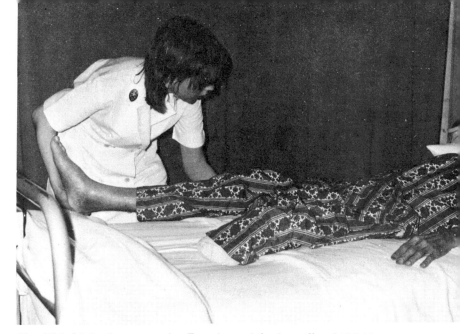

Plate 8/2 Left below-knee amputation. Extension work for the unaffected (right) leg, showing strong isometric work to emphasise supportive function

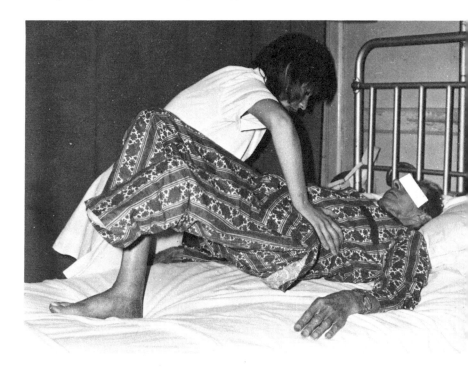

Plate 8/3 'Bridging', extension at the pelvis

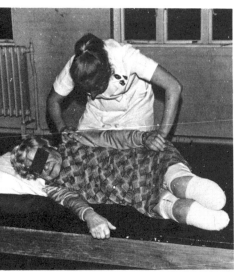

Plate 8/4

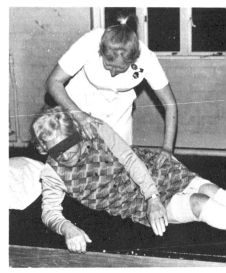

Plate 8/5

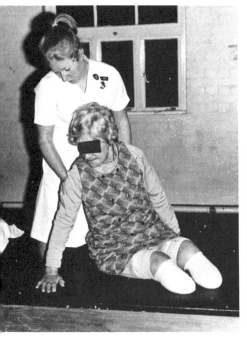

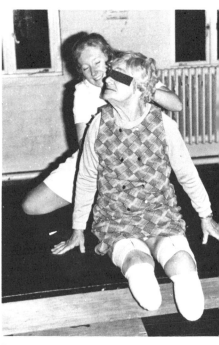

Plates 8/4, 8/5, 8/6 Rolling to sitting
sequence with guided resistance

Plate 8/7 Resisted sitting balance

are useful in helping to retain the supportive function of the leg, and this isometric work together with resisted isotonic exercises can be started the day following operation. During the next few days, as the patient's general condition improves, these exercises are progressed. When the sutures are removed from the stump and firm bandaging has been commenced, standing and walking in the parallel bars and on crutches is encouraged, emphasis being placed on hip extension.

TO STRENGTHEN AND MOBILISE THE TRUNK

'Bridging' exercises (Plate 8/3) and rolling exercises (Plates 8/4 and 8/5) can be commenced on the first day, and on about the third day when the patient is able to sit on the edge of his bed, resisted sitting balance work is given (Plates 8/6 and 8/7). As soon as the patient is able to go to the physiotherapy department, the resisted trunk exercises are progressed on mats together with reciprocal leg activity, and sitting balance improved. Attention is also given to the upper trunk and upper limbs and weight and pulley systems are useful for this, (Plates 8/8 and 8/9). Group work can be of value although elderly patients benefit more from individual treatment sessions, and two of these sessions daily in the physiotherapy department with perhaps occupational therapy as well is usually an adequate programme for these patients.

INDEPENDENCE IN FUNCTIONAL ACTIVITIES

At all times the patient must be encouraged to be as independent as possible. His treatment programme should progress in the physiotherapy department as soon as he is fit enough to leave the ward, usually about the fourth day. He should dress himself in the morning (sometimes it is necessary for the occupational therapist to give dressing practice) and he should wear a good walking shoe on the unaffected leg. Basic wheelchair independence is taught including transfers from bed to chair and from chair to lavatory, and he should be able to wheel himself around the ward and if possible to the physiotherapy department.

CONTROL OF OEDEMA

When the sutures have been removed (between 14 and 21 days after amputation) firm stump bandaging must be commenced. The purpose of this is to disperse the terminal oedema which is always present, particularly in the above- and below-knee stumps.

It is essential that the oedema is reduced as quickly as possible so that the stump assumes its ultimate size quickly and the limb fitting programme is not delayed. Firm bandaging conditions the stump to constant all-round pressure which the patient will experience when wearing a prosthesis.

Above-knee or through-knee stumps require 5 yards (4·5 metres) of 6 inch (15cm) wide 'Elset S' or crêpe bandage.

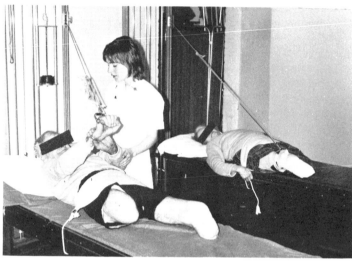

Plate 8/8 Weight and pulley work. Left: bilateral upper limb extensions for trunk. Right: extension, abduction, medial rotation pattern of right leg

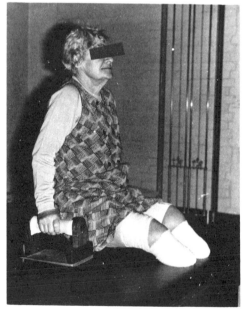

Plate 8/9 Extensor 'push-ups' for upper limbs

ABOVE-KNEE OR THROUGH-KNEE STUMP BANDAGING (Fig. 8/1)

1. With the patient in the half-lying position, place the end of the bandage anteriorly at the inguinal fold, the patient or assistant holding the two corners with his thumbs.
2. With the bandage at half stretch take it distally over the end of the stump and up the posterior aspect to the gluteal fold, the bandage is then held here by the patient's fingers. The next turn is taken again over the distal end of the stump slightly laterally and then returned anteriorly to the starting point, this turn again being held by the patient's thumbs.

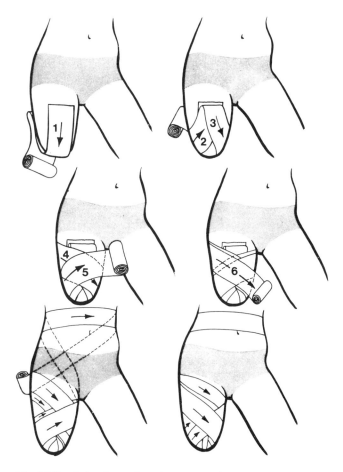

Fig. 8/1 Bandaging for an above-knee amputation

3. Once more the third turn passes distally over the end of the stump, this time slightly medially. It is now passed proximally and laterally across the posterior aspect of the stump. It is held at this point and then brought diagonally downwards and medially across the anterior aspect (turn 4) and a turn is now taken firmly around the back of the stump at the distal end (turn 5).

4. Figure of eight turns are now continued around the stump working proximally until the whole of the stump has been covered and the turns taken well up into the groin.

5. A fixing turn is made by taking the bandage from the posterior aspect of the stump up over the buttock and then forward around the waist. It is best to have the patient turn on to the other side for this. As the turn is brought around the patient's back, he is asked to extend the stump. The bandage is then brought down again to the anterior aspect of the stump.

6. The rest of the bandage is used on one or two more turns on the stump, and fixed by two safety pins high up postero-laterally on the pelvis.

BELOW-KNEE STUMP BANDAGING (Fig. 8/2)

1. Place the end of the bandage anteriorly just below the tip of the patella, the patient or the assistant holding the two corners with his thumbs. With the bandage at half stretch take it distally over the end of the stump and up over the posterior aspect of the popliteal space. The bandage is held here by the patient's fingers.

2. The next turn is taken again over the distal end of the stump slightly laterally and then returns anteriorly to the starting point, this turn also now being held by the patient's thumbs.

3. Once more the third turn passes distally over the end of the stump, this time slightly medially. It is now passed proximally and laterally across the posterior aspect of the stump. It is held at this point and then brought diagonally downwards and medially across the anterior aspect (turn 4) and the turn now taken firmly around the back of the stump at the distal end (turn 5).

4. Figure of eight turns are now continued around the stump working proximally until the whole stump has been covered.

5. It is important not to put too much tension on the bandage or too many turns over the tibia as pressure sores can easily occur.

6. The bandage is finished by two or three turns above the knee. If the stump is short or the tibial shaft very superficial, the stump should be bandaged in extension and the knee joint included.

When the suture line of the below-knee amputation lies anteriorly, the turns of the bandage should be made in such a way that the bandage assists in approximation of the skin flaps and does not have the reverse effect.

Stump bandages should be reapplied at least three times a day or more frequently if necessary. The patient should be taught to apply the bandage himself and if this is not possible, his wife or closest relative should be taught to do it for him. It will be essential for the stump to be bandaged until the patient is wearing his definitive prosthesis all day, at least three to four months.

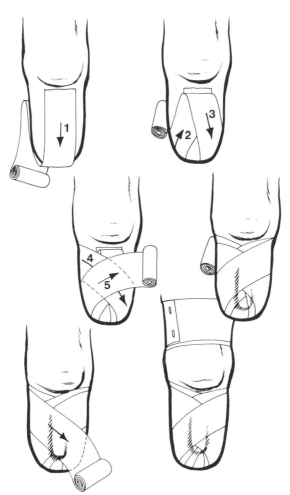

Fig. 8/2 Bandaging for a below-knee amputation

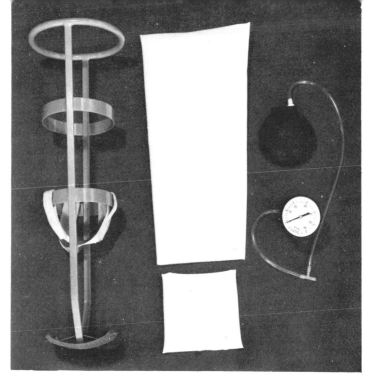

Plate 8/10 The component parts of the pneumatic pylon (PPAM AID)

EARLY AMBULATION

It is most important, particularly for the elderly, to encourage the patient to stand and walk as early as possible. In this way balance and postural reactions are maintained and improved and the walking pattern retained. It is of course also essential to keep the elderly patient as mobile as possible. The first temporary prosthesis or pylon which is made for the patient is not usually available until approximately four to six weeks after amputation. Recently a mobility aid has been developed which does not have to be made and fitted for the individual and can be put on the patient as early as five to seven days postoperatively. This is the Pneumatic Post-Amputation Mobility Aid (PPAM AID). The equipment consists of an outer plastic inflatable sleeve, a small inner plastic bag which is invaginated on itself, a metal frame with rocker base and a pump unit with gauge (Plate 8/10).

The patient walks partial weight-bearing in the parallel bars, and if suitable progresses to elbow crutches. The PPAM AID is not worn outside the rehabilitation department. Oedema in the stump is kept under control in the PPAM AID which is applied over any dressings, bandages, trouser legs or other clothing (Plate 8/11).

Referral to the Limb Fitting Centre

As soon as the wound is healed the surgeon refers the patient to the regional Limb Fitting Centre. He is examined by a Medical Officer and if the stump is satisfactory he will be measured for his first temporary prosthesis, the pylon. This will take two or three weeks to make and in the meantime the patient is usually discharged from hospital. It is important that his physical condition be maintained and improved, and it is usually necessary for these patients to attend the physiotherapy department of their nearest hospital on an outpatient basis. A young active patient will probably be able to carry out a home programme on his own and for him, outpatient treatment will be unnecessary.

Prosthetic Stage

As soon as the patient takes delivery of his pylon, arrangements are made for him to continue his rehabilitation with it, either in the

Plate 8/11 Patient walking partial weight-bearing on PPAM AID

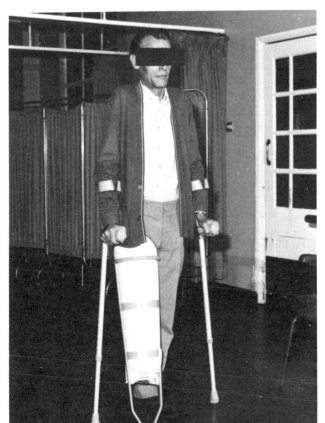

physiotherapy department of his original hospital or in the department at the Limb Fitting Centre. The patient must learn not only to walk safely and well but also to be able to put the pylon on independently, to stand up from a chair, climb stairs, walk up and down a slope, on rough ground and possibly manage public transport.

It is advisable for the patient to attend daily if possible for a whole or half-day session. Elderly patients frequently experience difficulty in tolerating the prosthesis, and unless they wear this regularly for the greater part of the day their performance on an artificial limb is certain to remain limited. During all stages of treatment, it should be remembered that many of these patients have undergone amputation for vascular conditions and therefore the other leg is likely also to be involved. It is important to observe the other leg and to make sure that any lesions of the foot are dressed and sufficiently protected by adequate footwear when commencing gait re-education (see chapters on Peripheral Vascular Disease in *Cash's Textbook of Chest, Heart and Vascular Disorders for Physiotherapists*).

In teaching the patient a good gait pattern on his pylon, it is necessary to bear in mind the fact that the patient will of necessity have to walk with a stiff knee. Accordingly hip up-drawing on the side of the pylon must be stressed and the patient taught to bring the pylon forward without circumduction. All pylons have a type of knee mechanism which will only take the patient's weight if locked in extension. The knee lock can be released on sitting down. When the patient sits in a chair he puts his weight on the sound leg, releases the knee lock and sits down. On standing, he pushes on the arms of the chair, and with his weight on the sound leg and with the rocker base of the pylon on the ground, he extends his stump as he stands, so locking the joint. Alternatively, the patient can be taught to lock the pylon before standing and to release the lock only after he has sat down. On climbing stairs, the patient puts the sound leg up first and brings the pylon on to the same step. To descend, the pylon is lowered first, the sound leg following.

The pylon is suspended on the patient by a pelvic band and shoulder strap. There is a rocker base instead of a foot, which facilitates weight transference and good even gait (Plate 8/12).

Although no allowances are made for cosmesis, the pylon is usually acceptable to the patient because it is functional and takes only two weeks to manufacture. It is lighter than a definitive prosthesis and because of the rocker base it is relatively easy for the patient to walk well. Usually two walking sticks are the only aids required once the patient has learned the correct gait between parallel bars.

After one or two weeks the patient is normally discharged from

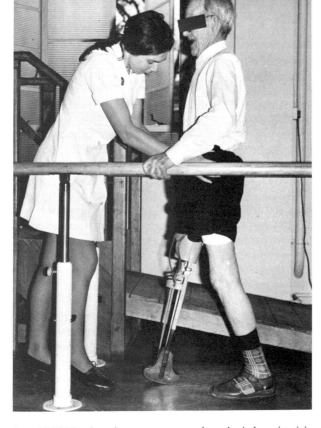

Plate 8/12 Right above-knee amputee on pylon, physiotherapist giving resistance at pelvis for weight transference

outpatient treatment and he continues using his pylon at home, wearing it daily, for the whole day. Some patients at this stage are able to return to work.

The patient is reviewed by the Medical Officer in four to six weeks' time, and if the stump has sufficiently reduced in size (bandaging is still being continued at night), a cast and measurements are taken for the definitive prosthesis. At present, this will take up to three months to manufacture, with at least one fitting. On completion of the prosthesis, the patient is called up to the Limb Fitting Centre and if all is satisfactory, he takes delivery of the limb. He then reattends at an outpatient department as he did with his pylon, for final rehabilitation.

Again it will be necessary to teach the patient how to put on his new artificial limb and carry out all functional activities. His gait may be altered, for if he is an above- or through-knee amputee he may have been given a free-knee mechanism and he must learn to control the prosthesis accordingly. In this case, during the swing phase the prosthesis is brought forwards by hip flexion to heel strike, the stump is then extended strongly against the posterior wall of the socket of the prosthesis which will ensure that the limb is fully extended and so stable enough to take the patient's weight for the stance phase.

Stairs are negotiated in the same manner as with the pylon. A below-knee amputee will have to accustom himself to controlling his prosthesis with his normal knee joint and musculature which probably will have become weak during the time spent on the pylon. Frequently the elderly amputee will be given a knee lock on his prosthesis, resulting in more stability.

It is advisable both with the pylon and the definitive limb to start the patient in the parallel bars, teaching the basic fundamentals of gait with good weight transference, and then to progress to walking with two sticks. Occasionally two tetrapods will be necessary. The patient should be encouraged not to look down at his feet when walking, although this is inevitable in the early stages as it will compensate for the total loss of proprioception in the joints of the amputated part of the limb. He must learn as soon as possible to feel with the remaining joints the positioning of the prosthesis in the gait sequence.

A patient should never be allowed to walk with crutches while wearing his prosthesis as he will tend to bear weight on the crutches and not on the artificial limb. Very occasionally it may be necessary to teach the patient to walk with a frame, although this should only be done when he has proved unsuccessful with other walking aids. It is not possible to attain a good gait when using a frame and the patient will always be dependent on this rather bulky aid.

Elderly patients, particularly those living on their own, should be taught how to get up from the floor should they have a fall. This is best done by showing the patient how to pull himself across the floor to some stable piece of furniture, e.g. sofa, armchair, bed, and then to get himself from the floor onto this. Double amputees are best advised to remove their prostheses first.

THE BILATERAL AMPUTEE

Occasionally as a result of trauma it will be necessary to amputate both lower limbs immediately. Unilateral amputees with vascular disease should be regarded as potential bilateral amputees within three years, depending upon the severity of the condition. It can be seen therefore, that it is not uncommon for the physiotherapist to be called upon to rehabilitate these severely disabled patients.

The pre- and postoperative treatment of the bilateral amputee

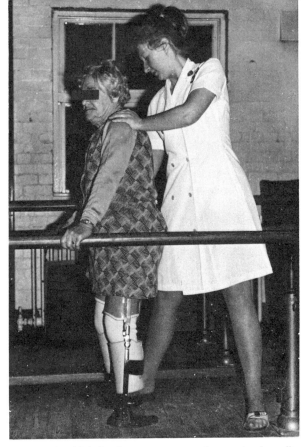

Plate 8/13 Double below-knee amputee on pylons, resisted standing balance in parallel bars

follows that of the single amputee, although obviously he will be unable to walk on crutches or in the parallel bars. Particular attention must be paid to strengthening and mobilising the upper limbs and trunk, and care taken to prevent flexion contractures of the hips developing while the patient waits for his pylons. These patients will all require a wheelchair and a suitable model must be ordered for the patient while he is in hospital. All wheelchair activities must be taught, including transfers, possibly with the use of a sliding board.

The temporary pylons that the patient receives, rocker pylons, are very much shorter than the patient's normal legs, being 18 to 24 inches (45 to 60cm) high for the above-knee amputee and proportionately shorter for the through- and below-knee amputee. These short pylons lower the patient's centre of gravity and make balance easier. The patient takes weight on both ischial tuberosities and so in effect is

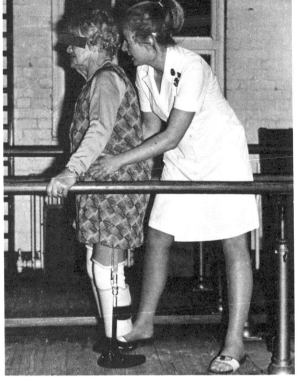

Plate 8/14 Resistance at pelvis to emphasise hip extension. Note the rocker bases extend posteriorly to prevent patient losing balance backwards. This is particularly important if there is any hip flexion contracture

walking upon two stilts. He does not have a normal foot on the ground feeding in sensory information and helping with balance. It will be appreciated that these patients require a longer period of prosthetic rehabilitation, frequently four to five weeks of daily attendance. (Plates 8/13, 8/14, 8/15, 8/16.)

When the patient is mobile and competent on his pylons, he is reviewed by the Medical Officer who will decide whether the patient will be able to manage definitive prostheses, or whether he should remain in his wheelchair, walking on his pylons only in the house. If he receives definitive prostheses, these will tend to be shorter than his normal legs, but nonetheless, cosmetically acceptable. A further period of rehabilitation will be necessary on these.

Very occasionally a patient will not be fitted with prostheses, either as a single or as a bilateral amputee. He may have multiple disabilities including hemiplegia, blindness or rheumatoid arthritis, his social conditions may make it unrealistic for him to be mobile on prostheses, or he may himself elect not to be fitted. These patients will need to be rehabilitated to a wheelchair existence and adaptations in the home will have to be made where necessary.

Immediate Postoperative Fitting of Prosthesis

In some hospitals and centres a slightly different postoperative routine is employed. While the patient is still under anaesthetic, the surgeon applies a rigid plaster of Paris socket to the stump over the dressing. To the end of this is incorporated a metal fitment to which can be attached a length of tubing and a prosthetic foot. The advantages of a plaster of Paris 'wrap' are firm control of the stump oedema with early maturation or shrinkage of the stump. The patient stands two to three days after surgery, but takes only minimal weight on the prosthesis. Other strengthening and mobilising exercises are given as previously described.

After 14 days the plaster is removed and the sutures taken out,

Plate 8/15 Double above-knee amputee on short rocker pylons. Note the need for a wide base

Plate 8/16 Climbing stairs – the rocker is placed on the edge of the step and the patient extends the hip on that side as he pulls with his hands on the rails

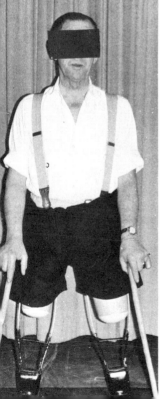
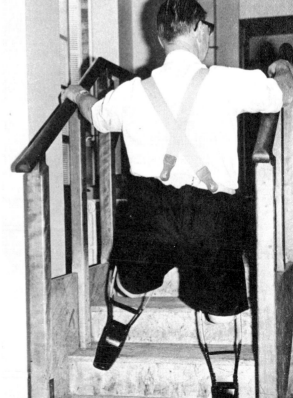

another plaster together with the prosthetic appliance is applied and rehabilitation continued. The patient progresses to walking on the prosthesis with elbow crutches, still only taking minimal weight on that side. At no time does the patient take full weight on this prosthesis, and he continues to walk with elbow crutches. After a further 14 days the plaster is removed and if the stump is satisfactory a cast is taken for a prosthesis.

With this method, earlier fitting of a definitive prosthesis is normally possible and the patient is rehabilitated in a shorter period of time. However, a closely co-ordinated team of specialists in the rehabilitation of amputees is necessary, and in order to reduce the risk of infection, patients need to be cared for in specialised units. It has been found that general surgical wards are not suitable for this regime.

Controlled Environment Treatment (CET)

Another method of postoperative management of the amputee involves the use of the CET machine (Plate 8/17). Immediately following amputation, the stump is placed in a transparent plastic sleeve with a non-constricting seal proximally. Distally a length of hosing links the sleeve to the machine. The machine delivers sterile warmed air under intermittent positive pressure and so maintains an optimum

Plate 8/17 Patient receiving controlled environment treatment (CET)

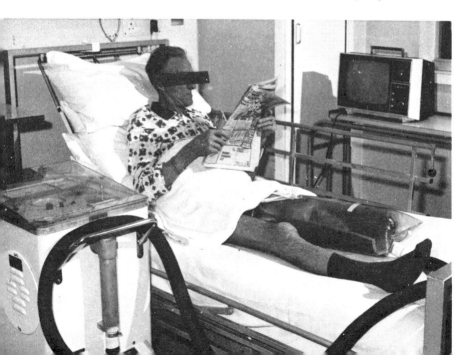

environment for wound healing within the plastic sleeve. No dressings are necessary so healing and tissue reaction can be observed. The patient can exercise within the sleeve, can stand and hop in parallel bars or on crutches and be reasonably mobile while attached to the machine.

After 10 to 14 days the equipment is removed and usually a plaster of Paris socket is applied with foot piece so that the patient can walk partial weight-bearing, and the oedema kept under control. Alternatively the PPAM AID will be used in sessions in the rehabilitation department. A cast and/or measures for a pylon are taken at 21 days and the patient continues his rehabilitation as normal.

UPPER LIMB AMPUTATIONS

Patients who undergo amputation of the upper limb do so most commonly as a result of trauma from accidents at work or road accidents, and these patients therefore tend to be in the younger age-groups and are of employable age.

The suddenness of the accident and the psychological shock of losing an arm cannot be underestimated. The physiotherapist can do much to help the patient in this respect as she will be treating the patient from the day following the operation, and much will need to be done to prepare the patient for wearing and using a prosthesis.

The aims of physiotherapy are as follows:

1. To strengthen and mobilise the entire shoulder girdle.
2. To prevent contractures.
3. To strengthen the muscles controlling the stump and maintain full range of movement in the joints.
4. To control oedema of the stump.
5. To maintain a good posture.

On the day following amputation, exercises to the shoulder girdle and unaffected arm are commenced. The patient will depend upon good mobility of this region for the control of his prosthesis.

The stump must remain in a good position and this must be supervised by both nurses and physiotherapists. The contracture most likely to develop in the above-elbow amputee is one of flexion, adduction and medial rotation at the shoulder, and frequently there is the danger of a frozen shoulder developing. The contracture most likely to occur in the below-elbow amputee is that of flexion at the elbow.

A few days following amputation, active exercises for the muscles controlling the stump can be started and gradually progressed to strong resisted exercises when the sutures are removed.

After the sutures are removed on the fourteenth day, firm stump bandaging is commenced in the same way and for the same reasons as for the lower limb amputee (see p. 143). A 3 inch (75mm) wide 'Elset S' or crêpe bandage is used.

A constant check on the posture of the patient is necessary to ensure a level shoulder girdle and good position of the head and neck.

Four to five days postoperatively, a leather gauntlet can be applied over the bandage. Into this gauntlet simple tools such as cutlery in below-elbow stumps or a pencil or paintbrush can be fixed, and the patient encouraged to use his stump. Where possible early use of the stump for functional activities diminishes the risk of the patient becoming 'one-handed'.

Prosthetic Stage

As soon as the sutures are removed the patient is seen by the Medical Officer, at the regional Limb Fitting Centre, and measurements are taken for a prosthesis.

At present it is not possible to fit the patient with a temporary prosthesis as in the case of the lower limb amputee, and the patient must wait two to three months for the manufacture of his definitive prosthesis. Sometimes at this stage the patient will be given a discarded 'second-hand' prosthesis of which the appropriate parts including the socket are remade, and arm training with this temporary prosthesis is commenced at the Limb Fitting Centre.

Usually the arm training units in the Limb Fitting Centres are staffed by occupational therapists, emphasis obviously being placed upon independence and training in functional skills and work and recreational activities.

A patient can be fitted with a heavy working arm, a light working arm or a dress arm which is purely a cosmetic prosthesis. In the first two cases, control of the prosthesis and of the terminal device is by straps which pass posteriorly across the patient's scapular region and which are activated by protraction of the scapula and extension of the stump (Plate 8/18).

Numerous terminal devices are available, but all patients will be given a split hook (Plates 8/19, 8/20) which can be used for many activities and is the most commonly used device, and a cosmetic hand. The occupational therapist will assess the patient and depending upon his work and hobbies he will be supplied with the relevant devices.

It is essential that the patient return to work or be trained for

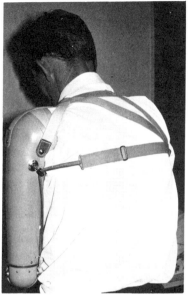

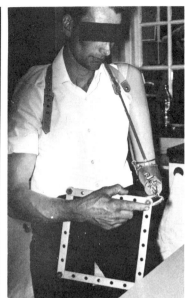

Plate 8/18 Posterior view of
above-elbow prosthesis showing
leather operating cord (inferior)
attached to the appendages.
Protraction of scapulae to operate
terminal device

Plate 8/19 Anterior view showing
strap to operate elbow lock

Plate 8/20 Close-up of split hook

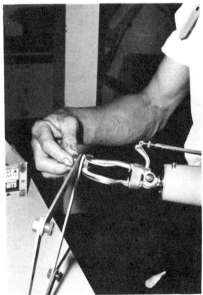

alternative employment as soon as possible, and normally these patients, once over the initial shock, are well motivated to do so.

BIBLIOGRAPHY

Anderson, M. H., Bechtol, C. O. and Solars, R. E. (1959). *Clinical Prosthetics for Physicians and Therapists*. Charles C. Thomas, Illinois.
Gillespie, J. A. (Ed.) (1970). *Modern Trends in Vascular Surgery*. Vol. I. Butterworths.
Humm, W. (1977). *Rehabilitation of the Lower Limb Amputee*. 3rd edition. Baillière Tindall.
Klopsteg, P. E. and Wilson, P. D. (1969). *Human Limbs and their Substitutes*. Hafner Publishing Co., New York.
Little, J. M. (1975). *Major Amputations for Vascular Disease*. Churchill Livingstone.
Murdoch, G. (Ed.) (1970). *Prosthetic and Orthotic Practice*. Edward Arnold.
'Symposium on Limb Ablation and Limb Replacement' (1967). *Annals of the Royal College of Surgeons of England*, **40**, 4.
Vitali, M., Robinson, K. P., Andrews, B. G. and Harris, E. H. (1978). *Amputations and Prostheses*. Baillière Tindall.

ACKNOWLEDGEMENTS

The author thanks Mr. M. Vitali, F.R.C.S., Principal Medical Officer, The Limb Fitting Centre, Roehampton and Miss M. A. Mendez, M.A.O.T., District Occupational Therapist, Roehampton Health District for their help in the preparation of this chapter. Thanks are also expressed to the Photographic Department, The Limb Fitting Centre, Roehampton for their help with the illustrations and to the secretaries who helped with the typing.

Miss P. A. Downie, F.C.S.P., overall editor of the book, is most grateful to Seton Ltd. of Oldham for allowing the use of Figs. 8/1 and 8/2 and the text of their leaflets on below-knee and above-knee stump bandaging.

Chapter 9

Injuries to Soft Tissues – I

by M. K. PATRICK, O.B.E., M.C.S.P.

While the ensuing chapter deals with trauma and its effects on soft tissues, it must be remembered that these tissues can show inflammatory changes as a result of other pathological causes. These conditions are discussed in other chapters.

The principle of treatment for all will be to establish the cause of the tissue abnormality and then to deal with it.

The aims of local treatment are: prevention of further tissue damage; reduction of effusion; prevention of loss of range of movement; prevention of muscle atrophy; regaining full power and function; and restoration of confidence in the affected part or limb.

PHYSICAL EXAMINATIONS

When a patient presents himself after an injury with a shoulder pain, knee pain or back pain it is essential to determine which structures have been damaged and to what degree. The treatment will be based on these findings.

The history of the injury that the patient gives will reveal the time of the incident and how it occurred. The physical signs and symptoms indicate the results of the mechanical failure. It is by understanding these that the tissue damage can be determined. It is obvious that if a knee is found to have spasm of the hamstring group of muscles and atonia of the quadriceps, with local spasm around a large haematoma of the thigh, that the latter is the site of the lesion. However, when large 'joints' are involved the massive reaction to injury can make it difficult to decide exactly which tissues are damaged.

The tests are made by a doctor initially, but it is important that the physiotherapist should understand them and be able to repeat them if necessary. Some of the physical tests that are carried out are actually diagnostic, but most of them are indications. When they are 'positive' together with physical signs, a gradual picture is built up. Other tests will be tried and found not to be positive and so the field of diagnosis is narrowed until either a definite lesion can be pinpointed, or a general diagnosis made. It is important for the physiotherapist to understand the significance of these tests. While the total tests are legion the most common ones are discussed here with the examination of the area.

EXAMINATION OF THE SHOULDER

A shoulder cannot be examined for a lesion, in isolation. It is essential to consider the shoulder girdle and whole upper limb as well, since they are all functionally interrelated, and any impairment of the action of one part often disturbs the harmony of movement of the whole region. The cervical spine must also be examined, as some muscles acting on and influencing the shoulder region take their attachment from the cervical spine. The nerve roots of the cervical and brachial plexuses provide the myotomes and dermatomes to the arm and shoulder region.

History

It is often better to obtain the history before the patient is asked to undress, then the clinical picture that the examiner is forming from the history can be checked against the observation of the patient as he undresses.

Attention should be paid to the onset of symptoms, method of injury, the forces involved and the signs and symptoms that the patient has observed. Previous injuries, painful episodes or loss of movement should also be noted. Patients do not always readily associate their previous pain as being relevant. The large range of the shoulder joint and girdle movement makes it particularly vulnerable to the effects of wear and tear, and it is not uncommon to find that the middle-aged and elderly have some limitation of range. A woman may admit that she has been unable to raise her arm to do her hair, or a man may say he has pain when carrying a heavy weight. Any previous treatment they may have had, and their response to it, may be significant, as may the nature of their work and hobbies over the years.

Observation

Observation should begin as soon as the patient arrives. The patient's general posture should be noted. Some patients will hold the arm close to the body and support its weight at the elbow with the other hand. This is usually a sign that the patient is in great pain.

When the patient undresses it is important to watch not only the movements but the expression on the patient's face to verify his reaction to any pain that may have been experienced. The actual removal of clothes normally involves rotation of the shoulder joint and girdle, as well as a rhythmical sequence of movement which is particular to the person. Any pain or limitation of range in the region can interrupt this sequence and it becomes laboured. If, however, undressing is relatively easy, it is possible that the lesion is of nerve root origin rather than in the shoulder region, since it is the traction strain of the weight of the arm on the nerve root which causes the pain.

Once the patient is suitably undressed he should be observed in the relaxed standing position. The posture of the head, neck and shoulder girdle and the contours of the areas are compared for any deviation from the normal. An elevated shoulder may be associated with an increase in muscle tension due to pain, but it could be the result of changes which have developed over the years as a result of occupational habit. The rest of the examination is conducted with the patient sitting.

Atrophy is most readily observed in muscles such as the lateral rotators of the shoulder, and either part or the whole of deltoid. Judgement has to be based on comparison with the unaffected side. Gross alteration of contour such as occurs with dislocation or displaced fractures is readily seen. Swelling is unusual in the shoulder region as the capsule is loose and can accommodate any increase in synovial fluid that may occur.

Following a direct injury a localised haematoma may be observed, but bruising from damaged blood vessels at a deeper level may be considerably delayed. This is because the deeper structures are tightly compressed by overlying muscles, and the blood and other exudate tracks downwards through the relatively loose fascia to appear distal to the site of the injury.

Palpation

This must be carried out gently and carefully to ensure that the patient remains as relaxed as possible. A sound understanding of normal anatomy and considerable experience is needed, before a precise interpretation of the findings of palpation can be made. A generalised palpation is carried out to ascertain the temperature of the area, the mobility and elasticity of the skin, the degree of muscle tone and area of maximum tenderness.

Specific palpations, in association with particular movements, are then undertaken to localise the pain and tissue structure involved if muscle relaxation can be obtained.

ACUTE JOINT INFLAMMATION

The examiner compresses the shoulder between flat hands placed on the anterior and posterior aspects of the shoulder joint area. An increase of pain will be experienced by the patient if there is an acute inflammatory state, when tension is increased within the joint.

BICIPITAL TENDONITIS

When the shoulder muscles are relaxed the intertubercular sulcus (bicipital groove) can be palpated. Localised tenderness is found. This is made worse when the patient is asked to supinate his forearm and flex his elbow against resistance.

SUBACROMIAL (SUBDELTOID) BURSITIS

Deep palpation just lateral to the lateral border of the acromion process of the scapula will elicit tenderness in the subacromial bursa if it is inflamed. This bursa is susceptible to trauma due to its position under the subacromial arch. Passive compression of the bursa can also be carried out by placing one hand under the flexed elbow and the other over the acromion process. The humerus is moved passively upwards, thus compressing the bursa, and this causes acute pain if the bursa is swollen.

SUPRASPINATUS TENDONITIS

This tendon can be palpated when the arm is adducted and rotated medially, thus bringing its area of attachment on the upper margin of the greater tuberosity out from under cover of the acromial arch. The examiner then places a finger transversely across the tendon and pain is elicited if there is tendonitis present.

JOINT LINE PALPATION

This can be palpated anteriorly and posteriorly, but only if the muscles are fully relaxed. In the elderly, whose muscle tone is less, it is often possible to elicit joint line tenderness which is very specific and localised, indicating chronic osteoarthrosis.

ACUTE CAPSULITIS

The region of tenderness is much larger than that in the chronic osteoarthrotic patient. If the arm is moved passively in a lateral direction, with some traction on the humerus, an increase of pain will be felt by the patient with an acute lesion of the capsule.

STERNOCLAVICULAR AND ACROMIOCLAVICULAR LESIONS

These joints may show a slight swelling or feel warm on palpation if there is an acute traumatic lesion of either joint. If these signs are not obvious the joints can be 'sprung' to assist in the identification of soft tissue damage. This is performed by placing the fingers over the appropriate end of the clavicle near the joint and depressing it. The joint movement creates stress on the soft tissues and causes acute pain if damage is present. This 'springing' is especially helpful when examining a patient whose injury occurred a week or more ago. The pain from this type of lesion follows the dermatome of the nerve root, but it may only be apparent at certain points. For example a fifth cervical nerve root irritation nearly always produces an area of pain and tenderness at the insertion of deltoid. Similar painful and tender areas can be identified just above the superior angle of the scapula, or at the elbow near the origin of the common extensor muscles of the forearm. (This is often confused with a tennis elbow.) If it is thought that the lesion is of cervical origin, then the usual tests for root pain should be carried out, e.g. does nerve stretching cause pain.

Movement

From the history, observation and palpation, the examiner will have built up a picture of the lesion that he thinks has occurred. It only remains to test the appropriate movements to conclude the examination. Since pain and its resulting muscle spasm are so often such paramount features of shoulder lesions it is advisable to carry out all movements on the unaffected side first. Then the patient is likely to co-operate better in demonstrating similar movements on the affected side. All of these movements must be carefully recorded for comparison of one shoulder with the other, and at a later stage to assess progress. The point at which pain is experienced should also be carefully noted. When the patient is asked to raise his arm, he should be observed from the rear and the examiner's thumb placed on the inferior angle of the scapula, the forefinger on the posterior rim of the glenoid cavity, the other fingers on the arm. Movement of the arm, and the point in movement at which the scapula moves, can be felt. Resisted movements should be tested to ascertain if there is any muscle weakness. Again the unaffected side is tested first and used as the comparison.

Passive movements of the injured shoulder are often not possible because of the acute pain and muscle spasm which is present. Usually if a passive movement can be made without causing pain, whereas a similar movement performed actively causes pain, it is reasonable to assume that the muscle, or the structures being compressed by the muscular contraction, are damaged. In the shoulder region this is not altogether true. If a pain-free passive movement can be performed it is usually a sign that the lesion is not in the shoulder region, but is that of a nerve root irritation, since in shoulder lesions there is usually too much muscle spasm to allow a passive movement of any great range to be performed.

Painful Arc Syndrome

This is the name often given to describe an injury to the rotator cuff. When the patient is asked to raise his arm above his head through abduction, the first 50° to 70° of movement are usually pain-free. When attempting further movement the patient may be seen to elevate his shoulder instead of producing pure abduction – reversed scapulohumeral rhythm (Fig. 9/1). If the patient persists with the movement the pain usually fades after a further 30° to 40° of the painful arc. This pain is caused by a lesion of the rotator cuff muscles (infra- and supraspinatus, subscapularis and teres minor) at their point of attachment to the capsule, which is compressed under the

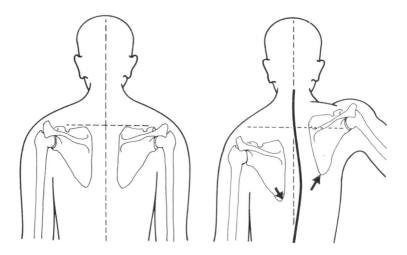

Fig. 9/1 Reverse scapulohumeral movement. Attempting abduction of the arm results in elevation of the scapula instead of rotation

acromial arch in this particular range of movement. A further test for this lesion is to ask the patient to take up the inclined walk standing position. Then, while retaining that trunk posture he is asked to elevate the arm. This is usually pain-free as the weight of the arm acts as a traction force on the shoulder joint and relieves the compression on the affected structures.

FROZEN SHOULDER

This is usually the result of a chronic state of this rotator cuff lesion, which has not been treated, thus allowing a chronic capsulitis of the shoulder joint to develop. Few patients willingly inflict pain on themselves and therefore they avoid the painful arc of movement. They use the arm only for actions which involve a small range of pain-free movements of the shoulder and this range gradually becomes less as the capsule becomes thickened and adherent. In a few weeks there can be a complete loss of range which is difficult, if not impossible, to regain fully.

An established frozen shoulder may well be pain-free as all movements in the joint have ceased. Assessment of this condition should be made from the rear of the patient, from where it may be seen that the shoulder girdle rises as the arm abducts and no movement between the scapula and humerus can be detected because the structures move as one (Fig. 9/2). A further test is to ask the patient to stand with his arms

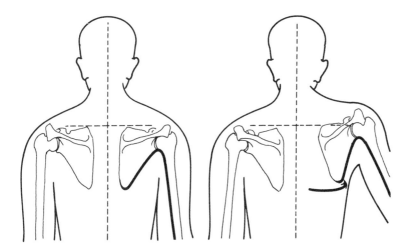

Fig. 9/2 Frozen shoulder. Attempted abduction of the arm results in 30° of lateral movement of the scapula. The distance between the humerus and the inferior angle of the scapula remains the same

by his side, then to bend both elbows to a right angle. Keeping his upper arms close to his chest wall outward rotation is attempted. The frozen shoulder will only move a few degrees, and this is not true shoulder joint rotation. It is made by the action of trapezius and the rhomboid muscles retracting the scapula.

Consideration of all the findings and history should enable the examiner to make a differential diagnosis and so select the appropriate treatment. However, in the acute stage of shoulder lesions this may not be possible, and a diagnosis indicating an area of damage rather than a specific structure may well have to be made.

Mobility is the chief requirement of the shoulder region, but while full range movement is the aim of physiotherapy, this may well have to be compromised in order to obtain a pain-free, functional arm, especially if the patient is in the older age-group.

EXAMINATION OF THE KNEE

History

The time spent talking to a patient about how and when the incident occurred is most valuable. It will become obvious which tissues are likely to have been damaged, and to what extent, from the patient's remarks. A sensible patient can help greatly in the assessment of his injury. For example, a footballer may say that he was dribbling the ball in a forward direction, when he was tackled by another player. Immediately he attempted to pivot with his knee slightly flexed, but his foot was held in the tackle and so he sustained a rotational strain of his knee joint. This indicates that it is more likely to be a cartilage injury than a medial ligament tear, as the latter normally occurs when the leg is straight.

The descriptive terms that the patient uses must be fully understood so that they can be used both for the records and for forming a clinical judgement of the injury. 'Gave way' or 'letting down' can mean a temporary loss of muscle power so that the patient actually fell, or that the knee feels momentarily weak when making a certain movement. Sometimes the patient says he thought the lower leg 'was coming off'. This is the impression that the patient has when there is an abnormal amount of movement of the tibia on the femur due to the laxity of the cruciate ligaments. This movement is actually only a few centimetres, but can be seen on examination.

'Locking' in medical terms means a state when the knee is held in some degree of flexion, usually about 10° to 15°, by a mechanical derangement, usually a cartilaginous obstruction. A degree of manipulation, whether by the patient himself or another person, will be needed to unlock the knee joint. Many patients use the term 'locking' to describe a painful reluctance to move, combined with muscle spasm; or a momentary spasm of pain which checked movement.

'Lumps' or 'swellings' are terms used indiscriminately to describe either bony, soft tissue or fluid alterations that the patient feels when palpating his knee. Only by careful questioning can such remarks be helpful in diagnosis. A patient who has dislocated his patella seldom remarks on the patella being displaced, but complains of a lump which appears on the side of his knee. This is really the exposure of the medial condyle of the femur. Other patients are good historians and can clearly indicate where and how they feel a loose body, or a tag of cartilage which moves so that it can only be felt at certain times, or after certain movements.

Observation

It is useful to watch a patient unobtrusively as he enters a cubicle and gets onto an examination couch. The position of the knee joint when it bears weight, whether the patient 'swings' the leg up on the couch or has to assist it with his hands, the expression on his face at the time, all help to make a clinical assessment. The degree of flexion that the knee is held in while walking may gradually lessen as the patient relaxes on the couch. Any skin discolouration or alteration in contour should be noted.

Palpation

This allows the patient to get accustomed to his painful joint being handled, and if it is done with care, he will relax more easily since he does not feel so apprehensive. To the examiner it is an opportunity to feel the swelling and warmth of an inflammatory lesion and to feel the alteration in muscle tone when tenderness is present, thus helping to determine the site of the lesion.

Movement

Usually the patient is asked to demonstrate the degree of flexion and extension he is able to perform. A comparison of the muscle power of the unaffected and affected leg is made. Thereafter much of the examination is passive movement performed by the examiner to form the diagnosis. Many of these tests are performed on the sound leg first. This not only allows the patient to know what is going to be performed, but more importantly it gives a comparison of movement. All joints have some laxity and it is reasonable to assume that normally it is equal in a similar joint of the same patient, unless there is some obvious reason why this should not be so.

Ligament Damage

TIBIAL COLLATERAL LIGAMENT

Medial ligament damage is tested with the knee extended (*not* hyperextended) and the joint is stabilised by the palm of the examiner's hand being placed on the lateral aspect of the knee with the fingers supporting the knee posteriorly. The other hand which is placed on the medial aspect of the lower tibia then abducts the tibia on the femur. If there is damage to the ligament the movement will be more than normal and pain will be felt by the patient, either on the medial condyle of the femur or along the upper tibia, depending on which end of the ligament has been damaged. The pain and muscle spasm are usually too great for this test to be conclusive diagnostically for a complete rupture of the ligament, and it may have to be repeated under an anaesthetic.

FIBULAR COLLATERAL LIGAMENT

Lateral ligament damage is tested by a similar method with the supporting hand held medially and the tibia adducted on the femur.

An alternative test can be performed with the patient in prone lying. The affected knee is flexed to 90°. The patient is then asked to relax and the operator holds the leg at the ankle and gives a slight lift which opens the knee joint (i.e. traction). The tibia is then rotated and if pain is experienced by the patient it is indicative of collateral ligament damage. (Only a few patients with severe damage will be able to flex their knee to a right angle in the acute stage.)

CRUCIATE LIGAMENT DAMAGE

When an anterior cruciate ligament is torn off violently it often removes a flake of bone and this is visible on an X-ray. The test for laxity is only possible if the patient can relax his knee completely. It is not conclusive evidence of a complete rupture. The hip and knee are flexed to 90°. The foot is rested on the couch and stabilised by the examiner lightly sitting on it. The examiner's hands are then placed around the tibial condyles so that the thumbs are either side of the tibial tubercle. The upper end of the tibia is then rocked forwards and back and the range is assessed against that of the other knee.

LIGAMENTUM PATELLAE DAMAGE

The leg is relaxed in the extended position and palpation will reveal the 'gap' either below or above the patella. (See muscle rupture, p. 185.)

DAMAGE TO THE MENISCUS

When the knee is flexed to 90°, palpation of the joint line will often elicit acute pain over a tear of the rim of the cartilage, or the tag may be felt. The test as for cruciate ligament laxity is performed, and may elicit pain which could indicate that a torn section of the meniscus is folded backward into the joint, causing strain on the anterior cruciate ligament. A 'springing' of the knee joint, that is, gentle forced hyper-extension of a knee that is held in slight flexion by spasm, can be helpful as an aid to diagnosis of a tear of the posterior horn of a cartilage, but it is performed with care as it may well be putting strain on the cruciate ligaments, which may be already under strain by the internal derangement of the joint.

McMurray's Test

This is to confirm a meniscus lesion. The knee and hip are fully flexed. The examiner's hand is placed posteriorly round the knee joint so that the thumb and forefinger are on the joint line. The heel is gripped by the other hand and the tibia is rotated outward. A low-pitched clunk indicates a medial cartilage tear. The rotating of the tibia inwards would be performed to test a lateral cartilage. If no sound is obtained the procedure is repeated with the knee in less flexion. The less flexion needed to obtain the sound, the further inwards the tear. If no sound can be obtained then the manipulation is repeated when moving the knee through flexion or extension. It is often impossible to be certain where the tear is, or whether there is one, until an operation has been performed.

An alternative test is similar to that described for collateral ligaments (p. 170). Again the patient is lying prone and flexes the knee to 90°. The operator holds the ankle and the patient is asked to relax. Pressure is then exerted to close the knee joint (compression) and the tibia is rotated. This grinding action causes pain if there is damage to the meniscus.

Patella Tap

This test is used to establish if there is fluid in the knee joint. The knee is supported in a relaxed extended position. The operator then places his hand above the knee joint. This hand is then moved distally while exerting some posterior pressure, so that any fluid within the capsule is compressed. While the position of this hand is maintained, the other is used to depress, or tap the patella against the femur. A knocking sound can be heard and felt when there is an effusion in the joint. Sometimes there is too much, or too little fluid to elicit the tap. An alternative procedure is to place both hands across the knee, one above and one below the patella. The fingers should be on one aspect and the thumbs on the other. Pressure is then exerted on the side of the joint by the fingers and if there is an effusion, the fluid will move away from the pressure and can be felt by the thumbs on the opposite side of the joint. The fluid's movement can also be observed.

EXAMINATION OF THE LOW BACK
History

Careful questioning of the patient is essential. It is important to understand what he means by the terms he uses to describe his pain and how it occurred, and to find out about previous incidents of trauma that he may not think of mentioning. For example most people over 40 have suffered some pain in the back before the incident which finally brings them to hospital. Questioning will elicit which time of day this was usually at its worst, and whether it stopped them from working, etc. A pain on waking is often an indication that there is a lack of mobility in the spine. Such pain 'wears off' as the patient moves about. Increasing pain and stiffness as the day progresses indicates a more inflammatory state which is caused by increasing protective muscle spasm.

A person who gives a history of a blow on his back will have local swelling, tenderness, etc., associated with a contusion at the site of the injury. The examination will be to determine the severity of injury and to exclude complications such as bony damage or damage to internal organs.

Observation

The way a patient walks or moves himself on arrival is always watched carefully since it is the only really free movement he will make. This observation is continued to include how he gets himself on or off a plinth, but this is not such valuable evidence as his first free movements. Thereafter he will be performing actions on request and these may not give a true picture.

POSTURE

This is always a most valuable guide to the severity of nerve root irritation. Unless there is a medical reason to make it impossible, the patient should always be examined standing. Any alteration of lumbar, thoracic or cervical curves should be observed from both the side and the rear of the patient. Any scoliosis and the relative position of the shoulders to the hips should be assessed from the back of the patient. The distribution of the muscle spasm should also be noted.

Palpation

Palpation of the back is an important part of the examination, because much can be deduced from the distribution of increased muscle tension. The patient stands with his back to the examiner, who places her flattened hands over the lower lumbar region. The difference in tension of the erector spinae muscles on each side can then be detected.

By gentle palpation, the whole lower back can be examined in order to ascertain the distribution of muscle spasm and its effect on the position of the vertebral column. The most usual pattern of muscle spasm is such that the vertebrae adjacent to the lesion are deviated to that side, with a compensatory muscle spasm above and on the opposite side, resulting in scoliosis.

Tenderness should be carefully noted. In many lesions, while the pain may be diffuse, there will be an area of localised tenderness which indicates the precise site of the lesion.

Movements

FORWARD FLEXION

The patient is asked to bend forward without bending his knees, and the muscle spasm evoked is carefully noted. If one knee were allowed to bend, the distribution of muscle spasm in the back would be altered and the effectiveness of the test nullified. During forward flexion, it is usual for the examiner to put her hand sideways over the spine so that the thumb and little finger touch the patient over the sacrum and upper lumbar vertebrae. Contact is maintained as the movement is performed and any alteration in distance between the digits is noted. If the distance shortens, which is rare, it would indicate extra spasm, and lengthening would indicate a degree of movement occurring in the lumbar spine. Such movement is not usual in an acute lesion. If the lesion is of lower lumbar origin, the hamstrings will go into spasm.

The ability to 'touch the toes' has no bearing on the progress or severity of the condition. Some patients will be able to touch their toes while their upper lumbar muscles are in severe spasm; others with no spasm will never be able to demonstrate this action. It is only a guide to the length of the hamstring muscles, and many chronic back sufferers will have gradually stretched the hamstrings to compensate for loss of lumbar flexion. While this forward flexion is being attempted the patient is asked to indicate when and where pain is produced; this helps to determine the mechanism involved in the production of pain.

HYPEREXTENSION

Extension of the spine is then requested into the hyperextended position. In an acute lesion of the lower lumbar region this can seldom be performed as a postero-lateral disc protrusion commonly occurs. However, if the disc had protruded anteriorly, hyperextension would be the post-traumatic stance and forward flexion would probably only be to the upright.

LATERAL FLEXION

This is not usually affected except that muscles involved in the action may be in spasm.

Lasègue's Sign

When this was originally described by Lasègue he said that the patient should be lying relaxed in a supine position. The affected leg was then passively raised so that the hip and knee were each in flexion to 90°. Then, keeping the hip still, the lower leg was raised to the straight position. If pain was experienced the test was described as positive. Today this test is usually adapted to a passive straight leg raising which is performed slowly and carefully. During the first 30° of this movement no lumbar spine movement occurs, thereafter there is some movement, particularly at the level of L5 and stretching of the nerve root occurs. The nerve root movement is at its greatest when the leg is raised to between 60° and 80° (Fig. 9/3). The clinical interpretation of this sign is that if the pain is severe the lesion is likely to be the fifth lumbar nerve root.

Charnley is of the opinion that this test does not necessarily indicate a disc protrusion unless the back is stiff. He suggests a modification of the test which is passive straight leg raising until there is pain. Then flex the knee until the pain goes, and press sharply in the popliteal

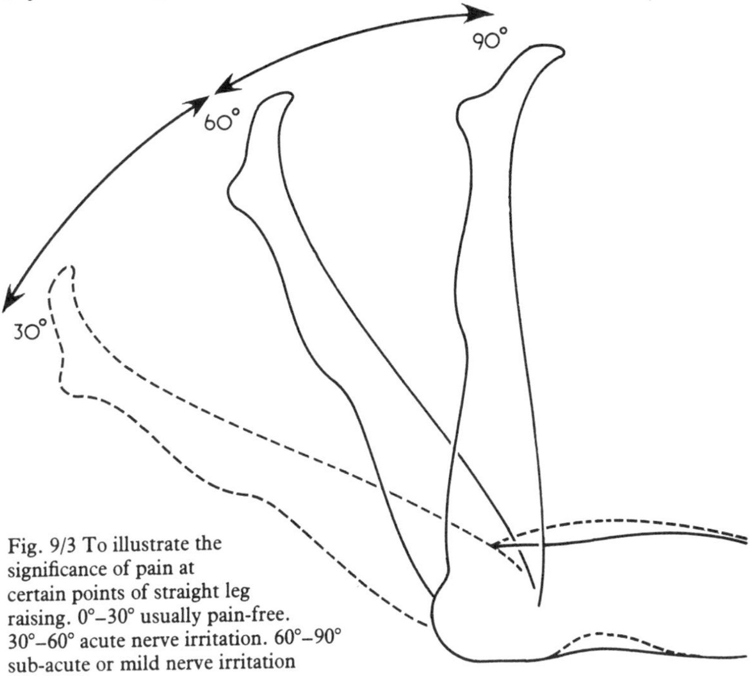

Fig. 9/3 To illustrate the significance of pain at certain points of straight leg raising. 0°–30° usually pain-free. 30°–60° acute nerve irritation. 60°–90° sub-acute or mild nerve irritation

fossa without moving the hip or knee. If pain is elicited by this finger pressure it is a nerve root pain and not a muscular one.

Fajersztajn's Sign

This was described by an Austrian neurologist who found that when the non-affected leg is passively raised, pain is felt on the affected side. Woodhall and Hayes (1950) were able to describe why this occurred. It is because when the leg is raised the lower lumbar nerve roots on the opposite side emerge a little from their foramina, shifting a little towards the middle line and to a lesser extent towards the anterior wall of the spinal canal, causing a stretching of the nerve if there is a disc protrusion.

There are many variations of these tests which are based on this mechanical principle.

Third lumbar nerve root lesions are tested by lying the patient prone and passively flexing the knee towards the buttock. Any pain felt is the result of compression of the nerve root due to its loss of mobility.

The second lumbar nerve root is tested by the patient standing and raising the affected leg forwards with the knee flexed to 90°. This action has the greatest nerve root movement for L2 and to add to the stretch on the nerve the trunk is flexed forward. This test is repeated with the other leg and will, to a lesser extent, cause pain on the affected side.

Muscle Power

Loss will be assessed by static contractions. While each nerve root supplies more than one muscle, each muscle has a predominant nerve root supply. Clinically it is usually found that the involvement of the third lumbar nerve root results in weakness of the quadriceps action, the fifth lumbar nerve root the extensors of the great toe, and of the first sacral nerve root the gastrocnemius.

Sensory Loss

Sensory loss will be assessed, but this, while following the pattern of the appropriate dermatome, is very variable from one patient to another. However, a reasonable guide is that L4 nerve root affects the area around the antero-medial aspect of the knee, L5 nerve root the dorsum of the foot, especially the great toe, and S1 nerve root the heel and lateral aspect of the foot.

Reflexes

These will also be tested. The loss of the patellar reflex would indicate an L3 nerve root and the loss of the plantar reflex an S1 nerve root involvement. See Table.

SYNOVITIS

This term is used to describe an inflammation of the synovial membrane of a joint. When the synovium is injured excessive synovial fluid is secreted into the joint cavity. The quantity is dependent on the amount of trauma that has occurred, but it is not uncommon to find that the capsule is fully distended by this effusion. If the trauma has caused damage to blood vessels, the effusion will be bloodstained.

The most usual way to damage the synovium is a twisting strain on a

Nerve root	Reflexes Knee jerk	Ankle jerk	Muscles pre-dominantly affected	Areas of most usual sensation alteration
L3	–	+	Quadriceps	
L4	+	+		Antero-medial aspect of knee
L5	+	+	Extensor of great toe	Dorsum of foot and great toe
S1	+	–	Gastrocnemius	Heel and lateral aspect of foot

joint, and this occurs most readily when the joint is flexed. It can be due to a direct blow. In either case other soft tissue damage may have occurred at the same time.

Let us take as an example traumatic synovitis of the knee which may have occurred as a result of an accident on a rugger field two hours previously.

CLINICAL FINDINGS

The knee joint is grossly swollen, clearly outlining the limits of the synovial membrane.

The leg is held in slight flexion (20°) so that the tension on the capsule and ligaments is reduced to a minimum. There is considerable muscle spasm of the hamstrings with inhibition of the quadriceps.

On palpation the joint is warm and the swelling is found to fluctuate. It is exquisitely tender.

Any movement of the joint causes great pain. It is for this reason that the player with a severe synovial injury cannot continue playing and is often carried off the field.

INVESTIGATION

It is essential that a very thorough investigation is made. An X-ray should be considered to eliminate the possibility of damage to the joint surfaces. Assessment for ligamentous damage may be prevented by the extreme pain, and examination under anaesthetic with X-ray control will have to be considered.

TREATMENT

Only very occasionally is the joint tension so severe that the effusion needs to be aspirated. The danger of infection is so high that this is seldom performed and then only with full aseptic precautions.

When all other major damage has been excluded the knee is usually supported by a pressure bandage. While this may be able to prevent further effusion it will not aid the resolution of the existing one. It should not be retained for more than three days.

Ice therapy is most helpful, as is deep heat for assisting in the quick absorption of the effusion.

Muscle activity, within the limits of pain-free movement, should be started at once.

While the joint is warm and tense, that is, showing the signs of acute inflammation, excess movement would result in exacerbation of the lesion. However, the muscle contractions will help to control the effusion and prevent muscle atrophy which occurs very quickly in the quadriceps due to the inhibiting factor of the spasm of the hamstring group. The rule should be for the patient to be taught a few simple exercises to do at home for five minutes in every hour. It must be remembered that the athlete or sportsman will always overdo exercises and suitable warnings should be given. The most important exercise, and one that should be performed frequently, is full extension of the knee joint to the locked position. This involves the vastus medialis muscle in the last part of the movement. This muscle atrophies quickly and is more difficult to re-educate at a later stage of treatment, so that it is important to restore its function immediately.

At first all exercises should be performed in the non-weight-bearing posture. No walking should be allowed on a knee that exhibits a quadriceps lag on straight leg raising; but of course the patient will be allowed to walk with crutches, taking no weight on the affected leg.

It must be remembered that the sportsman will soon become generally out of training when he is restricted to non-weight-bearing exercises and a general 'whole body' programme of exercises should be given as well as specific knee exercises. There is, for instance, no reason why he should not go swimming or use a static rowing machine with the affected leg left to the side.

Weight-bearing exercises will probably begin at about two weeks if the injury has been severe. These will be progressed to form the basis of an early full training programme. It is essential that absolutely full fitness and confidence is restored before play is allowed.

PROGNOSIS

The function and power of the knee should have been fully restored, so that the player can participate in his sport again within three to six weeks depending on the severity of the injury.

TENOSYNOVITIS

This is an inflammation of the tendon sheath which can be caused by a sudden wrench or a direct blow, though it usually occurs as a result of over-use. The effusion thus caused reduces the lumen of the sheath so making it more difficult for the tendon to run freely. This is an acute tenosynovitis which can, if repeated, become a chronic state in which the continuous process of fibrotic repair makes a thickened sheath, with tiny fibroid nodules, often referred to as melon-seed bodies. This loss of normal lumen makes all movements of the tendon painful.

Any tendon sheath can be affected, but some are more vulnerable to the effects of over-use than others, because of the mechanics of their anatomical action. An example of this is the common sheath for extensor pollicis brevis and abductor pollicis longus which have an angular pull as they pass around the radial styloid. Acute tenosynovitis of this sheath is known as de Quervain's disease.

De Quervain's Disease

Women are affected more often than men. The patient will probably give a history of having just started a new job in a factory. The work involves a light gripping action, which has to be repeated constantly several times a minute. After two days at this work she woke to find she could not move her thumb because of the pain.

CLINICAL PICTURE

There is a localised sausage-shaped swelling over the inflamed tendon sheath, which is very warm and tender.

Any movement of the tendon within the sheath causes pain. The pain may be so great that movement appears impossible. It has often been found that these patients have a low pain tolerance and will be disinclined to move any part of the hand or even the forearm.

IMMEDIATE TREATMENT

The thumb and wrist are rested on a cock-up splint. This is to restrict movement rather than prevent it.

To obtain a quick absorption of the inflammation, ultrasound and ice therapy, or short wave diathermy may be used. No movement of the tendons involved is encouraged for the first two days.

PROGRESSION

Once the very acute pain has subsided, unresisted movements are added. At first these will only be performed for a minute several times a day, using the splint for rest at other times.

After about seven to ten days, free gentle use of the hand will be encouraged with gradually shortening periods of rest on the splint. It is often useful to retain the splint for use at night for rather longer than it will be required for use during the day.

Before the patient is allowed to return to her job, a simulated gripping device must be found for her to practise upon. This serves several purposes:

● It can determine whether the inflammatory state has resolved.
● It can be used to check that the patient is performing the action of gripping properly. It is often found that these patients are only using the thumb to make the grip against statically held fingers. By encouraging them to share the work-load by actively flexing the fingers, further incidents may be prevented. A repetition of similar trauma may lead to a chronic inflammation of the tendon sheath.
● It will prove to the patient that she can have confidence in her ability to use her hand effectively at work.

Sportsmen seldom get de Quervain's disease but they do get tenosynovitis affecting the biceps, or the flexors of the fingers. This latter can either affect the common sheath in the region of the carpal bones, or more likely, in the digital synovial sheath.

Chronic Tenosynovitis

This is usually treated with an infiltration of hydrocortisone and a resting plaster, which is retained until there is complete resolution at about 10 to 12 days. Occasionally transverse frictions are requested after the plaster has been removed. Persistent lesions may require an operation to relieve the symptoms. It is seldom that these patients require physiotherapy as they use their limb normally once the pain has subsided.

BURSITIS

Bursae are small membranous sacs lined by synovium, which are sited to prevent frictional wear on tendons at joints. This friction could be between two tendons, but more usually it is between a tendon and a bone. True bursae are found at certain joints such as the elbow, heel and knee, but it is also possible to form a bursa over a joint which has become damaged or deformed and presents a new area of friction for a tendon. These are called adventitious bursae, but their reaction to injury is the same as that of a true bursa.

An acute bursitis is caused by a direct blow such as a fall on the knee or shoulder, or it can be the result of too much activity, especially of an unaccustomed action. Many bursae can be injured and cause little discomfort to the patient, since pain only occurs if pressure is put on to the inflamed bursa. For example, olecranon bursitis is almost painless until the elbow is leant upon. However, the subacromial bursa, when inflamed, is acutely painful due to the pressures put upon it during movements of the shoulder joint.

Subacromial Bursitis

A middle-aged patient wakes up to find he has a very painful shoulder. The day before he had been decorating a ceiling, a job he is not accustomed to doing.

CLINICAL PICTURE

He will be holding his arm close to his body, usually supporting the elbow with his other hand.

Any movement will cause great pain and he will have difficulty in removing his clothes.

It will be found that he has spasm of the adductor and medial rotator muscles of his shoulder, with a very tender area along the lateral border of the acromion.

The area will feel warm, but little swelling will be present as the damaged tissues are confined within the bursa and this is deep to the middle fibres of deltoid.

IMMEDIATE TREATMENT

After suitable investigation to eliminate other pathology, his arm will be rested in a sling under his clothes. Physiotherapy will aim at relieving the pain and reducing the inflammation.

PROGRESSION

It is important to retain shoulder movements. After the very acute phase is over, assisted movements must be given. These are progressed to full active movements as the inflammation resolves.

The anatomical construction of a shoulder is so complex that it is often impossible to decide which structures are damaged. However, the treatment is the same for all soft tissue lesions of the shoulder rotator cuff.

While a sling may be worn for a few days, it must not be retained for longer, especially in the older age-group, or range will be lost which it may not be possible to regain. For this reason full range movements must be aimed for at a very early stage. Ice therapy will usually relieve the pain and muscle spasm to enable proprioceptive neuromuscular facilitation (P.N.F.) techniques to be used to build up the power and range of movement. Functional activity is given as soon as possible.

REFERENCE

Woodhall, B. and Hayes, G. J. (1950). 'The well leg raising test of Fajersztajn in the diagnosis of ruptured lumbar intervertebral disc'. *Journal of Bone and Joint Surgery*, **432**, A4, 786.

BIBLIOGRAPHY

See end of Chapter 11.

Chapter 10

Injuries to Soft Tissues – II

by M. K. PATRICK, O.B.E., M.C.S.P.

INJURIES TO MUSCLES AND TENDONS

These injuries range from a simple strain to a complete rupture of the muscle or tendon. Within this range come some of the most common injuries sustained by athletes and sportsmen as well as the general public.

Strain of Muscle

Normal muscle is able to respond to the demands made upon it and is capable of a graded contraction directly proportional to the stress. It is only capable of this response if all the components of the neuro-muscular mechanism are working in a co-ordinated manner. If a sudden stretching force is applied to a muscle unexpectedly, the response may not be sufficiently co-ordinated and the result may be a rupture of a few muscle fibres or a minor tear in the connective tissue framework of the muscle.

Such injuries happen to athletes and sportsmen at the beginning of the season before they are fully trained, or to members of the general public who try to perform an action beyond their muscle strength. The effect of the damage will be seen at the weakest point in the muscle, and usually in muscles which work over two joints. The terms 'strain', 'tear' or 'pull' of muscle are commonly used to indicate a relatively trivial injury. The amount of haemorrhage that occurs will be directly proportional to the vascularity of the muscle and inversely proportional to its tone. The haematoma lies in the extracellular and interstitial spaces.

CLINICAL FEATURES

The patient presents with a muscle which has a localised tender swelling at the point of injury.

Protective muscle spasm and pain will be demonstrated proportional to the severity of the injury.

These will cause limitation of movement.

TREATMENT

Ice therapy (that is a pad soaked in ice-cold water, not direct ice), is the first-aid treatment for this injury. Usually strapping is applied to the area more for reassurance than support, since the bleeding will be controlled by the compression that occurs as the intramuscular tension builds up. Physiotherapy is not required for the acute lesion, but may be needed to encourage the patient to regain confidence in the limb. Normally clotting takes place in a few hours and in about three days full activity can be undertaken without fear of further tissue damage.

Contusions

These are the results of a crush injury, or a direct blow or kick. The blood and lymph vessels in the connective tissues of the muscle framework are ruptured and their contents released into the surrounding tissues to form a haematoma. The result is similar to that described for muscle strain except that with extrinsic violence there is subcutaneous as well as deep connective tissue damage. The sheath of the muscle may well be ruptured, allowing a muscle hernia to develop. The example will be taken of a footballer who has received a kick on his thigh over rectus femoris about 22·5cm (9in) above the knee joint and slightly lateral to mid-line, two hours previous to examination.

CLINICAL FEATURES

The leg will be held in slight flexion due to the protective spasm of the hamstrings. The quadriceps will show inhibition and loss of tone except in the vicinity of the injury where muscle fibres will be in spasm. There will be a marked swelling over the site of injury which will be both warm and tender.

TREATMENT

Ice-cold pads applied over the site of injury are the first-aid treatment for these lesions and may be continued for several days if required.

Strapping is applied, usually either over a cotton cylindrical bandage, or reversed, so that it does not adhere to the skin. The leg should be elevated to assist drainage while physiotherapy is given and the patient instructed to elevate his leg at home. Ultrasound therapy given to the area proximal to the haematoma aids rapid resolution. Static (isometric) quadriceps exercises are most important in that they restore the tone to the muscle and aid the reabsorption of the haematoma.

PROGRESSION

Due to the dangers of further damage to the blood vessels knee movements are usually delayed for 24 to 48 hours in severe injuries. Thereafter gentle knee movements are encouraged, watching always for any increase in bleeding. This would be indicated by an increase in both pain and swelling. These exercises are performed with a supporting bandage on.

The maximum effect of ultrasound and ice therapy is obtained during the first week. If further treatment is necessary then short wave diathermy may be given. At this stage there should be discolouration of the skin distal to the injured area. If there is not it may indicate that the haematoma has become 'trapped' by the organisation of the exudate peripherally, thus preventing its drainage. This can soon lead to ulceration and medical advice should be sought, as aspiration may be necessary.

Usually progress is quite fast after the first 10 days and is similar to that of muscle strain. The type of exercise is more fully described under synovitis of the knee (p. 176).

The long-term complication of severe haematoma is calcification within the muscle. If this causes weakness or loss of movement, the calcified mass may be removed surgically some months later.

Rupture of a Muscle

A complete rupture of a muscle belly rarely occurs except as a result of laceration, and the surgeon will have to consider the need or desirability of suture. Spontaneous repair will not take place as the two parts of the muscle contract, leaving a wide gap. Partial ruptures are more common and have been described under contusions (p. 184). A complete rupture can occur as a result of a direct blow on a contracted muscle, or by forced stretching of an already contracted one.

Such a complete tear of the belly of a muscle can occur in a very fit young athlete, and the belly of the rectus femoris is most often affected. A similar strain in an elderly person would result in a tear of the quadriceps femoris tendon immediately above the upper pole of the patella. In those who are neither elderly nor highly trained athletes, the rectus pull would tear the tendon below the patella.

Let us take as an example a young athlete who has sustained a complete rupture of rectus femoris an hour previously.

CLINICAL FEATURES

A flexed knee due to the spasm of the hamstrings which are only weakly opposed.

A large swollen area over the site of the injury which is very warm and fluctuates on palpation. This is a haematoma and is tender.

The upper section of rectus is contracted upwards and the lower section downwards to form hard 'knots' of muscle, leaving a palpable gap between them.

IMMEDIATE TREATMENT

The two ends of the muscle are brought together and repaired surgically.

The leg is supported in a back splint for 10 to 21 days. During this time static quadriceps exercises are given and active knee flexion is usually encouraged after the tenth day.

PROGRESSION

This is as for partial tear or severe contusion, once the surgeon has agreed to the starting of knee flexion and weight-bearing.

Rupture of Tendons

The causes of these injuries are the same as for ruptures of the muscle tissue.

A completely torn tendon will not repair itself spontaneously. Whether the surgeon decides to effect a surgical repair will largely depend on the age of the patient and the disability caused by the injury. For example, it is not uncommon for the tendon of the long head of the biceps to rupture in the over-70 age-group. This is seldom operated upon since the disability is a weakening of flexion of the elbow, but not a loss of the action, and does not usually warrant surgical intervention. However, complete rupture of a tendo-calcaneus causes great disability and the tendon is usually sutured. Let us look at two common examples of tendon rupture.

AN ELDERLY MAN WITH A RUPTURED LONG HEAD OF BICEPS TENDON

The patient will probably explain that he suddenly found difficulty in using his arm when he was trying to put his arm inside the sleeve of his coat. A history of traumatic incident can seldom be given.

CLINICAL APPEARANCE

The belly of the muscle will have contracted down into a hard knot, leaving a clearly defined 'space' where it would normally lie. This is even more clearly demonstrated if the elbow is flexed against slight resistance.

If it is truly the tendon that has ruptured, as is usual in the elderly, there is little swelling or bruising since the exudation is minimal. If, however, the tendon ruptures at the union with the muscle, the blood content of the exudate is increased.

IMMEDIATE TREATMENT

Rest in a large arm sling will be given, but active movements of the shoulder and elbow must be encouraged at once or range will be lost, and this may never be fully regained. A full range of movement of shoulder, elbow and radio-ulnar joints must be given, even if they have to be assisted or passively performed once on the first day. Relaxation of muscle spasm is needed to obtain pain relief and this is best obtained by resisted movements of the antagonist group. Heat is usually helpful. If there is a large haematoma or effusion then the techniques previously described under contusions (p. 184) may be tried.

The sling must be removed totally by the second or third day or flexion contracture of the elbow will develop as the torn muscle becomes adherent. To prevent spasm the hand can be carried some of the time in a coat pocket or the elbow rested on a chair-arm or table. Active use of the arm should be practised in the physiotherapy department to show the patient that it can be used normally. It is advisable to keep these patients in the department for most of the day in the first week after injury so that they can have repeated short activity sessions. If left at home they tend not to use the arm.

Full but weakened function should be obtained in two to three weeks.

A MIDDLE-AGED MAN WITH A RUPTURED TENDO-CALCANEUS (ACHILLES TENDON)

A fit, middle-aged man has torn his tendo-calcaneus when doing a sudden unco-ordinated muscle movement involving a powerful plantar-flexion of the foot. Most commonly this is done in sport, but it can be done by stepping on to the edge of a kerb instead of fully on to the pavement. The foot, instead of being stopped at 90°, is forced into full dorsiflexion. The calf muscle makes a violent contraction to try to counteract the dorsiflexion, but is unable to take the strain.

CLINICAL APPEARANCE

The belly of the gastrocnemius will be contracted upwards, but cannot retract far because the aponeurosis of the posterior aspect of the tendon is united to the soleus muscle, gradually forming a single tendon. However, a clearly defined gap in the tendon is palpable about 2·5 to 5cm (1 to 2in) above the insertion into the calcaneum. Occasionally this is masked by a chronic thickening of the area or a local swelling.

Plantar-flexion of the foot is performed weakly and only in a non-weight-bearing posture, by the posterior tibial muscles.

TREATMENT

The tendon is surgically repaired. The lower leg is put in plaster with the foot plantar-flexed.

PROGRESSION

After about three to four weeks the foot is brought up to a right angle, and walking with crutches is permitted. At four to six weeks a removable cast is often used so that active non-weight-bearing exercises can be given and non-weight-bearing walking with crutches has to be resumed. At about six to eight weeks full weight-bearing walking is allowed. The patient should be warned at this stage not to allow his foot to be suddenly forced into dorsiflexion.

Graduated exercises are given to build up the power of the calf muscles which will have atrophied considerably. The final result depends on the patient's willingness to practise exercises, and his confidence in his own ability. Some patients make a very good recovery and are able to raise the body weight onto the ball of the affected foot. Others are not able to do this. A poor result is in part a reflection on the therapist who should have been able to build up the patient's enthusiasm and confidence throughout the rehabilitation period.

Partial ruptures of tendons are said by some surgeons to be impossible, that is, the tendon either tears completely or does not tear at all. Other surgeons say partial ruptures can occur but do not require treatment beyond reassurance and perhaps an injection of local anaesthetic.

Peritendonitis

One of the most common injuries in athletics is peritendonitis of the tendo-calcaneus. When this is seen it is often an acute exacerbation of a chronic state and may exhibit stenosing or crepitus. The former will require operation, but the latter should resolve with rest. It is important that the rest period is at least ten days, during which time no heel raising should be performed. A pad in the heel of the shoe to elevate the heel, and walking with a shortened stride, will help to reduce the strain on the tendon. Any pain, however slight, should be taken to indicate that the activity must be reduced.

The physiotherapy needed is ultrasound and ice therapy, or short wave diathermy during the rest period, to help speed the resolution of the inflammation. Thereafter a carefully controlled introduction to movement of the tendon should be made. Running and jumping exercises should not be attempted during the first three weeks. Full training should be delayed until there is no pain on plantar-flexion in weight-bearing or jumping. This is probably five or six weeks after the incident. Any attempt to hurry back to athletics before the condition is completely resolved will result in a recurrence which is not only painful, but undermines the confidence of the athlete in his future ability.

LIGAMENTOUS DAMAGE

Normally a joint is stabilised by the muscles which control its movements, but if a strong external force is applied to the joint, particularly if it occurs unexpectedly as in an accident, the ligaments will be stretched. The individual fibres of the ligament will either tolerate the stress or rupture. The proportion of the fibres ruptured determines the clinical findings, the treatment required and the terminology used to describe the injury.

Williams and Sperryn (1977) classify ligamentous damage as follows:

'Stretched ligament': an occasional fibre ruptured.

'Mild sprain': a small proportion of fibres ruptured.

'Severe sprain': about half the fibres are ruptured.

'Complete rupture of the ligament': all fibres ruptured.

It must be remembered that other soft tissue damage must have taken place in all but the mildest of injuries, and probably in these too. The doctor and physiotherapist must assess the total clinical evidence and base treatment on their findings.

STRETCHED LIGAMENT

This might be presented by a patient who complains of having stumbled, and in preventing his fall has taken the force of the body weight on the medial border of the hand. The ulnar collateral ligament is stretched.

CLINICAL FINDINGS

A small swelling over the ulnocarpal joint, the pain of which limits movement, particularly radial deviation.

TREATMENT

Usually Elastoplast strapping for a week and full activity is all that is required.

MILD SPRAIN

This might be presented by a housewife who says that while she was making a bed her thumb was caught in a sheet as she tucked the bedclothes in, and it was forcibly hyperextended. She may well have ruptured a few fibres of the palmar ligament of the metacarpophalangeal joint.

CLINICAL FINDINGS

The thumb is held in slight flexion.

The metacarpophalangeal joint is very slightly swollen on the palmar aspect and very tender over the area of the damaged ligamentous tissue.

While all movements are possible, hyperextension of the thumb (i.e. a repeat of the direction of injury) causes acute pain.

IMMEDIATE TREATMENT

Ultrasound therapy or short wave diathermy is given to the affected area to help resolve the inflammation. Strapping in the form of a spica is applied to give support. The patient is encouraged to use the hand fully.

PROGRESSION

This should be fast, the strapping being removed at seven to ten days and full power and function recovered within two weeks.

SEVERE SPRAIN

A youth has sustained an inversion injury to the ankle on a rugger field.

CLINICAL FINDINGS

The foot will be in slight plantar-flexion with some protective spasm in the peronei.

There will be an egg-shaped localised swelling over the anterior talofibular ligament. This ligament is the most vulnerable because of the natural rotation of the forefoot.

The site of the lesion will be warm and tender.

Within a few hours of the injury the swelling will become less clearly defined and may well spread across the dorsum of the foot, and postero-laterally around the ankle.

Inversion will be severely limited by pain and muscle spasm.

Other movements will be performed in small range only.

X-ray investigation should be carried out to exclude bony injury.

TREATMENT

Since the ligament is not completely torn, conservative treatment will be required. The speed of starting physiotherapy is very important. Ultrasound and ice therapy should be given at once with the limb elevated. These are followed immediately by the application of a stirrup-type Elastoplast strapping which holds the foot in eversion. Since the strapping has to be removed frequently, it is usual to shave the limb first. Walking, with two sticks if need be, should be started at once, but the patient should only take short strides in order to eliminate a limp. After the first few steps the pain eases off. It is very important that walking is practised for short periods throughout the day. Progress in activity should be made quite quickly, but care must be taken to ensure that weight-bearing on an inverted foot does not take place for several weeks. For this reason the boy should be advised not to play rugger for two months if the injury has been severe.

COMPLETE RUPTURE OF A LIGAMENT

This might be presented by a pedestrian, who was struck on the lateral aspect of his leg by a car bumper. At the moment of impact the leg was fully extended. The force was such that it momentarily forced open the medial aspect of the knee joint and the tibial collateral ligament ruptured.

CLINICAL FINDINGS

The leg will be held in slight flexion due to the protective spasm of the hamstring muscles.

Within an hour of the incident there will be an effusion of the whole knee joint.

Localised tenderness over the site of the lesion will be very marked in the early stages. This becomes masked with the passing of time and the increase of the general effusion.

All movements will be grossly restricted by pain and muscle spasm, making it difficult to determine the site of the actual lesion.

X-ray investigation will be required. This may show the elevation of a flake of bone from the tibia or femur if the rupture has occurred at either of these points. It is often necessary to examine the knee while the patient is under an anaesthetic. The knee joint is given manual stress to open the joint to determine if a complete rupture has occurred.

TREATMENT

Surgery is required to repair the ligament. The leg will then be enclosed in a plaster cylinder from groin to ankle. This is retained for four to six weeks. The patient is usually kept non-weight-bearing for the first 10 to 21 days depending on how easily the surgical repair was made. After this walking is permitted. Once the plaster is removed knee movements are begun. The knee is usually supported by a back-splint (i.e. posterior half of the plaster cylinder) until the therapist is sure that the muscle power is sufficiently restored to protect the ligament from stress. Full range of movement and power should be restored in two to three months from the time of the injury.

Sprung Back

Young fit sportsmen do not suffer disc lesions as a result of their activities unless there is a major catastrophe such as the collapse of a rugger scrum, or a novice weight-lifter attempting too heavy a lift. They do, however, sustain repeated minor trauma, which can lead to early disc degeneration. This is particularly true of high and long jumpers, hammer and disc-throwers. They are frequently subjected to flexion stresses manifested as muscle spasm which usually resolve spontaneously after a few days, particularly if they can 'relax' the tense muscles. For this reason heat and massage are sometimes given.

The term sprung back is often used in sport. It is really a sprain of the lumbar intervertebral ligaments. This can be so severe that there is instability (which is demonstrable on stress X-rays), allowing a disc protrusion. The repeated attacks of low back pain or sciatica that follow can mean the end of sport participation. Sprung back in its milder form is treated as any other ligament strain.

DAMAGE OF MENISCI AND MENISCECTOMY

The menisci of the knee joint serve several purposes. They act as 'shock absorbers' in the straight leg posture as when walking, and as 'rockers' for the rolling action of the femoral condyles during flexion or extension. They are usually injured by a rotation strain on a flexed knee while it is weight-bearing.

It is very unusual for a child to tear a cartilage, but it is possible. The young and middle-aged form the majority of patients who suffer from this injury in its traumatic form, that is to say the patient can give a definite history of sudden pain, loss of power and range, with 'locking' of the joint (see p. 168). In the over-60 age-group a meniscus can be torn without the patient being able to give a history of any definite injury. This is because the cartilage is somewhat degenerative and possibly has had many previous minor injuries. Finally a minor incident completes a tear, or moves an already torn tag (which may well have been folded back within the joint), into a position where it cannot be tolerated. In this age-group the cartilage, either in its entirety, or just the torn slip, will have to be removed, since spontaneous repair is unlikely.

In younger people it is not thought advisable to remove menisci unless they have given rise to several previous episodes and have become an intolerable handicap, or if the 'locking' does not respond to manipulation. If the meniscus is removed the knee joint is mechanically imperfect, for the replacement cartilage that grows does not have the correct contours for the rolling action of the condyles of the femur, and so the knee is slightly less stable because hyperextension can take place. This defect is largely overcome by good muscle power when the patient is young, but later in life it often gives rise to further problems.

CLINICAL PICTURE

Immediately the incident takes place the knee which was bent at the time of injury, will 'lock'. This is a combination of muscle spasm caused by pain as well as the actual mechanical obstruction of cartilage. Sometimes the knee will only stay in this position for a few minutes. Gradually the muscle spasm lessens and the knee recovers its normal degree of laxity so that it can slowly be eased to a more straight position. In some cases the knee cannot be straightened until it has been manipulated under an anaesthetic.

The knee will lack full extension and any attempt to 'spring' it to the extended or hyperextended position will cause pain and increase the muscle spasm in the hamstrings.

An acute synovitis of the knee joint will develop slowly over a period of a few hours (see p. 176).

TREATMENT

Once the knee has been unlocked it is then rested for at least 24 hours in a compression bandage or on a back-splint. Static quadriceps exercises are started quickly to restore the lost tone of the muscles and to help to control the effusion by their compression action. As soon as the acute inflammation has subsided, muscle and joint activity is gradually increased. Full power and function must be obtained before the patient is discharged.

If full range and power cannot be obtained it may indicate that a 'tag' of torn cartilåge is rolled back in the intercondylar notch, causing a strain on the anterior cruciate ligament when the knee is fully extended. This prevents the quadriceps muscles from performing their full action and the vastus medialis muscle will atrophy very quickly. If full flexion is not possible, this may indicate a posterior horn tear. These patients may well be ordered 'provocative exercises', i.e. exercises devised to reproduce similar strains to those which occurred at the time of the incident. These exercises are chosen to subject the knee joint to rotational stress with the knee in flexion and under load. Before these are given, it is important to explain to the patient the purpose of the exercises, otherwise if the knee does 'lock' and operation is decided upon, he may feel that the therapist was to blame. This could lead to a lack of confidence in the therapist's ability which would be detrimental at a later stage of rehabilitation.

AFTER MENISCECTOMY

The routine of postoperative treatment will depend on the surgeon. Usually the knee is supported in a compression bandage for at least a few days. Knee movements may be started on the second day, or not until the tenth day. The patient may be allowed to resume partial or complete weight-bearing at any time from a few days to 10 days postoperatively. However, before the patient is allowed to bear weight it is important that he has good control of his quadriceps muscles and can perform straight leg raising without a quadriceps lag. Progress is usually uneventful, with full power and range at six weeks. It is important to remind the patient that the power of the quadriceps must be maintained or further incidents may occur.

The degree and type of rehabilitation required will depend on the age, activity and occupation of the patient. Miners, and others who work in flexed positions, are particularly at risk and require a very strong knee before a return to work can be allowed. In sport a meniscus lesion is a hazard of footballers and others, and careful, graded training must be undertaken before the resumption of competitive sport. Circuit training is a useful method of developing strength and endurance (see p. 204).

DISLOCATIONS

Any joint may suffer a dislocation, that is one bone may be displaced out of its normal joint position. By their anatomical construction some joints are less stable than others and therefore dislocate more readily. This is especially true of the shoulder joint which has poorly adapted articular surfaces and no true ligaments to support the capsule. The hip joint, on the other hand, which is a similar type of joint, has deep acetabulum and strong ligaments and is not easily dislocated, except that a flexed hip dislocates relatively easily because the capsule is thin posteriorly and the head of the femur is not well supported in this position. This is an increasingly common injury in car accidents when the knee strikes the dashboard.

Categories of Dislocation

1. A complete dislocation when the dislocated bone is lying completely out of its normal position.
2. A subluxed, or partial, dislocation where the bone is out of its normal position but still in partial contact with the opposing joint surface.
3. A spontaneously reduced dislocation. This occurs when the bone has been dislocated momentarily and has sprung back into its normal position again.

When a joint is dislocated there must be soft tissue damage. The amount of this damage depends on two factors, the distance the bones have been separated and the structure of the joint involved.

For example, a shoulder joint which is not held rigidly by ligaments can, if the force is not too severe, be dislocated with a minimal stretching of the soft tissues, causing only slight damage. However, in a violent dislocation of the shoulder, when the humeral head is widely separated from the glenoid cavity, very severe soft tissue damage will be sustained. The capsule will be torn, ligaments stretched, even an avulsion fracture of the greater tuberosity may occur. Blood vessels, nerves and cartilaginous structures may also be damaged.

CLINICAL PICTURE

The physiotherapist is not required to diagnose or reduce dislocations.

However, the abnormal anatomical appearance of the joint affected would make the diagnosis obvious to her. This is especially true of shoulder dislocations. A close appraisal of the shoulders will reveal a gap, perhaps masked by an effusion, where the head of the humerus ought to be. It is often easier to feel this rather than to observe it. Subluxations are not always easily identified without an X-ray. In the elderly, who have a weak musculature, the inability to move the shoulder is often incorrectly attributed to soft tissue damage, when in fact they have a subluxed joint. Redislocation or subluxation can easily occur in these elderly patients and it is important for the physiotherapist to check for any malalignment each time the patient attends for treatment, especially in the first 10 days.

Effusion into and around the joint will always be present immediately after reduction.

There will also be some warmth, indicating the inflamed state of the joint. These two signs will vary according to the amount of soft tissue damage and are a very rough guide to the time that recovery is likely to take.

TREATMENT

The immediate treatment for completely dislocated or subluxed joints is reduction to replace the bone into its normal position. The quicker this can be done the less the signs of damage will be, as the soft tissues are no longer stretched. A finger joint that is dislocated and reduced within minutes of the injury will only be slightly swollen and tender for a day or two, but if it is left dislocated and the patient makes his way to hospital for a reduction, perhaps with a time lag of over an hour, then the finger will be very swollen and painful for perhaps as long as 10 days after the injury.

Obviously some joints cannot be reduced quickly. The reduction of the hip joint, for example, requires an anaesthetic to overcome the muscle spasm which follows the injury. It may be necessary to wait for several hours before it is safe to give the anaesthetic. The soft tissues around the joint which are being stretched while the joint is disorganised respond to this by pouring out exudate so that there is a large effusion and great pain on any movement, however slight.

The shoulder dislocation often happens on the sports field. 'Instant reduction' used to be carried out by another player but this practice has now been discontinued since a hastily performed reduction could well be a bad reduction, which caused more damage than the original injury. The availability of a 24-hour Accident and Emergency Service has made medical care readily available. Many of these patients have little pain or swelling after reduction.

The elderly person, who may fall at home onto the outstretched hand and dislocate his shoulder, may not realise what injury he has sustained. He is aware only that his shoulder is painful if he moves it. These people often wait to go to the doctor's surgery later in the day and from there to hospital. The delay before reduction may be many hours. By this time there will be a gross effusion and full recovery of function is often delayed by weeks.

Movement of the affected joint immediately after reduction is not advisable. However, it is important to ascertain that the joints adjacent to the injury move normally. Any lack of movement should be considered carefully to see if it might indicate a nerve injury – alteration of skin sensation would also indicate this.

Immediately after reduction, i.e. on the day of the injury, there should not be any alteration in the skin colour distal to the injury. If there is any, a check should be made of the pulses to ascertain if the blood vessels are damaged. If there is any doubt medical advice must be sought at once.

Movement should be encouraged the following day. Any gross effusion, or complications such as nerve involvement, will be treated as for any other similar lesion. Except for the elderly, or patients with severe injury, physiotherapy is seldom needed for more than a few days. Ice therapy and P.N.F. are the most effective aids for regaining normal movements. The only complication that might occur is the formation of adhesions due to lack of full range movements.

INTERVERTEBRAL DISC LESIONS

The term 'disc lesion' is used to describe the effects of degeneration, rupture, 'slipping' or bulging of the disc as well as nerve root pain. Intervertebral discs are firmly attached to the surfaces of the bodies of the vertebrae above and below them, as well as to the anterior and posterior longitudinal ligaments. They are shaped to fit the opposing vertebrae and consist of an outer annulus and an inner nucleus. The annulus is made up of concentric lamellae, the outer layers of which are primarily fibrous and the inner ones fibrocartilaginous. The fibres of the annulus interlace with each other and resist the forces of rotation. The nucleus pulposus is placed nearer to the back than the front of the disc. It changes in structure from a soft mucoid gelatinous substance in the first decade of life to a soft fibrocartilage in later years; this is difficult to distinguish from the annulus.

The depth of the disc in comparison to the depth of the adjacent vertebrae determines the amount of movement possible between the segments. This vertebral body/disc ratio is greatest in the cervical region and least in the thoracic.

In the young adult the discs are so strong that it is more likely, when violence is applied to the spine, for the vertebra to be affected than for a healthy disc to be damaged.

The ageing process, coupled with wear and tear occasioned by movement (maximal in the cervical and lumbar regions), causes the rupture of some of the fibres of the annulus, and when this has occurred the disc can become internally or externally displaced. Since the annulus is weaker in construction posterolaterally, this is the usual area to show the first signs of degeneration.

The shape of the disc contributes to the curvature of the spine. The lumbar and cervical curves develop as secondary curves and are therefore convex forwards. To allow for this the discs in these regions are wedge-shaped, thicker in front than behind. Flexion compresses the anterior surface of the disc. This will tend to cause further backward displacement of nuclear material through the cracked fibres of the annulus where the structure has been previously weakened. This can lead to a posterior protrusion of the disc into the vertebral canal.

In the lumbar region there is extra compression on the discs because of the greater body weight transmitted through them and because the vertebral body/disc ratio is less. These factors, together with the shape of the disc and amount of movement of the spine, tend to make a disc lesion more common in this region. External protrusion often creates pressure on the nerve roots giving rise to radicular pain. If the nucleus pulposus becomes internally deranged, it will give rise to the acute muscle spasm (without radicular pain) of 'lumbago'. These changes are usually gradual, occurring over a period of years, minor trauma giving only minimal physical signs or symptoms. Ultimately a relatively trivial incident causes the final trauma which produces the 'acute' disc lesion.

In the cervical region, the degeneration of age and 'wear and tear', coupled with its extreme mobility, may also cause adhesions to form between nerve roots and their sheaths. Any excessive flexion therefore, stretches the adhesions and an inflammatory state is created, giving rise to radicular pain, even without disc protrusion. In addition the normal compression force of gravity upon the discs is increased by muscle tension. This is why neck pain is often aggravated by mental tension which tends to be manifested as abnormal hypertonia in the muscles of the neck, particularly longissimus cervicis and capitis and the trapezius muscles. This increases the pressure on the discs and tends to restrict the normal blood flow.

The lumbar region is repeatedly subjected to stress, especially during forward flexion. As the discs degenerate and become less elastic they also become somewhat flattened and thinner. This creates a small amount of laxity in the capsules and ligaments of the intervertebral joints. The natural angle of inclination between L4 and L5 and at the lumbosacral junction makes them particularly liable to a shearing stress, thus increasing the 'wear and tear' on these discs. The relative 'slackness' of these joints in middle age makes them particularly liable to disc protrusion.

Acute Intervertebral Disc Lesion

A middle-aged man tried to lift a weight which was too heavy for him, from the factory floor when in the 'stooped' position, that is, flexed with his legs straight. This resulted in right postero-lateral herniation of the disc between the fourth and fifth lumbar vertebrae, which gave rise to the irritation of the right fifth lumbar nerve root. Since this root forms part of the right sciatic nerve, this will also be affected.

CLINICAL PICTURE

The patient will probably arrive at the hospital on a stretcher. While his pain makes him think he cannot stand, it is unlikely to be true.

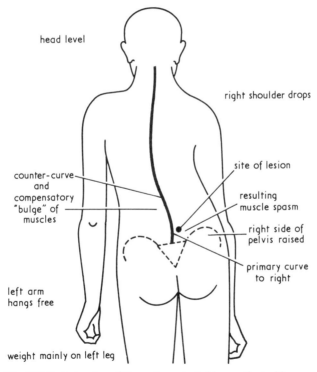

head level

right shoulder drops

site of lesion

counter-curve and compensatory "bulge" of muscles

resulting muscle spasm

right side of pelvis raised

primary curve to right

left arm hangs free

weight mainly on left leg

Fig. 10/1 Posterior view of the posture adopted by a patient with a right-sided nerve irritation from a postero-lateral disc herniation, between C4 and C5

When standing it will be seen that his lumbar curve is 'flattened', which is the result of protective spasm preventing forward flexion of the lumbar spine. The erector spinae muscles on the right immediately adjacent to the lesion will be in very severe spasm causing the pelvis to be raised on the right (Fig. 10/1). At about the level of L1 there is the beginning of a counter-curve to the left, making a very marked scoliosis. There may be a rotation of the lumbar vertebrae as a result of these abnormally violent muscle actions. The widespread protective spasm of the upper left lumbar muscles can be so great as to create a 'bulge' which, at first glance, may well be thought to indicate an injury in this area. This curvature is further exaggerated if forward flexion is attempted, and the left shoulder and arm will be seen to be in a line further to the left than the left hip. Tenderness is usually diffuse in the first few hours, but careful palpation will elicit an acutely tender area over the lesion. Pain will be generalised in the back and radiate down the leg following the pattern of the fifth lumbar dermatome (see p. 327).

IMMEDIATE TREATMENT

Complete bed rest is essential for the true disc protrusion. Every means to reduce the muscle spasm should be used, e.g. analgesics, ultrasound therapy and possibly even continuous traction. It is maintained until the patient has a passive pain-free straight leg raise to 60°, which indicates a healing of the annulus.

CONSERVATIVE TREATMENT

If after bed rest, etc., the muscle spasm is greatly reduced, then a graduated scheme of activity is introduced. Isometric exercises for power and endurance are given to the back extensor and abdominal muscles. Mobility exercises may be started only when the signs of nerve root irritation have subsided. Sometimes a plaster corset may be applied; this is only meant to inhibit forward flexion of the lumbar spine. Therefore extension exercises should be given, and the progression is similar to that for the surgical patient.

Surgical Treatment

LAMINECTOMY

If the signs and symptoms persist, after suitable investigation, it may be decided to perform a laminectomy. After this operation isometric back extension and abdominal exercises are usually started within a few days. These exercises are progressed both in duration and resistance. Whether forward flexion exercises are ever given depends on the surgeon. Many feel a fully mobile spine is essential if further back pain is to be avoided (see also p. 343).

ADVICE TO PATIENTS

All patients who have had disc lesions should be advised by the therapist concerning the following:

● Correct methods of lifting
● Care in activities which require sudden muscular contraction, e.g. removing a heavy object from a high shelf
● Awareness of the importance of good posture in sitting, e.g. selection of a chair which fits the patient
● Need for good muscle tone of both back extensor and abdominal muscles.

PROGNOSIS

This is very dependent on the patient's attitude to his injury. To many people a back injury remains a psychological barrier to activity for the rest of their lives. In fact 'backs' are one of the chief causes for work loss in this country.

REFERENCE

Williams, J. G. P. and Sperryn, P. N. (Jt. eds) (1976). *Sports Medicine*, 2nd edition. Edward Arnold.

BIBLIOGRAPHY

See end of Chapter II.

Chapter II

The Physiotherapist's Approach to Athletic and Sports Injuries

by M. K. PATRICK, o.b.e., m.c.s.p.

The 'athlete' has a different approach to his injury than almost any other patient who comes for physiotherapy. The injury is often a soft tissue lesion requiring similar treatment to the same lesion in a 'non-athlete', but the person is different, because for years he has devoted himself to this particular sport, often with great dedication, to the exclusion of almost everything else. His personal state of fitness is something of which an athlete is always aware and strives to improve. If he stops training following an injury, he soon feels generally unwell and becomes depressed about himself and his capabilities. When he is injured he is apprehensive about his injury and the effect it will have upon his future performance. It may be easy to think of him, mistakenly, as a hypochondriac.

The athlete also has a special problem in relation to his return to his particular sport, where individual performance will be noted to the inch, or the tenth of a second of time. The footballer or cricketer returning to a team does not have this extra worry. It is possible for him to resume his sport while not at the peak of his fitness as his first appearance will be in association with other players. The mental strain is therefore less for him and it should be possible to get such a player back to his team more quickly.

Causes of Injury

The injuries that these athletes and sportsmen suffer fall into two main categories, those with a known cause and those with no definite cause.

INJURIES WITH A KNOWN CAUSE

These are more obvious, because the patient has fallen or been struck by a missile, like a cricket ball. In some sports there may be a sudden violent physical contact with another player, such as occurs in football. The resultant injury is likely to recur, or at least, it is not possible for the physiotherapist to ensure that it does not do so. It is, in fact, the result of a hazard rather than a stress of sport. These are not situations which the sportsman can train himself to avoid completely. Naturally, training will include sharpening the performer's reflexes so that the injury can be minimised wherever possible. The injuries that result from these hazards of sport vary from the trivial to a major lesion.

INJURIES WITHOUT A KNOWN CAUSE

These injuries often appear to occur at a particular moment, but are really the result of a number of minor lesions which have been disregarded. Most athletes suffer some pain or discomfort while performing. It is often the ability to perform in spite of the pain which distinguishes the champion from the 'also ran' performer. No athlete will readily admit that he is injured and he will always hope that the pain will wear off in a few days. This means that these patients will often present themselves at a hospital when the lesion is no longer really acute. From the physiotherapist's point of view, this is a disadvantage as so often treatment given at the time of the injury would have resolved the condition, whereas a week or more after the lesion, definite changes are occurring which may be difficult to reverse.

The lesion is often due to a fault in the athlete's technique which is causing repeated minor traumata resulting in a chronic irritation of soft tissues. Muscle groups act and react in patterns of movement which normally cause no stress. If, however, the performer fails to 'carry through' the movement and performs a 'snatch-like' action, then there is considerable strain on the muscles. This is particularly true of the pain which occurs at the origin of the flexor and extensor groups of muscles in the forearm. Tennis or badminton players, javelin throwers and golfers often suffer from a chronic inflammation of the appropriate group of muscles at the elbow.

Each sport has its own pattern of movement, and therefore its own pattern of stress on the soft tissues of the body. The object of training for a sport is to build up the power and endurance of muscles so that they may perform an action repeatedly without suffering any strain. The joints must become supple but remain well controlled, if ligaments are not to be damaged. Theoretically, it would seem possible to train to a point of perfection where no stress injury could occur. In fact this is not possible, as an athlete does not train to produce a rhythmical performance. He trains to get to his 'personal best', which is a combination of technique and endurance. In competition, he will often have to force himself on to do more than the 'best' for which he has trained.

Approach to Treatment

Each sport or athletic activity can provide lesions which are predictable, since they are the direct result of the pattern of stress created by the action performed. While some of these are very obvious, others are not. Any physiotherapist who intends to become seriously involved in the treatment of athletic or sports injuries, should make a careful study of the mechanics of the sport. She should also watch the sport carefully to become familiar with its hazards and to observe the mental and physical stresses of the players under competitive conditions.

All physiotherapists are well aware that they treat the patient, not the lesion. Their technique and approach has to vary with the patient's age, fitness, and mental state. It has already been stressed that the trained athlete has a particular mental approach to injury. Consequently, he needs attention paid to three aspects of his treatment: resolution of the effects of trauma; retraining in strength and endurance; and regaining of confidence in his affected limb, and its fitness for activity. When he has achieved this, he will be able to retrain for his particular sport.

Although the diagnosis will have been made before the patient is referred for treatment, the actual method of treatment used will have to be determined by the physiotherapist. In addition to the usual appraisal of the signs and symptoms, there should be a discussion with the patient as to how and when the injury occurred and which sport was involved. It may not be possible for the patient to give a particular incident as the cause of the trauma, but the athlete is so aware of his body's performance that he will know how he thinks the stress occurred.

In the first few days although the treatment will be directed primarily at resolving the acute soft tissue lesion (see Chapters 9 and 10) the athlete's general physical state must not be ignored. Usually the injury, unless it was the result of a hazard, involves the part of the body used most in the sport and therefore normal training has to be discontinued. It follows, therefore, that a general scheme of exercises must be devised to keep the athlete in as near peak condition as possible. The best way to do this is by circuit training.

Circuit training is a familiar part of almost every athlete and sportsman's normal training schedule. It remains only for the physiotherapist to discuss with the patient what exercises his normal circuit contains and to adjust these to avoid damage to the affected area.

Circuit training is a part of the normal way of life of an athlete and does not require to be performed in a hospital. While the patient is having daily treatment for his acute lesion one session of circuit training can with advantage be performed there. This gives the physiotherapist the opportunity to check that the 'circuit' is safe. Later, when it is desirable to increase the muscle activity of the affected limb, the circuit is adjusted. Both the power and endurance of muscles are built up in circuit training, and so the athlete can see for himself that the injury which stopped him performing is really 'cured' and his confidence in his limb and his own ability to perform are restored.

It has been found that many athletes who have had a history of repeated small incidents of pain in a particular muscle or tendon are reassured if it is suggested to them, at the time of discharge from the hospital, that they might like to come for 'checks' from time to time. It is implied that it is the 'circuit' that is to be checked, but both the physiotherapist and the athlete know that this gives a reason for the athlete to return if he is worried about his old injury. This prevents a chronic state occurring, because the sportsman would be unlikely to make a formal appointment with a doctor to discuss a vague pain. The physiotherapist would of course seek medical advice for the patient if it was required. A further advantage is the prevention of more serious trauma, since it is a well-established fact that a sportsman who is unsure of his physical fitness is 'accident-prone'. His concentration is diverted to thinking about himself instead of the action he requires to make.

BIBLIOGRAPHY

Dyson, G. H. G. (1977). *The Mechanics of Athletics*, 7th edition. Hodder and Stoughton.
Morgan, R. E. and Adamson, G. T. (1961). *Circuit Training*, 2nd edition. G. Ball and Sons.
Williams, J. G. P. and Sperryn, P. N. (Jt. eds. 1976). *Sports Medicine*, 2nd edition. Edward Arnold.
Williams, John (1978). *Injury in Sport*. Bayer, U.K. Ltd. Pharmaceutical Division. (Free of charge.)

Chapter 12

Multiple Injuries

by M. K. PATRICK, O.B.E., M.C.S.P.

Road traffic accidents are producing many more patients with major multiple injuries. Due to the better understanding of the problems of immediate aid, more of these patients are surviving. While it is estimated that 80 per cent of the patients who sustain a traumatic rupture of the thoracic aorta die before or soon after admission to hospital, it is rare for accident patients to die of exsanguination (Porter, 1972). While head and chest injuries are the major problems for the physiotherapist, the internal abdominal injuries, such as ruptures of the spleen, liver or kidneys may be of greater importance when the patient is first admitted. After the surgeon's immediate care, whatever the extent or multiplicity of the injuries that the patient has sustained, the care of the chest must be the first consideration of the physiotherapist. To enable this to be carried out efficiently, the patient's position must be changed frequently. Many trauma surgeons will carry out lengthy surgery to obtain fixation of the fractured limbs so that the patient can be turned.

Chest Injury

Fractures in the chest wall can vary in severity from a fracture of one rib, which will cause little trouble in a young man, to multiple fractures of ribs leading to a completely flail chest wall, but a single broken rib in a patient who has acute bronchitis is a severe complication and he may well be admitted to hospital for intensive chest physiotherapy.

Physiotherapy for patients with fractures of the chest wall can present many problems. Fractures of the ribs are very painful and it is important that the patient with even the most trivial rib fracture is given analgesics. Unless the pain is controlled the pulmonary ventilation will be decreased. This can lead to an alteration in pulmonary ventilation rate (increased speed, decreased depth of respiration). As hypercapnia may ensue, the physiotherapist must understand the significance of the measurements of blood gases as well as the techniques of chest physiotherapy. There is a natural reluctance to give any percussion to an already crushed chest and indeed it would be wrong to do so in severe injuries. To feel the fractured bone ends grinding against each other is a distressing and worrying experience to the physiotherapist who is not familiar with this type of injury. If the patient is unconscious, pain is not a problem, but this also means that the greatest care must be taken while treating the patient as the lung can be lacerated by the bone ends.

A patient with chest injury must have his airway kept clear and good ventilation of his lungs. How this is achieved depends on the severity of the injury and the general state of health of the patient. Most of these patients will be conscious and many will be unable or unwilling to cough. Adequate analgesics must be given to reduce the pain and in many instances it is better to arrange for this to be given in anticipation of the physiotherapist's visit. Support at the site of the fracture, by the physiotherapist's hands, will greatly help the patient to co-operate in coughing. If the patient is unable to cough a suction catheter will often stimulate the cough reflex, and the fracture site should be supported in anticipation of this coughing.

The flail chest is caused by double fractures of the same ribs, and is now very common, often caused by violent impaction with the steering-wheel of a car. Paradoxical breathing (that is, the flail section is blown out on expiration and sucked in on inspiration) is often a feature of such injuries. This paradoxical breathing has a neutralising effect on the lung ventilation and atelectasis quickly develops. The airway must be kept clear, especially in the unconscious patient. After blood or air in the pleural cavity has been drained, some form of fixation of the flail chest is essential. This can be done by plating or wiring of the ribs so that the thorax can move normally in respiration, or by giving positive pressure ventilation through an endotracheal tube, thus ensuring that the pressure of the lung tissue supports the fractured ribs from within. It is reasonable to assume that at least 10 days are required for some union of the fractured ribs to take place. The endotracheal tube can be left in situ for up to 14 days, and this would seem to be the easiest method of support. It is the most commonly used form of treatment, but it has its own complications and dangers. Cross-infection and tracheal stenosis cause a significant morbidity, if not mortality rate (Porter, 1972). Some cardiothoracic surgeons advocate that surgical fixation of the seriously damaged chest wall should be undertaken at a relatively early stage, since prolonged artificial ventilation is not desirable. If the clavicle is fractured as well as the upper ribs, it must be surgically reduced and fixed or a permanent deformity and limitation of chest movement will result.

The techniques that the therapist uses for these seriously ill patients are largely determined by the particular injury. It may only be possible, in the early stages, to assist the lung drainage by the position of the patient and use of the suction catheter to clear the airways. More active percussion may be necessary later. The patient will be gradually weaned off the respirator as soon as he has adequate pulmonary ventilation without assistance (Brown, 1979).

Head Injury

Head injuries are now recorded at the rate of 100 000 a year. Fortunately most are relatively trivial and leave no disability. However, 60 per cent of road accident deaths are the result of head injuries (Proctor and Lockhart, 1972). Of those that survive, about 1 000 a year are left with severe disablement which may be physical, intellectual, emotional or a combination of any of these. Ethically this is a very real problem to all members of the staff who are involved with these patients. While the ultimate decisions are made by the medical staff, many physiotherapists are deeply concerned with their part in keeping patients alive when they have already suffered cerebral death. This may have occurred as a result of the anoxia which develops when there is intracranial damage.

Initially the physiotherapist is concerned with keeping the chest functioning effectively. Often the patient is restless, even violent, when unconscious. Suitable medication helps to reduce this. Later, when the patient's level of consciousness is rising, it is often very difficult to carry out chest physiotherapy, as the patient will attempt to get out of bed or to clutch at anyone who touches him. It is usual for these patients to be nursed in an intensive therapy unit where the staff ratio is higher than in normal wards, so that nursing staff can help to control the flailing limbs and the more violent activities of the patient while the physiotherapist ventilates the chest. Later the patient suffers disorientation and confusion and may well be very uncooperative. Fortunately, these two stages usually pass off relatively quickly.

When the patient recovers consciousness he may be partially paralysed and unable to speak. Then follows a time when he suffers great changes of mood and frustration, and the physiotherapist, together with her colleagues, starts the often prolonged rehabilitation of the patient as a 'whole being'. Often there is so much intellectual damage that rehabilitation is greatly hampered. Regrettably, those who do overcome great physical disability are often unable to find employment. However, centres for these patients are now operating, such as that in Birmingham, and show that, given a slow introduction to the factory situation, some can re-establish their confidence and are capable of normal work. All too many head injury patients spend the rest of their lives in mental, geriatric or younger chronic sick institutions. Renfrew (1977) discusses the physiotherapy for these patients.

Stab Wounds

Stab wounds are becoming more common in many of our cities. These, too, are now so much better understood that they present less of a problem to the surgeon (Porter, 1972). To the physiotherapist they are post-multiple surgery patients. Many of these stab wounds are into the chest and the principal treatment is chest ventilation.

Burns

Burns may also be a feature of multiple injuries and Boardman and Walker (1979) discuss the role of the physiotherapist in the treatment of burns. The surgical methods of treating these have greatly reduced the scarring which was the cause of so many contractures in the past.

Whatever the extent of the injuries, chest ventilation is the first priority of the physiotherapist, and later, when survival is assured, the rest of the patient's injuries are treated by the appropriate methods.

REFERENCES

Boardman, S. and Walker, P. M. (1979). *Burns*. Chapter included in *Cash's Textbook of Medical Conditions for Physiotherapists*. 6th edition. (Ed. Downie, P. A.) Faber and Faber.

Brown, S. E. (1979). *Intensive Care*. Chapters included in *Cash's Textbook of Chest, Heart and Vascular Disorders for Physiotherapists*. 2nd edition. (Ed. Downie, P. A.) Faber and Faber.

Porter, N. F. (1972). 'Advances in the Care of the Injured'. *The Practitioner*, **1252**, 209.

Proctor, H. and Lockhart, P. (1970). '*Head Injuries: problems of the crippled survivors*'. Chapter included in *Modern Trends in Accident Surgery and Medicine*. (Ed. London, P. S.) Butterworths.

Renfrew, E. L. (1977). *Head Injuries*. Chapter included in *Neurology for Physiotherapists*. 2nd edition. (Ed. Cash, J. E.) Faber and Faber.

Chapter 13

Fractures

by M. K. PATRICK, o.b.e., m.c.s.p.

A fracture is a break in the continuity of bone. Most fractures occur as a result of violence.

Classification

Fractures are classified according to the pattern of the resulting bone damage. Most of the terms are self-explanatory, such as impacted (when the broken bone ends are rammed together after the fracture has occurred), and spiral or oblique (which indicate the direction of the fracture line). Some fractures involve joint surfaces or are associated with dislocations, or produce the avulsion of a piece of bone when a tendon is violently stressed.

The comminuted fracture is one in which the bone is fragmented into several pieces (Plate 13/1). Children have more pliable bones and sustain greenstick fractures, which are similar to the break that would occur if a green stick were bent.

Fractures are described as simple or closed if the skin is not broken. If the skin is broken, then they are called compound or open fractures and can be complicated by infection of the soft tissues or bone ends. This may occur at the time of the accident or afterwards. The skin may be broken either by an object penetrating the skin from without, or by a spike of the fractured bone protruding through it.

COMMON FRACTURES

Causes

The vast majority of fractures are sustained as a result of direct or indirect violence. It is the stresses applied to the limb at the moment of impact that determine which bone, or bones, fracture and this may not be at the point of impact.

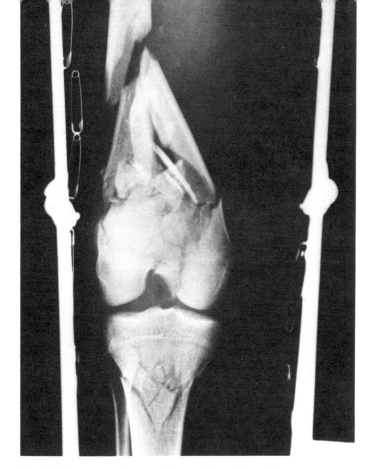
Plate 13/1 Comminuted fracture of upper tibia and lower femur

DIRECT VIOLENCE

This may occur when a limb strikes an object and fractures. This often occurs in road accidents when the occupant of the vehicle either strikes a part of the structure of the car, or is thrown out and strikes another object.

The limb may be struck by an object as happens when a footballer is kicked and sustains a fracture.

There may be a crush injury such as a finger being caught in a closing door, or the calcanei may be crushed by jumping, or falling from a height onto one's heels.

INDIRECT VIOLENCE

A fall onto the outstretched hand accounts for most fractures of the upper arm.

Fatigue or stress fractures occur, as their name suggests, as a result of repeated stress. The 'march fracture', so called because it was frequent among army recruits, is the most common. It involves a fracture of the shaft or neck of the second or third metatarsal bone. Athletes who run on hard tracks or roads can sustain stress fractures of the fibula or tibia, but these are comparatively rare.

PATHOLOGICAL FRACTURES

These fractures can occur in any age-group. While the fracture may occur as a result of minor trauma, the predisposition of the bone to give way under stress has been a gradual process of change in the structure of the bone, occurring over many months or even years. The patient may give a history of having stumbled and broken his leg. He attributes the fracture to the stumble, but it must be remembered that a bone with advanced changes in its structure could easily have fractured while the patient was asleep in bed.

The treatment for these patients will depend on the cause of the change in bone pathology. In the young it can be due to a cyst or benign tumour, but in the older age-groups it is frequently a systemic condition such as a lack of calcium ions ensuing from a nutritional or hormonal disturbance, or Paget's disease. The possibility of a malignant tumour must also be considered. If the disease is systemic, other fractures may be sustained and the physiotherapist must be very careful in the re-education programme, which should be slower than normal, as re-fracture is not uncommon.

It must always be remembered that soft tissues will be damaged in all fractures. The site of the soft tissue damage may be well away from the site of the fracture as well as immediately adjacent to it. This is particularly so in the case of indirect violence, for example a fall on the outstretched hand can result in a fracture at the wrist and damage to the soft tissue around the shoulder joint.

Signs and Symptoms of Fractures

Immediately after a fracture there is pain and muscle spasm. There will also be a degree of swelling and heat which varies with the way the fracture occurred and with the soft tissue damage which has been sustained. For example, if an object strikes the thigh with sufficient force to fracture the shaft of the femur, there will be a severe contusion on the aspect which was struck, plus soft tissue damage on the opposite aspect where the periosteum is torn and the bone ends project into the muscles. The thigh muscles are very vascular and so the resulting haematoma will be considerable and the area will be hot as well as swollen.

If, however, the fracture is an undisplaced one of the scaphoid, caused by falling on an outstretched hand, while there will be pain and tenderness at the fracture site, there will be minimal, if any, visible swelling. The soft tissue contusion on the palm of the hand, where it struck the ground, would not normally be great, and the haemorrhage from the bone would be slight and contained within the periosteum.

Displacement, causing alteration in body contours, or the position or attitude of limbs, can be a very marked sign of a fracture. It is confirmed by X-ray evidence. When there is a fracture the bone ends must move, but they can return to their original position (undisplaced fracture), or be driven into each other (impacted fracture). More usually they are displaced. The degree of displacement depends on the number of muscles and their power and direction of pull on the bone fragments, as well as the degree and direction of the stress which caused the fracture. Usually this displacement has to be reduced in order to obtain normal, or as near normal as possible, re-alignment of the fragments. This is done because union will only occur if the fragments are in apposition and the limb can only be functional again if its architecture is correct. It must also be remembered that while jagged bone ends are protruding into soft tissues they can cause further damage, either by pressure or by laceration. This extra damage could involve not only the muscles, but blood vessels and nerves. It is for this reason that even the most seriously injured patient will have his fracture reduced as soon as the essential life-saving procedures have been carried out. Only when the fractures are securely held can the nursing and physiotherapy procedures needed by these patients be given safely and adequately.

Repair

The repair of the bone is similar to the repair of other connective tissues. It differs only in the activity of specialised cells which lay down new bone, and in the calcification of the matrix. The specialised bone-forming cells are derived from the periosteum and endosteum of the damaged area. Some reticulo-endothelial cells from the bone marrow also seem to have the ability to take on an osteogenic function. The type of activity of all these cells depends on the stimulus which is provided. Too much movement at the fracture site stimulates the production of fibrous tissue. For bone to be laid down, the fracture area must be relatively immobile.

STAGES OF FRACTURE REPAIR

The stages of fracture repair which will be considered are: 1. haematoma formation and organisation; 2. subperiosteal proliferation, procallus; 3. callus formation, woven bone; 4. consolidation, lamellar bone; and 5. remodelling.

It should be remembered that these stages fuse with each other, and that more than one stage may be going on at the same time in different parts of the fracture site.

HAEMATOMA FORMATION AND ORGANISATION

Bone is a highly vascular tissue. When cortical bone is broken, the vessels of the Haversian systems are ruptured, and a few millimetres of ischaemic bone will therefore die. This dead bone is gradually absorbed over a few days, leaving a gap between the cortical bone ends. Cancellous bone has a more open meshwork, and less necrosis occurs.

Between both types of bone, profuse bleeding occurs at the time of fracture, and a haematoma will form, which is usually contained by the periosteum. The haematoma forms the basis for the type of repair which would occur in any wound. New capillaries penetrate the haematoma, fibres are laid down and granulation tissue is thus formed. This should be regarded as a temporary repair process as the granulation tissue does not form the basis of the true bony repair.

SUBPERIOSTEAL PROLIFERATION – PROCALLUS

Simultaneously with the formation of granulation tissue (by the second or third day after the fracture), there is proliferation of cells in the area immediately adjacent to the damaged periosteum and endosteum. These cells may lay down primitive bone, or occasionally, small areas of cartilage. The combination of the subperiosteal collar thus formed and the soft granulation tissue makes a weak link between the broken bone ends. This is known as provisional callus, or procallus.

It is essential that the fracture site is protected from major stress at this time. The body is capable of this without assistance, by the interaction of the pain/muscle spasm cycle. Muscle spasm keeps the bone ends together until healing has occurred, and provided that there is good bony alignment, a reasonable result will be obtained. However, the certainty of good repair and maintained alignment, with pain relief, can be better obtained by the use of artificial aids such as plaster casts or internal fixation.

CALLUS FORMATION – WOVEN BONE

The area of activity of the cells which formed the subperiosteal collar gradually extends. Provided that the fracture site is kept relatively immobile, the cells lay down an osteoid material in a calcified matrix. The osteoid trabeculae show no particular pattern, hence the term 'woven bone'. When the woven bone extends between the bone ends and thus bridges the fracture site, it is visible on X-ray. This does not mean that the repair is strong enough to withstand the stress of weight-bearing or heavy activity, or that the woven bone extends fully through the area previously occupied by the haematoma. It will take time for this to occur. The granulation tissue is absorbed as the woven bone extends.

CONSOLIDATION – LAMELLAR BONE

The simultaneous activity of osteoblasts and osteoclasts gradually replaces the woven bone with lamellar bone. This is the type of bone which will withstand the strains and stresses of weight-bearing. The trabecular pattern is similar to that found in normal bone and has a 'ply' arrangement. When lamellar bone has been formed, full bony union is said to have occurred, and the fracture repair is complete.

REMODELLING

Although lamellar bone is strong, the appearance of the bone may be far from normal. Excess bone may be present at the fracture site, or the bone ends may have healed without perfect alignment. These imperfections are gradually adjusted, as the bone is constantly remodelled by continuous osteoblast and osteoclast activity.

GENERAL PRINCIPLES OF TREATMENT

Basically, all treatment is performed hoping for a complete recovery to normal function. It is the surgeon's hope that he can obtain and maintain perfect alignment of the fractured bone ends. The physiotherapist hopes for full range and power. Often the results that have to be accepted are less than this, not because of the failure or lack of skill, but because the two aims are not always compatible. It is, therefore, worth considering what is acceptable, and why.

Upper Limb

This is a non-weight-bearing limb, which needs range of movement and dexterity. Neither of these are of use if the nerve supply to the hand is absent, for the arm moves to allow the hand to act.

Some degree of loss of length of bones or deformity can be accepted, as long as the retained range is functionally useful. If immobilised for more than two or three weeks, both the shoulder and the elbow will develop soft tissue changes which result in permanent loss of range. In the over-60 age-group, these changes occur in a week, if there is soft tissue damage to the joint. Therefore, early movement takes precedence over the need for good bone alignment. The early rehabilitation programme is planned for range of movement and followed by a power-building programme.

Lower Limb

This is a weight-bearing limb. Any shortening or deformity which occurs will affect the gait and posture of the patient. Therefore, every effort is made to obtain and maintain correct bone alignment while union is taking place. In order to achieve this, it may be necessary to immobilise the limb in plaster for many months, and perhaps to adopt more than one procedure of treatment (e.g. a bone graft, or plating operation when union has failed to take place after the limb has been in plaster for several months). Long periods of immobilisation may well result in some permanent loss of joint range.

The primary aim of the rehabilitation programme after lower limb injury is controlled movement, since stability is of the greatest importance. The patient will soon learn to accommodate to any loss of joint range. A patient may have an arthrodesed hip or knee joint and is able to regain functional activity; but a patient who has a knee joint that does not fully extend is at a great disadvantage because the quadriceps cannot work efficiently.

In the ankle joint, loss of dorsiflexion can be accommodated by raising the heel of the shoe, or loss of plantar-flexion may be overcome by shortening the stride. The subtalar joint is usually painful if its range is not full. This patient finds himself unable to walk on any surface, other than a perfectly flat one, without great pain, and this may well be so intolerable that the joint has to be arthrodesed. This operation, while relieving the pain, leaves the patient with a severe disability, and such an altered gait pattern that a very careful and often prolonged rehabilitation programme has to be undertaken.

SUPPORTS FOR FRACTURES

These are not always necessary, but if they are used, they can be applied either externally or internally.

External

LARGE ARM SLINGS

Impacted fractures of the upper limb are often rested in a large arm sling. This may well be worn under the clothes for the first few days, but should not be retained there for longer than 7 to 10 days, because the shoulder joint, especially in the elderly, soon loses its range of movement.

The 'collar and cuff' is designed to provide a slight traction (the weight of the arm) on the shoulder joint while restricting the movement of the joint.

STRAPPING

Some fractures do not require reduction. For example, fractures of the outer toes will unite spontaneously. They are seldom grossly displaced and the tendons will support the fractures. They do not require any further support, but sometimes a collodion bandage is applied, more for the reassurance of the patient than any other reason. Fractures of the shaft of the middle phalanges of the fingers are similarly supported by the tendons. It is usual to apply two narrow bands of strapping, one distal and one proximal to the fracture, enclosing the finger next to the one injured, which is thus used for support.

Fractures of the distal phalanx are often displaced because of the muscular attachments. These are usually supported on the palmar aspect, on a small 38mm (1½in) gutter splint which is held in position by strapping. The advantage of this light support is that functional use of the limb can be resumed at once.

PLASTER CASTS

The majority of fractures are reduced and supported in a plaster cast. This cast is not meant to hold the fractured bone ends rigid. It would be impossible for the cast to do so because of the bulk of soft tissues between it and the bone. It is meant to support the limb and prevent gross displacement recurring as a result of severe muscle spasm or external force.

In order to give greater stability to the fracture the joints adjacent to it may be included. Indeed, it is said that the joints immediately above and below should be included, but frequently one of these may be excluded. For example, a forearm plaster for a Colles fracture does not normally include the elbow joint. If the elbow joint is not immobilised, some pronation and supination can take place. However, an elbow joint soon stiffens when it is immobilised. This could produce a major disability following a relatively trivial injury of the wrist which did not require perfect alignment for functional use.

The lower limb function is weight-bearing, and therefore good anatomical alignment is essential. For this reason, it is usual to treat severe fractures of the lower leg in a long plaster (groin to base of toes). This is retained at least until some union has taken place when the knee joint may be freed so that it can be mobilised.

THOMAS'S SPLINTS

It is sometimes necessary to give prolonged traction to a fracture, to reduce the overlapping bone ends and then to maintain them in apposition. For this technique, there are several types of frame. These splints can either be designed for the support of injuries to the upper leg, in which case they are full-length, and based on the principle of the Thomas's splint, or they are modified for the treatment of the lower leg – Braun's splints.

Internal Fixation

This term is used to describe the fixation of a fracture by an operative procedure in which a metal support is used. This may be a medullary nail, which is within the bone; or a plate, screws or wire bands applied to the bone. Some surgeons will not use internal fixation unless other non-operative procedures have failed, or there is some other over-riding reason. This is because of the hazards of the technique (e.g. bone sepsis, tissue/metal reactions, fatigue fractures of the metal, etc.). However, in recent years, many of the problems associated with internal fixation have been better understood, and overcome. The advocates of the Swiss A.O. technique of compression plating (Arbeitgemeinschaft für Osteosynthesefragen, Fig. 13/1) feel that compression is essential for the success of internal fixation.

ADVANTAGES OF INTERNAL FIXATION

Fractures with severe displacement may be very difficult to reduce without an open operation. To maintain the corrected position prolonged traction may be required, or it may be quite impossible without an operation and internal fixation. Unless the broken bone ends are kept in close proximity to each other no bony union can take place. The fixation does not of itself speed up the repair processes, but it does make it possible.

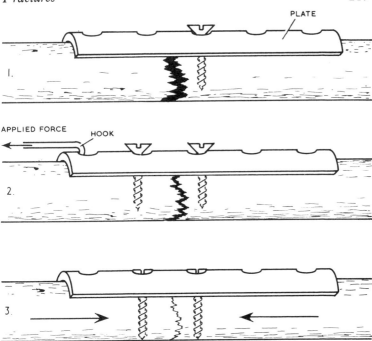

Fig. 13/1 Compression plating. 1. The first hole is drilled approximately 1cm from the fracture. The plate is applied and the screw inserted so that the head just touches the plate. 2. The fracture is then reduced accurately and the compression force applied. The second hole is drilled as far as possible from the fracture site through the next hole in the plate. 3. Pressure of the head of each of these screws against the flange of the hole will further compress the fractured fragments. (Further screws are then inserted into the remaining holes)

Another reason for internal fixation can be the desire to mobilise the patient quickly. This is especially true of the elderly patient with a fractured neck of femur, who could well become a chronic invalid if he were required to stay in bed for 12 weeks while his fracture united.

The Smith-Petersen pin for the fractured neck of femur was one of the first means of internal fixation to be universally adopted. A few weeks after the operation the patient was able to walk in a weight-relieving caliper. Over the years a great deal of progress has been made in improving operation techniques, and new metals have become available, so that today there are many different types of nails, pins, plates, screws and prostheses available to the surgeon as methods of internal fixation for many types of fracture.

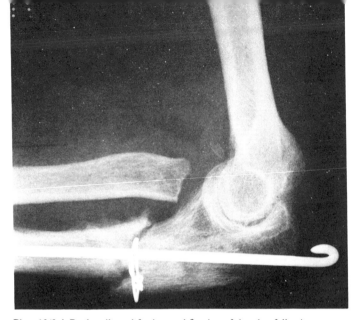

Plate 13/2 A Rush nail used for internal fixation of the ulna following a Monteggia's fracture of radius and ulna. The head of the radius has been excised

PLATING

If a plate is applied at once, there is a danger that a 'gap' might be created between the bone ends as reabsorption takes place. If this 'gap' becomes too wide, the periosteal and endosteal bone-forming cells (osteoblasts) will not be activated, and a fibrous union will be formed. For this reason, plating is usually delayed.

No plate, pin or screw is designed to take full weight-bearing until it is supported by a bony union. The purpose of the fixation is to try to maintain the proximity of the bone ends. After most of these operations, a plaster cast, or other support, is still required. In medullary nailing and A.O. compression plating, the limb is free for non-weight-bearing exercise.

MEDULLARY NAILS

The use of nails inserted into the medullary cavity to support fractures, especially spiral or comminuted fractures, was described by Rush in 1955 (Plate 13/2). These are often used in fractures of the humeral shaft, since they allow for careful early movement of the shoulder joint. They are used rarely for fractures of the femoral shaft, since they are not sufficiently rigid in the fixation. However, they are used in pairs, in tibial fractures, especially as a delayed procedure for fractures that do not seem to be uniting. A supporting plaster is usually applied.

Küntscher advocated a much stouter nail which gave greater rigidity. These are often used for middle-third fractures of the femur, especially if the patient is of slight build, because weight-bearing can be started as soon as the surgeon feels there is a bridging callus formation. There is a tendency for these patients, who are quite pain-free, to feel that the leg is normal and subject it to too much stress. Some surgeons, therefore, keep their patients on sticks longer than they appear to need them. Certainly, a small proportion of the patients who have these nails inserted have non-union, or refracture a few months later. This is thought by some to be due to the damage to the medullary circulation caused by the nail. The physiotherapist should watch for any loss of joint range or complaint of pain, as this is often a sign that excessive stress is being put upon the fracture site and that malunion is occurring.

INTERNAL FIXATION WITH COMPRESSION

In the Swiss A.O. method of fixation with compression, the operative procedure aims at an accurate alignment of the bone fragments with a rigid fixation of the fracture, at the same time preserving the vitality of the soft tissues and bone (Fig. 13/1). A few days after the operation, the patient is pain-free, and the limb has no external support, so that non-weight-bearing exercises can be started at once.

REPAIR OF BONE

When internal fixation with compression is used, there is a different process of repair, since there is no movement, and no space between the bone fragments. If the fixation is rigid so that shearing and torsional forces cannot act, no major reabsorption of the bone ends takes place. However, any minute bone fragments or spicules which are denuded of their blood supply will be quickly absorbed by the scavenger cells (osteoclasts). This takes place as the healing process is proceeding.

Any part of the periosteum which might be trapped between the bone ends and which is therefore subjected to compression will continue to form osteoblasts. That is, its osteogenic layer, in the presence of an adequate blood supply, will form bone cells. The fracture haematoma is reduced by the compression, but the blood supply of the bone ends is normally adequate for repair to take place.

The bony union that takes place shows no radiological evidence of callus. If there is such evidence, it indicates that the fixation has not been perfect and that some movement at the fracture site has taken place. The radiological evidence of union is the presence of trabeculae across the fracture line.

TREATMENT OF FRACTURES BY THE PHYSIOTHERAPIST

While some fractures are more commonly encountered than others, each of these will have variations which make the surgeon decide on a particular regime of treatment. Some will have been reduced, some supported in plaster or splints, others will be left free. These decisions will have been made before the patient is referred for therapy, and they will affect the treatment only in detail.

It is important to remember why the fracture is being treated. It is not to obtain perfect bone alignment which looks excellent on X-ray. It is to restore to the limb as full a function as possible. Often a compromise has to be reached and the best alignment that can be achieved without the risk of permanently affecting the range of movement of an adjacent joint has to be accepted.

Fractures that do not Require Major Support

Many of these fractures are of minor bones, or of ones which would lead to joint stiffness if immobilised.

A fracture remains a fracture until it is fully united, whether it is supported in a plaster cast or left free, and the physiotherapist must select suitable activity, at each stage. For example, a patient with a fractured metacarpal can reasonably be expected to try to grip a small ball on the day after his injury, but he should not be asked to carry and stack bricks. An elderly patient with an impacted fracture of the neck of the humerus will require assistance when asked to raise his arm in the early stages of rehabilitation.

It is important to apply common sense, as well as professional expertise, to the choice of activity. The degree of functional activity normal for the patient is the aim. By talking to the patient about his hobbies, mode of living, and work, the physiotherapist can ascertain the patient's normal use of his affected limb. The young man with fractured metacarpals, who is a bricklayer, requires mobility of movement rather than power. It is this mobility which he is likely to lose quickly and permanently if the rehabilitation programme is not planned properly.

Fractures in Plaster

When a patient with a fracture in plaster is referred to the physio-therapist for treatment, the rehabilitation programme should include maintenance of mobility of all joints which are not enclosed in plaster and isometric exercises for all muscle groups enclosed in the plaster.

After the plaster is removed, the regaining of lost joint movement and muscle power are the primary aims of treatment. It is in the first few days of this section of the rehabilitation programme that the physiotherapist must watch for signs of non-union. This shows as swelling, heat and tenderness and even reddening of the skin over the fractured area, indicating an acute inflammatory state. Normally a patient will attempt to move stiffened joints and resume normal function of the affected area with encouragement. If he does not, it is often a sign that union is not quite complete. During the first week after the plaster has been removed there is no long-term advantage in 'forcing on' with activity, rather it should be an attempt to get the patient to start using the limb normally, and once this is achieved mobility and strength quickly return.

Fractures of the Lower Limb Treated by Prolonged Traction (e.g. Thomas's splints)

The amount of exercise that can be given is limited by the fixation. If skin traction to the lower leg is the method used, then foot and ankle movements are given with especial care to watch for any paralysis due to pressure on the peroneal nerve, and for pressure sores over the tendo Achilles. Knee movements are often very delayed in this fixed traction technique and it is seldom used today. The disadvantage of the prolonged traction method is the stiffness of the knee, which may take as long as two years to recover full range.

More usually a Steinmann's pin is inserted through the tibial condyles and sliding traction is given by means of a stirrup. Foot and ankle movements and isometric contractions are given at once. Knee flexion, within the confines of the splint, is permitted as soon as clinical union has taken place.

A Braun frame is seldom used in this country for the treatment of fractures of the femur. However, it is used for fractures of the tibia, especially those which have had open surgery. It is used more as a resting splint than as a means of applying traction. The amount of physiotherapy that is given depends on the particular fracture being treated and on the method used.

Fractures Treated by Internal Fixation

Early activity is nearly always requested for patients who have had internal fixation applied. It must be remembered that no weight-bearing or resistance that could cause a strain on the plate, screws or pins is given until bony union is established.

Smith-Petersen pins and other devices to stabilise hip fractures, medullary nails and A.O. compression plates are all used to allow immediate freedom of movement. The exercises chosen are in keeping with the fracture and the musculature of the patient. The frail elderly patient who has had a hip fracture may need help to lift her leg for the first few days, whereas the young fit man should have sufficient muscle power to perform this action.

When plating (non-compression) is used, the limb is usually enclosed in a plaster cast until clinical union has taken place. These patients are given exercises as for any other patient in plaster.

Compression plating and screwing by the A.O. method allows immediate free movement of the limb. Even if the fracture goes into a joint, active movements should be given immediately. The limb is elevated for the first few days. A tibial fracture is often rested on a Braun's frame to allow the initial inflammation to subside. Localised treatment for this is seldom needed as the generalised activity of the limb enables the inflammation to resolve spontaneously and quickly.

This A.O. method of treating fractures of the tibia enables the patient to have full joint movement at all times. There is a special caliper that is used to allow early walking while preventing weight-bearing on the fracture site (Plate 13/3).

Once weight-bearing is allowed some care should be taken for the first few days. It must be remembered that the patient has been in no pain for some weeks and feels able to do everything. There will be no evidence of callus on the X-ray. It is the presence of trabeculae across the 'old fracture line' that will determine whether union has been consolidated, plus the absence of pain on 'springing' the fracture, or on palpation. The physiotherapist should watch the fracture area carefully for the first signs of non-union which can be the *first* sign of swelling, redness or tenderness and note the most casual remark about pain. To wait and see 'how it is tomorrow' can be too late, as 24 hours of activity can loosen the metal fixation. It is essential to report these signs at once to the surgeon. It is better to be proved incorrect in one's suspicions than to miss an ununited fracture. This is of course true of all fractures, not only those which have metal implants.

Disability of a Fracture

It is always important to remember that a limb in plaster makes normal living more difficult, and sometimes impossible. A frail elderly patient with a wrist in plaster may be living alone. She may be unable to undress or dress herself. Even moving a kettle of boiling water may be too heavy for her with one hand. Care must be taken to

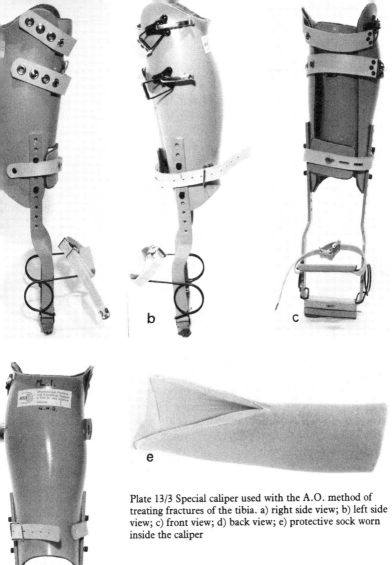

Plate 13/3 Special caliper used with the A.O. method of treating fractures of the tibia. a) right side view; b) left side view; c) front view; d) back view; e) protective sock worn inside the caliper

ensure that neighbours are asked to help, or the patient will soon show signs of debility from malnutrition and lack of personal care.

No elderly patient should ever be sent home non-weight-bearing on crutches or a frame, unless the home circumstances have been investigated to ensure that someone will call regularly to see that the patient is able to cope and has not fallen. It is worth remembering that many old people interpret 'non-weight-bearing' as meaning that they are simply not to walk on the limb. The writer has known many patients with hip fractures who thought doing housework on their knees was non-weight-bearing!

Progression of Treatment

This depends principally on the age of the patient. The elderly must be encouraged to keep their joints moving and, as far as the injury will allow, to keep 'on their feet'. Even a few weeks of bed rest will be disabling to them.

Children on the other hand will regain joint range and power with very little help, and even severe fractures with poor alignment will be remodelled, surprisingly well, in time. Young children should not normally be given regular treatment in a physiotherapy department. It is better to reassure and advise the parent and let the child make its own progress, with 'checks' at intervals. The biggest deterrent to this progress is an over-anxious parent, and at the 'check' visits it is often the parent who needs reassurance, rather than the child who needs physiotherapy.

Long-Term Care

When the patient has reasonable functional use of the limb and is confident in his ability, regular physiotherapy should be discontinued. The long-term recovery often takes many months, even a year for a major fracture. At this stage, the patient should be encouraged to take responsibility for his further progress. Normal use in daily living is all that should be needed to restore the part to full function. 'Check' appointments should be given so that the physiotherapist can be sure that progress is being made. Should it be found that the patient is losing range or power, an investigation as to the cause should be made, and perhaps a short, intensive course of treatment given.

REFERENCE

Rush, L. V. (1955). *An Atlas of Rush Nailing Techniques.* Meridian, Miss.

BIBLIOGRAPHY

Adams, J. C. (1978). *Outline of Fractures, including Joint Injuries*. 7th edition. Churchill Livingstone.
Apley, A. G. (1977). *A System of Orthopaedics and Fractures*. 5th edition. Butterworths.
Watson-Jones' Fractures and Joint Injuries. (Ed. Wilson, J. N.) (1976). 5th edition. Churchill Livingstone.

CHARTS OF COMMON FRACTURES

The following is a précis of the more common fractures that the physiotherapist can expect to see. When referring to this section, it is important to recall the previous detail that has been presented in the earlier chapters. For example, soft tissue damage will have occurred at the time of the fracture and may well influence the physiotherapy that is given, both in the early and late stages of rehabilitation.

Points to Bear in Mind when Reading the Charts

COLUMN 1

It is impossible to describe a typical fracture. The variations that can occur are legion.

COLUMN 2 USUAL AGE-GROUP

This is, as it says, an indication of the age-group which most frequently sustains this type of fracture. It must be remembered that almost any fracture can be sustained by a person of any age.

COLUMN 3 HOW INJURY OCCURS

This suggests the most usual but by no means the only way to sustain the fracture.

COLUMN 4 MOST USUAL METHOD OF FIXATION

The surgeon will consider many factors before selecting his method of treatment. While an internal fixation with a plate might be the choice for an adult, it would be unsuitable for a child, whose bones are still growing. One or two more common methods have been listed here for the guidance of the physiotherapist.

COLUMN 5 MOVEMENTS BEGUN

This is, of necessity, only a guide to the timing of progression. The surgeon will indicate his requirements, which will be based on local factors such as the general health of the patient, the degree of stability of the fracture, etc. The terms 'weight-bearing' and 'non-weight-bearing in plaster' indicate the time at which some weight can be expected to be taken on the limb.

Broad outlines only of treatment are given, and the reasons for them. It must be remembered that all injuries are different, as are the people that sustain them. The treatment must be given to meet the needs of the particular patient, *not* as they appear in any book.

Fractures   229

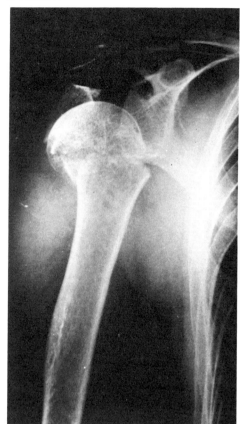

Plate 13/4 Impacted fracture
of neck of humerus

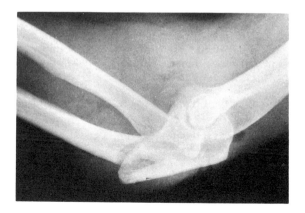

Plate 13/5 Monteggia's fracture of radius and ulna

FRACTURES OF THE SHOULDER REGION

Site	Usual age-group	How injury occurs	Most usual method of fixation
CLAVICLE – Outer third	Any	Fall on out-stretched hand	1. Sling for 10–14 days *or* 2. 'Figure of 8' bandages
SCAPULA – Glenoid – Neck – Acromion – Body	Adult	Direct blow or crush	Sling for a few days
HUMERUS – Gt tuberosity	} Adult	} Fall on out-stretched hand	Sling for a few days
– Gt tuberosity with dislocation of shoulder			
– Surgical neck (impacted) (Plate 13/4, p. 229)	Elderly		Sling for a few days
– Shaft	Adult	Direct blow	1. Operation. Rush nail and sling 3 weeks *or* 2. Guarding plaster 4–6 weeks

Notes

Normally an arm can move through an arc of 360°. This requires fr
movement of the shoulder joint and the shoulder girdle. With age th
range becomes slightly diminished. After injury it is very important
prevent further loss of this range, for it is difficult, if not impossible,
regain. Immediate, carefully assisted movements are therefore give
whenever possible.

Loss of range will reduce the functional use of the whole limb.

POWER
Full power can only be restored if the range is full. The easiest and safe
way to restore power is by normal usage.

COMPLICATIONS
Immediately after injury the only way a nerve lesion can be detected is t
loss or alteration in skin sensation. Blood vessel damage is observed
discolouration and swelling of fingers and hand. Test by pinching tips
the fingers and observing speed of blood return.

ovements begun	Complications	Results and comments
ımediately	—	Excellent. Large callus diminishes with time
ımediately	—	Excellent. Usually unites with fibrous tissue but this is not detrimental to function
ınmediately	—	Excellent in the younger age-groups
fter 24 hours	Axillary nerve lesion	The elderly nearly always lose range of shoulder movement
ımediate gentle ovements	—	Results vary. If the impaction leaves a poor bony architecture range may be very limited
ımediately avoiding tation ⎫ soon as practicable ⎭	Radial nerve or blood vessel damage	Good
		Stiff elbow and shoulder if patient is elderly

RACTURED CLAVICLE

his can be treated with a 'figure of 8' bandage; this does not support the acture. It can cause great discomfort in the axillae. It is used less often w. This fracture, if combined with a 'flail' chest lesion, is serious.

RACTURE DISLOCATION OF SHOULDER

his is a common injury in the elderly. Range must be maintained. This n be done if great care is taken to support the weight of the limb when the tient is performing movements. Axillary nerve lesion is fairly common. is not always easy to see whether deltoid muscle is working for several eeks, but the skin sensation of the C5 nerve will be altered. If the nerve is volved the need for maintaining the range of movement is still of the eatest importance. In most instances there is spontaneous recovery from e nerve compression.

RACTURED SHAFT OF HUMERUS

ood vessel damage is not common. If it occurs it is usually noted in the sualty department and dealt with there. Loss of extension of the wrist ay not be observed for a day or two after injury (radial nerve lesion).

FRACTURES OF THE ELBOW REGION

Site	Usual age-group	How injury occurs	Most usual method of fixation
SUPRA-CONDYLAR	Child	Fall	1. Collar and cuff 3 weeks *or* 2. Guarding plaster axilla to wrist 3 weeks
RADIUS – Head (undisplaced)	Any		Sling for a few days
– Head (with more than a third of articular surface involved)	Adult	Fall on out-stretched hand	Operation. Excision and sling 7–10 days
– Neck (undisplaced)			Sling for a few days
ULNA – Olecranon	Any	Forced flexion of the elbow Direct blow	1. Operation. Lag screw (compression) or wired and sling 3 weeks *or* 2. 3–4 weeks guarding plaster
– Monteggia's (fracture dislocation, upper third of ulna and dislocation of radius) (Plate 13/5, p. 229)	Adult	Direct blow (e.g. road traffic accident). Forced pronation	1. Operation. Ulna plated or nailed and wired or screwed (Plate 13/2, p. 220). Sling 3 weeks *or* 2. Axilla to metacarpal joint plaster 4–5 weeks

Notes
RANGE

Forearm rotation (Pro- and supination). The functional usefulness of t hand after an elbow injury is proportional to the degree of rotati regained. It is re-educated in functional activity only.

Flexion. The hand must reach the mouth; beyond this, flexion is n essential.

Extension. While full range movements are always the aim, an arm wi no extension beyond 90° can be functional, if the other movements a good.

Never attempt to increase the range by passive movements.

Movements begun	Complications	Results and comments
gentle activity when plaster or collar and cuff removed	Blood vessel or nerve lesion	Perfect in time, may take a year if damage has been severe
immediately		Full recovery
immediately gentle flexion/extension		90% of range recovered in middle-aged 75% of range recovered in the elderly
immediately	Radial nerve lesion (rare)	Good results
Elbow movements at 3-4 weeks (earlier for elderly patients)		Some range loss; often returns after use over some months
Elbow movements when plaster removed	Ulnar nerve lesion. Median nerve lesion (very rare)	Poor; now seldom used for adults because of joint stiffness
Elbow movements at 3 weeks		Results depend on post-reduction bone architecture
Elbow movements when plaster removed		Poor; seldom used, except for children, because of joint stiffness

POWER
Active use is the only safe way to increase the muscle power of an elbow. Any attempt to 'hurry' the recovery by weight-lifting, etc., will invariably result in loss of range and muscle spasm.

COMPLICATIONS
Blood vessel damage. While this is rare, it is extremely important to watch for signs in the first few days. A dead-white hand and forearm which is acutely tender must be reported at once. It could be a sign of Volkmann's ischaemia, which if dealt with immediately is reversible, but if delayed can result in permanent paralysis.

FRACTURES OF THE ELBOW REGION (CONTINUED)

A discoloured, swollen hand (venous congestion) must also be reported
It is usually caused by the plaster being too tight, or the deformity of th
limb impeding the venous return.

SOFT TISSUE DAMAGE
In elbow injuries this is often extensive, resulting in considerable swelling
In adults it tends to organise and give rise to permanent limitation of join
movements if it is not treated. Fortunately few elbow injuries of adult
need to be in plaster, so that ultrasound therapy can be given at once, eve
if movement is not permitted. Children are treated in plaster, sinc
operative procedures are avoided, but the stiffness resulting from the so
tissue damage is soon freed, once movement is allowed.

SUPRACONDYLAR FRACTURES
Either or both condyles can be fractured, causing considerable derange

FRACTURES OF THE FOREARM

Site	Usual age-group	How injury occurs	Most usual method of fixation
ULNA – Shaft	Any	Direct blow	1. Compression plating sling 3 weeks *or* 2. Plating and forearm plaster 4–6 weeks *or* 3. Axilla to metacarpophalangeal joint long plaster 6–8 weeks
RADIUS AND ULNA – Shafts	Any	Direct blow or fall	1. Compression plate to each bone and sling 4 weeks *or* 2. Plating of one or bot bones and plaster 4–6 weeks *or* 3. Axilla to metacarpal joint plaster 6–12 week (adult) 3–6 weeks (chilc

ment of the joint. This is primarily an injury of children. Swelling is considerable and a close watch must be kept to see that venous congestion does not occur and that the fingers are kept fully mobile. The immediate results are often not good but the bony architecture is improved in the later stages of bone repair and the range of movements improves as the deformity lessens.

FRACTURE OF HEAD OR NECK OF RADIUS
Early movement is essential for good results.

FRACTURED OLECRANON AND MONTEGGIA'S FRACTURE
In order to maintain the postoperative position movements cannot be given at once. When they are permitted remember to use triceps only 'smoothly' and gently until bony union has taken place, or the olecranon may be pulled off again.

Movements begun	Complications	Results and comments
Immediate gentle flexion of elbow Flexion and extension elbow 1–3 weeks Flexion and extension elbow when plaster removed	Non-union	Fairly good. Some loss of forearm rotation Poor, considerable loss of forearm rotation and some loss of flexion/extension of elbow. Improves over years in children. Seldom used for adults
Immediate gentle flexion and extension elbow	Non-union especially of ulna Non-union especially of ulna	Good results Fairly good if both bones are plated, some loss of forearm rotation
Immediately plaster removed gentle flexion and extension elbow	Cross-union	Poor, considerable loss of forearm rotation and flexion/extension. Improves over the years with children. Seldom used for adults

FRACTURES OF THE FOREARM (CONTINUED)

Notes

RANGE

Flexion and extension of the elbow and wrist are not affected unless the limb
is put into a long plaster. Usually only children are treated in plaster, since
operative procedures are avoided. These joints mobilise quite quickly.

Forearm rotations. These cannot be permitted until some bony union has
taken place. Rotations must be re-educated with great care, or non-union
or a re-fracture will occur. Usually these movements are only given as part
of a functional action.

POWER

This is quickly regained once firm union is established. The overall time
for complete rehabilitation is often shortened if 'strengthening exercises'
for the arm are delayed. The power of the hand in a 'gripping' action
should be encouraged from the beginning.

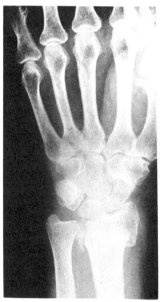

Plate 13/6 Colles' fracture. a)
Antero-posterior view; b) Lateral view

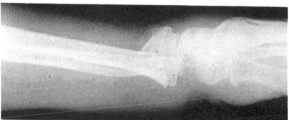

COMPLICATIONS
Blood vessels and nerves are sometimes damaged at the same time since these fractures are usually the result of direct blows and often occur in road traffic accidents. However, they are not complications in the normal sense of the word, in that they do not occur as a result of the fracture.

Non-union is the most likely complication, particularly of the ulna, which is slow to unite. Heat, swelling or tenderness over the fracture area or pain or sudden loss of forearm rotation should be regarded as possible indications of non-union or re-fracture.

PHYSIOTHERAPY
This must be directed towards encouraging use rather than attempting to 'hurry' recovery. These injuries are difficult to treat. Delaying movements may seem to be adding to joint stiffness, yet any attempt to force movements always meets with disaster.

Plate 13/7 Bennett's fracture of the first metacarpal

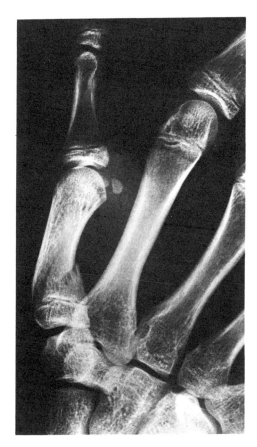

FRACTURES OF THE WRIST AND HAND

Site	Usual age-group	How injury occurs	Most usual method of fixation
RADIUS – lower end – Colles' (Plate 13/6, p. 236) – Smith's	Over-50	Fall on outstretched hand Blow on the back of the wrist	Short plaster 4–6 weeks (Colles' plaster) i.e. below elbow to knuckles with thumb free
SCAPHOID	Young adult males	Fall on outstretched hand	'Scaphoid' plaster 4–12 weeks (i.e. below elbow to knuckles with carpometacarpal joint of thumb enclosed)
METACARPALS	Young males	Direct blow (boxing)	1. None or strapping for a few days *or* 2. Colles' plaster 3 weeks
BENNETT'S 1st metacarpal (Plate 13/7, p. 237)	Any	Direct blow	1. Plaster for 4 weeks *or* 2. Operation, screwed or wired, plaster
PHALANGES	Any	Direct blow. Rotational strain	Girdle strapping 10–14 days (affected finger to next)

Notes

FUNCTION

Power and pincer-type grips are the primary functions of the hand. In order to perform these actions effectively, normal kinaesthetic sensation, good joint range and controlled muscle power are needed.

RANGE

The joints of the wrist and hand are a complex structure designed to perform very strong and very delicate movements. The actual range of movement of each joint varies with the individual, and comparison with the uninjured hand is the only guide to their normal range.

Since function is the essential feature of the hand, it is this, rather than particular joint range, which should be the aim. Shoulder movements should be carefully checked.

Movements begun	Complications	Results and comments
Use in plaster. Once plaster is removed all movements are given	Rupture of extensor pollicis longus. Causalgia (median nerve compression). Sudek's atrophy	Good function, but often considerable deformity. Contours improve with time
Use in plaster. Once plaster is removed all movements are given	Non-union. Necrosis, usually result of fracture not being immobilised immediately	90% unite, good results
Immediate use. Exercises when plaster removed		Loss of knuckle contours. Full function
Immediately after plaster removed		Risk of stiffness from plaster is great in elderly, therefore immediate use is sometimes ordered
Immediately. Normal use of hand		Function excellent. If articular surface is involved there will always be loss of joint range, which seldom impairs function

POWER
This is very important in the hand. All re-education should be designed towards power. Joint range is of no benefit if it is not controlled by strong muscle power.

COSMETIC APPEARANCE
This is often sacrificed in order to keep the functional range, e.g. fractured metacarpals usually result in the 'loss' of a knuckle because of a slight overlapping of the bone ends. To obtain a cosmetically perfect result would require an operative procedure which could result in a loss of metacarpophalangeal joint range.

FRACTURES OF THE WRIST AND HAND (CONTINUED)

COLLES' AND SMITH'S FRACTURES
A post-reduction 'slipping' of the bones often leads to a deformity, but this seldom interferes with function.

COMPLICATIONS
Late rupture of E.P.L. This is fairly common with elderly patients. It may happen at three weeks or three months after injury.

Causalgia. This is rare, and is caused by compression of median nerve Symptoms: hypersensitivity and exquisite pain, mainly over thenar eminence.

Sudek's atrophy. This is usually seen in patients who are fearfully unable or unwilling to use the hand. Clinically the hand is shiny, reddish in colour and swollen. X-rays show osteoporosis. It is almost impossible to regain

FRACTURES OF THE HIP AND THIGH

Site	Usual age-group	How injury occurs	Most usual method of fixation
UPPER FEMUR – Subcapital (intracapsular)	Elderly	Fall, quite often a minor one	1. Prosthesis *or* 2. Internal fixation
– Mid-cervical (intracapsular)	Elderly	Fall, quite often a minor one	Internal fixation – flanged pin or more usually a nail and plate
– Basal (intracapsular)	Elderly	Fall, quite often a minor one	
– Per-trochanteric (extra capsular)	Elderly	Fall	Internal fixation (nail and plate)
SHAFT	Young adult	Direct blow (e.g. road traffic accident)	1. Traction 3 months then caliper for 1 month *or* 2. Intramedullary nail or nails and plates or wires *or* 3. Plating and wire bands usually with groin to toe plaster *or* 4. Compression plating

movements if this syndrome has really become established, as the patient will seldom co-operate. It must be anticipated and prevented.

Persistent wrist pain (weeks after union) may be due to subluxation of radio-ulnar joint. Excision of distal portion of ulna may be necessary.

SCAPHOID FRACTURE
The application of a good plaster is essential. The thumb and index finger must oppose. Use of the hand in plaster is essential; very little physiotherapy is required.

COMPLICATION
Non-union occurs in less than 10 per cent of patients. Usually due to patient not reporting injury for several weeks. Early immobilisation is essential.

Movements begun	Complications	Results and comments
Immediately; partial weight-bearing 1 week to full weight-bearing	Avascular necrosis	Good if fixation holds and bony necrosis does not occur. The elderly may find non-weight-bearing difficult. Therefore weight-bearing may be allowed sooner than is desirable
Immediately; non-weight-bearing to full weight-bearing 10–12 weeks	Non-union	
	Avascular necrosis	
	Failure of fixation	
Immediately to foot; knee at 6–8 weeks; full weight-bearing 12–18 weeks	Non-union. Callus formation causing tethering of quadriceps	
Immediately; non-weight-bearing 2–3 weeks; full weight-bearing 10–12 weeks		Good results (if union achieved) in the young. Elderly patients may lose range in hip and knee
Dependent on external fixation; full weight-bearing at 12–16 weeks	Non-union Infection	
Immediately; non-weight-bearing 12–14 weeks		

FRACTURES OF THE HIP AND THIGH (CONTINUED)

Notes

UPPER FEMUR FRACTURES

These patients are usually elderly. Prolonged bed rest would often mean that the muscles atrophy and the joints stiffen. Generally their health would deteriorate. Therefore internal fixation is used. Early exercise and ambulation is encouraged.

RANGE

Usually these patients only want to be able to enjoy 'quiet' living, i.e. the ability to sit (90 per cent of hip flexion), to stand and walk (some extension of hip if possible), toileting (30 per cent abduction). A much greater range is desirable, but not essential.

POWER

Personal independence is only possible if the muscle power is sufficient to perform the action. Encouragement to keep practising sitting, standing or walking is very important. The quadriceps, hamstring and glutei muscle groups are the most important ones to maintain.

COMPLICATIONS

Intracapsular fractures. Avascular necrosis. In the elderly the blood supply to the head of the femur is mainly from the capsular blood vessels. A fracture severs this supply. Internal fixation is designed to keep the bone fragments in close contact and in the hope that a blood supply can be

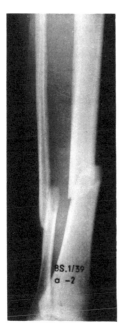
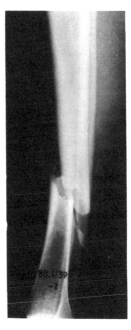
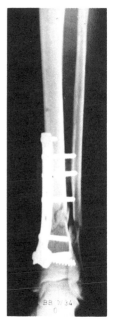

stablished. However, the fragments often separate and a slow necrosis ccurs resulting in a collapse of the bony union one or two years later.

Extracapsular fractures. Failures of fixation. A very accurate bone lignment is required if the stresses on the fixator are not to be too great. his is not always possible and the metal may work loose or break.

EMORAL SHAFT FRACTURES

hese are usually the result of accidents or severe violence. There can be a lean break or a very comminuted fracture. The type of fracture will etermine the method of fixation.

ANGE

nee movements are often limited after these fractures. This may be due) the involvement of the quadriceps muscle in the fracture callus. A uadriceps-plasty may be required at some future time to overcome this. If iis complication does not arise, knee range usually becomes normal.

OWER

he quadriceps muscle atrophies very quickly. It is important to encourge its use as quickly as possible after injury.

OMPLICATIONS

Von-union. This could be caused by over-traction, or a failure of the aternal fixation to keep the bone ends in close contact.

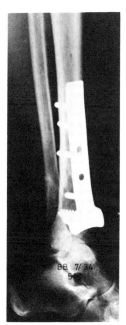

Plate 13/8 Fractures of the shafts of the tibia and fibula. a) & b) before treatment; c) & d) after treatment by compression plating

FRACTURES OF THE REGION OF THE KNEE

Site	Usual age-group	How injury occurs	Most usual method of fixation
SUPRA-CONDYLAR	Any	Direct blow	1. Traction 3 months *or* 2. Compression plating or screwing
PATELLA – minor without displacement – severe with displacement	Any	Direct violence or stress	1. Support bandage for few days *or* 2. Plaster cylinder (P.O.P.) groin to ankle for 3 weeks 1. Operation, wiring or screwing and P.O.P. cylinder *or* 2. Operation, excision of part or whole and P.O.P. cylinder
TIBIAL PLATEAU (Depression)	Adults	Fall	1. Plaster groin to ankle 8–12 weeks *or* 2. Operation. Elevation of fragments and metal fixation. P.O.P. groin to toe 6–8 weeks *or* 3. None (elderly)

Notes

FRACTURES OF THE FEMORAL CONDYLES OR TIBIAL PLATEAUX
Unless the bone architecture is restored after these fractures, the norma joint is deranged. Instability results in pain and loss of normal joint range The type of trauma which gives rise to these injuries usually will hav caused some degree of dislocation of the joint, often damaging the sol tissue very considerably.

RANGE
Full extension is the primary aim; without this the quadriceps muscle cannot act efficiently. A patient can learn 'to live with' a stiff straight kne

Movements begun	Complications	Results and comments
Immediately; 'static' exercises only permitted; weight-bearing 3 months	Tibial nerve and popliteal artery	Gross loss of knee movements
Immediately; weight-bearing 3 months		Some loss of knee movements
Immediately	Retropatellar arthritis Quadriceps lag	Young make full recovery, elderly lose some range and power
Immediately P.O.P. removed		
Partial weight-bearing in P.O.P. cylinder. Knee movements at –6 weeks		Knee stiffness
Knee movements as soon as plaster removed	Ruptured cruciate ligaments. Common peroneal nerve damage (in lateral plateau fracture) Osteoarthritis	If resulting depression is more than 1cm, malfunction and instability follow. Knee stiffness
Immediately; non-weight-bearing to weight-bearing 6 weeks		

but a loss of 10°, or more, of extension creates a weak painful joint and a poor gait. It is seldom possible to regain full range movements after these fractures in the middle or older age-groups, so that full extension is the most important movement.

POWER
Controlled movements of the knee joint are essential in walking, sitting and standing. Whatever movements are restored to the joint, these are only as useful as the degree of muscle power controlling them. Every effort to maintain the power of the quadriceps muscle must be made, even if the knee joint cannot be moved because of fixation.

FRACTURES OF THE REGION OF THE KNEE (CONTINUED)

COMPLICATIONS

Cruciate ligament damage. These ligaments sustain some degree of stretching from injuries which result in tibial plateau fracture. They may even be ruptured.

Any ligament of the knee joint is liable to damage according to the way the injury is sustained.

Common peroneal nerve damage. This can occur at the time of an injury which causes a fracture to the lateral tibial plateau or a fractured neck of fibula.

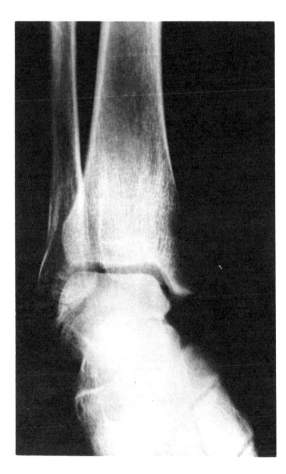

Plate 13/9 Fracture of lateral malleolus with no displacement of joint mortice

RACTURE OF PATELLA

The patella is a sesamoid bone in the tendon of the quadriceps. It alters the angle of pull of the muscle. Whenever possible it is repaired. It requires a very firm internal fixation after a fracture. If it is severely comminuted it is partly or totally removed (it often re-forms). After reduction the posterior surface must be smooth or retropatellar arthritis develops.

It is important to keep the quadriceps muscles as strong as possible. A 'lag' occurs if the patella is removed because of the change in the angle pull of the muscle. This 'lag', or loss of full extension, is a feature of most fractures of the patella in the early stages of rehabilitation and must be overcome if the knee is to regain full stability.

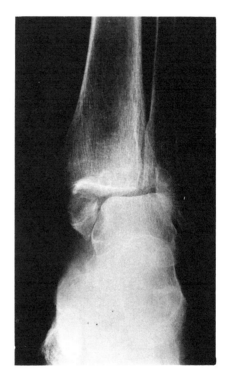

Plate 13/10 Pott's fracture of both malleoli, with disruption of joint mortice

FRACTURES OF THE TIBIA AND FIBULA

Site	Usual age-group	How injury occurs	Most usual method of fixation
SHAFT OF TIBIA (undisplaced)	Any	Direct violence	1. Groin to toe plaster 8–12 weeks, below knee P.O.P. for further 4 weeks *or* 2. Medullary nail
TIBIA AND FIBULA (shafts) (Plate 13/8, p. 242)	Any	Direct or indirect violence	1. Groin to toe plaster 10–14 weeks *or* 2. Plating and groin to toe plaster 10–14 weeks *or* 3. Compression plating
– Lateral malleolus (with little or no displacement) (Plate 13/9, p. 246)	Any	Inversion injury	1. Strapping *or* 2. Below knee plaster 4–6 weeks
– Medial malleolus	Any	Eversion injury	1. Below knee plaster 4–6 weeks *or* 2. Operation. Screwing and below knee plaster 4–6 weeks
– Both malleoli (with disruption of the mortice) (Plate 13/10, p. 247)	Any	Jumping from a height on to the heels	1. Below knee plaster (always for children) *or* 2. Operation. Screwing and below knee plaster 8–10 weeks *or* 3. Operation. Compression screws

Movements begun	Complications	Results and comments
Knee movements as soon as plaster shortened	Non-union	Good results in the younger age-groups
Knee and ankle movements 7–10 days; non-weight-bearing to full weight-bearing 0–12 weeks		
Knee and ankle movements when plaster removed; weight-bearing in plaster 8–12 weeks; full weight-bearing 12–16 weeks	Non-union	Slow, usually good results in time
Immediately; non-weight-bearing 12–14 weeks	Non-union, common peroneal nerve compression; Infection	Good results. Sometimes loss of full dorsiflexion of ankle
Immediately; weight-bearing		Excellent results
Weight-bearing in plaster; exercises when plaster removed		Excellent results
Walk in plaster at 2 weeks	Medial ligament damage leaving the joint unstable	Good if mortice is re-established
Exercises when P.O.P. removed	Osteoarthritis	Children do well. Results depend on the degree of perfection of the joint reconstruction. The older the patient the greater the loss of joint movements. Balance impaired
Immediate exercises, non-weight-bearing to weight-bearing 8–10 weeks		

FRACTURES OF THE TIBIA AND FIBULA (CONTINUED)

Site	Usual age-group	How injury occurs	Most usual method of fixation
CALCANEUM – simple	Adult	Jumping from a height on to the heels	Free
– involving joint surfaces	Adult		Below knee plaster 4–6 weeks
METATARSALS	Adult	Stress or weight falling on the foot	Below knee plaster 4–6 weeks
– 5th	Adult	Inversion injury	Strapping 1 week

Notes

FRACTURES OF THE SHAFT OF THE TIBIA AND FIBULA
There are many different types of fracture that can occur, from a simpl
transverse fracture of the tibia without displacement, to a severely com
minuted fracture of both bones.

COMPLICATION
Non-union. This is quite common, especially in young men. A secondar
operative procedure, such as a bone graft or internal fixation, may have t
be performed. While compression plating has reduced the percentage o
non-union results, it has its own complication of a 'drop foot'. It is difficu
to say whether this is a result of pressure on the common peroneal nerve b
the special walking caliper, or as a result of the operative technique. Ful
recovery of the nerve lesion may take several months.

FRACTURES OF THE ANKLE AND HINDFOOT
The function of the foot on the lower leg is to perform the actions require
for propulsion of the body over uneven surfaces and at varying speeds
The injuries that can be sustained vary from a simple strain to comple
fracture-dislocations involving one or more joints. Unless the bone an
joint architecture can be restored to normal, the function of the foot i
restricted and usually painful.

RANGE
Inversion and eversion are the most important movements to restore

Movements begun	Complications	Results and comments
Immediately; weight-bearing in 7–10 days		If there is a loss of subtaloid movement, the patient should not work above ground level again
Exercises when plaster removed at 6–12 weeks		
Weight-bearing in plaster		Excellent results
Normal use		

Without them walking on uneven surfaces is painful or even impossible.

Plantar-flexion is required to give the 'push off' range for the action of the calf and flexor hallucis longus muscles, which together make the normal gait. The loss of dorsiflexion can be accommodated by raising the heel of the shoe.

POWER
Controlled movement is more important than range. The whole body-weight rests on the forefoot during walking and running, and unless the ankle and hindfoot are controlled there is a great incapacity.

COMPLICATIONS
There are no specific immediate complications. However, these injuries are often disabling and result in patients being unable to resume their normal work again, e.g. calcaneal fractures which involve the subtaloid joint may necessitate a scaffolder giving up climbing.

Arthritis often develops where articular surfaces have been damaged. Ligaments may be partially or totally ruptured, giving rise to painful instability. Loss of normal joint architecture may make for either limited or unstable movements, which are often painful.

FRACTURES OF THE METATARSALS
These are minor injuries and repair well with no disability. Most can be treated by strapping and immediate use.

FRACTURES OF THE PELVIS

Site	Usual age-group	How injury occurs	Most usual method of fixation
1. SINGLE – Wing of ilium. Rami of either pubis or ilium	Adult	Crush injury or direct blow	Bed rest for 2–7 days
2. MULTIPLE – Two rami on same side with displacement	Adult	Crush injury or falling from a height on to one foot	Bed rest with skin traction on leg of affected side (2–3 weeks)
FOUR RAMI (butterfly fracture)	Adult	Crush injury	Operation. To stabilise fragments (wire or plates) and a pelvic sling
ACETABULUM – Posterior rim (and posterior dislocation of hip)	Adult	Blow on knee when leg is flexed and adducted	1. Reduction of dislocation. Traction for 4–6 weeks *or* 2. Large fragments screwed and traction for 4–6 weeks
– Comminuted (and central dislocation of hip)	Adult	Blow or fall on greater trochanter	Reduction of dislocation by traction from a pin in the greater trochanter 6–8 weeks (Reduction is not possible because of rotation of fragments). Traction for 6–10 weeks
– Iliopubic (and central dislocation of hip)			

Notes

PELVIC GIRDLE
A single fracture of the pelvic girdle (i.e. one ramus, or the winging of the ilium) does not significantly alter the stability of the pelvis. Early ambulation and exercise should be encouraged.

Multiple fractures (i.e. two rami on the same side, or all four rami render the pelvic girdle unstable. Therefore weight-bearing must be

1ovements begun	Complications	Results and comments
ed exercises; eight-bearing 2–7 ays		Good. Pain can persist for several weeks
hen traction moved gentle on-weight-bearing xercises; avoid raight leg raising in rly stages; partial eight-bearing 3–4 eeks. one until united; en gentle on-weight-bearing xercises; straight leg ising delayed for –8 weeks; walking at –12 weeks	Urethra or bladder damage	Slow but good
entle on-weight-bearing xercises when action is removed; eight-bearing 5–7 eeks	Sciatic nerve palsy, usually recovers quickly	Good
entle on-weight-bearing xercises when action is removed; artial weight-bearing –11 weeks; full eight-bearing 9–13 eeks	Osteoarthrosis inevitable. Possible damage to pelvic contents	Much better than one expects. The young make a very good recovery but often have osteoarthrosis later in life. If pain persists further surgery may be required

delayed until there is bony union. The strong pull of the muscles attached
o these bones makes displacement severe. Union is essential before
xercises are given. It must be remembered that straight leg raising,
specially if performed in the supine posture, is an advanced type of
xercise for these patients in view of the length of the lever. This type of
xercise should be delayed until the surgeon considers the bony union is
ufficiently firm to withstand the strain.

FRACTURES OF THE PELVIS (CONTINUED)

COMPLICATIONS
There is always a danger that the internal organs may have been damaged
at the time of the accident. The urethra and bladder are particularly
vulnerable. The final diameters of the pelvis are particularly important to
females of child-bearing age.

ACETABULUM
These fractures occur with dislocations of the hip joint. In the early stages
movements of the hip are not possible, because of the traction needed to
retain the reduction of the dislocation and the time necessary for the
capsular ligamentous damage to repair. When hip movement is permitted,
care should be taken to avoid reproducing the action which preceded the
dislocation as this may cause further soft tissue damage and even a redislocation of the joint. (E.g. a posterior dislocation occurs when the hip is

FRACTURES OF THE SPINE

Site	Usual age-group	How injury occurs	Most usual method of fixation
VERTEBRAL BODIES – Severe lesions with neurological involvement – anterior wedging (minor)	Adult	Flexion injury	1. Bed rest for few days *or* 2. Plaster corset
VERTEBRAL ARCH – transverse process – spinous process	Adult	Avulsion fracture due to violent muscle action	Continued activity

Notes

FRACTURES OF THE VERTEBRAE
Vertebral bodies. Minor crush injuries to vertebral bodies are usually best
treated by early ambulation and exercise. It is important to reassure the
patient that his injury is only a minor one, as the phrase 'broken back' or
'fractured spine' conjures up a very serious implication to most patients.

COMPLICATIONS
Persistent pain can be a feature and sometimes a fusion of two or three
vertebrae may be necessary to overcome this.
    The greatest complication is the patient's fear that he may be perma-
nently disabled.

flexed and adducted, and therefore these movements should only be performed with care.)

The speed at which exercise therapy is progressed is best left to the patient. Any pain he experiences should be considered an indication that the progression has been too fast. The young recover well; those within the older age-group are usually left with some loss of movement in the hip.

COMPLICATIONS

Osteoarthrosis is an inevitable long-term result. However, it is only an immediate problem with the elderly, many of whom already had some osteoarthritic changes present in the joint. Sciatic nerve palsy can occur with posterior dislocations, but this usually recovers quickly and spontaneously. Damage to internal organs may have occurred as a result of the compression force that was exerted at the time of the injury.

Movements begun	Complications	Results and comments
(see Chapters VIII–X, *Neurology for Physiotherapists*)		
Graduated extension exercises		Good result if only one vertebra is affected. Occasionally a fusion operation is needed if pain persists
Encourage movement		Good. Full recovery

VERTEBRAL ARCH

These fractures are often very painful since they are frequently aggravated with soft tissue damage. The best treatment for them is analgesics and normal activity. Bed rest tends to prolong the painful period. Local treatment may be given as for any contusion.

COMPLICATIONS

None, so long as the patient's natural apprehension can be overcome and free active movement re-established.

Chapter 14

Advanced Rehabilitation Following Trauma

by S. H. McLAREN, M.C.S.P., DIP. PHYS. ED. (LOND. AND LIVERPOOL)

This chapter on REHABILITATION concerns therapy of people by people and not by machine. There is obviously a place for treatments from highly sophisticated electro-medical equipment and, possibly, a niche for computerised statistics on patient numbers and types of remedial procedures available, but NOT in this chapter! Here is considered 'person to person' therapy – where the METHOD OF APPROACH to the injured human being and the TONE OF VOICE used are of paramount importance in the treatment regime.

In a more leisurely past (the so-called 'good old days') the individual with a problem could find a sympathetic listener and confidante in his home doctor or parish priest but now, sadly, pressure of work (frequently of the 'paper' variety) tends to close the door on this source of 'face to face' communication. The therapist should be able to fill this role in part – TIME should be allowed during the rehabilitation programme for conversation (p. 168). Often a vital glimpse of the patient's innermost soul may be gained and a reason elicited for his apparent excessive pain or a reluctance to return to his work situation or even to his family.

The previous chapters have dealt with the patients' regime both pre- and postoperatively and the charts on pp. 228 to 255 provide an excellent guide to the type of fracture the therapist may be expected to encounter. Also included are the various methods of treatment employed (both surgical and non-surgical) and the length of time required before each case is likely to be ambulant. With all this information to hand and the surgeon's permission to act it's 'all stations go' for the Advanced Rehabilitation stage!

THE END OF THE BEGINNING

Rehabilitation of the patient commences at the moment of accident. For example: A middle-aged man takes his dog for a customary walk along the usual route. Uppermost in his mind is a personal problem with which he is wholly preoccupied so that he crosses a familiar road without due care and attention into the path of an oncoming vehicle.

The first person on the scene should speak the truth to the injured man – 'You have broken your right leg but we will soon have you in St. Blogg's Hospital and on the road to recovery. We will contact your wife/mother with the news of your mishap as soon as possible and, don't worry, your little dog is quite safe and is in good hands.' The dazed, frightened victim now knows:

1. WHAT has happened to his limb and WHY he is experiencing pain.
2. WHERE he is going and
3. That his dependants are aware of his plight and, by no means least
4. That his much loved dog is perfectly safe.

With all these immediate problems 'solved' his mind is then more receptive to the re-planning of his temporarily altered life-pattern and, out of recent chaos, organised rehabilitation for his future has begun!

Causes of Accidents

Many people have accidents because they are:

a) physically exhausted
b) mentally depressed
c) suffering intense feelings of anger or
d) in a temporary state of euphoria.

All these conditions render the human body more prone to traumatic incident. The careless pedestrian, the bored machine operator, the frustrated car driver and the love-sick adolescent are all high on the list of homo sapiens most likely to 'meet with an accident going somewhere to happen'.

Advanced rehabilitation is not just a restoration of the patient to his or her pre-accident state – but to a much healthier, more VITAL life altogether (Fig. 14/1).

'Category' of Patient

It is the therapist's job to 'rehabilitate' but the methods and approach

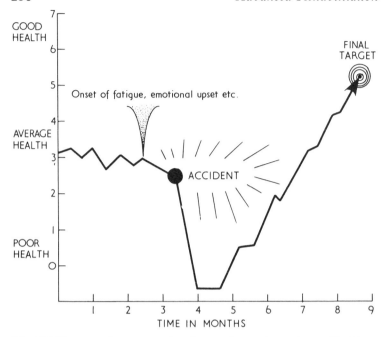

Fig. 14/1 Diagrammatic representation of restoration to a better degree of health following an accident

may vary with each type of patient. It has already been stated on p. 228 that 'treatment must be given to suit the particular needs of the patient'.

EXAMPLES

1. The amputee (Chapter 8) needs extra *time* to make the required psychological adjustment to an altered physical state.
2. The patient who has undergone surgery to arthrodese an ankle or knee joint must master a new technique of propulsion.
3. The patient who has had a joint replacement must also master a new technique of walking.

   Usually these patients have suffered a painful circulatory or arthritic condition for some considerable period of time before the surgical intervention and the type of rehabilitation required would be a continuation of the pre-operative treatment programme with progression as feasible.
4. Pre- and post-natal rehabilitation requires a somewhat different technique from the therapist – assuming that the condition in

which the patient finds herself is an anticipated event imposed upon her voluntarily!

These example patients have all experienced a doctor's surgery or a hospital department and are acclimatised. Not so the normally healthy victim of a road traffic accident (R.T.A.) who, in a state of surprised shock, finds himself compulsorily detained in a hospital bed with his leg residing in a warm damp plaster cast!

TREATMENT REGIME

'A MAN IS NOT FULLY REHABILITATED UNTIL HE IS AGAIN PAYING INCOME TAX'. There is therefore a great deal of work to be completed by both the victim of trauma *and* the therapist before the former is able to resume a normal, fully active life.

'THE DICTIONARY IS THE ONLY PLACE WHERE SUCCESS COMES BEFORE WORK'. It is therefore vital that the patient understands that ACTIVE PARTICIPATION in his own treatment programme is essential.

Patient Involvement

Rehabilitation is one continual process and must involve the complete person as a whole being. In many instances too much emphasis is laid on the injured part and the patient then becomes morosely absorbed by the presence of the fractured limb. It is the therapist's job to restore the patient's confidence in the affected part and *not* allow it to become the focal point of morbid fascination to that patient.

The success or failure of advanced rehabilitation depends almost entirely on the ATMOSPHERE in which it is conducted –

ENTHUSIASM IS CAUGHT AND NOT TAUGHT!

The ingredients for the making of a good rehabilitationist might well be:

a) An extrovert personality
b) A sense of humour
c) A delight in taking classes of patients for group exercise and
d) A commanding voice which will carry conviction!

SENSE OF HUMOUR – OR LACK OF IT

Frequently the patient's sense of humour has wilted or even disappeared by the time his plaster cast has dried out and restoration of the ability to laugh at tribulation – *and* at himself – is VITAL. A good therapist will be able to thread humour back into the treatment pattern.

> LAUGHTER IS A GOOD ABDOMINAL EXERCISE
> and
> HE WHO LAUGHS – LASTS!

To advance is to 'encourage the progress of . . .' and, from the outset, the patient should be involved in a forward-thinking regime. This pattern òf activity should be designed not only to prime him for his 'bread and butter' work but also to consider his free time expenditure of energy.

SOCIAL NEEDS

The patient may push a pen in an office from 09.00h to 17.00h Monday to Friday but lead an energetic golf playing, sailing, cycling, footballing, dancing or gardening life in the evenings or at the weekend. Any one of these activities requires a very high standard of stamina, co-ordination and general physical fitness. Into the majority of these extra-mural exertions creeps an element of competition . . . This is important and can be utilised with success when injected into the patient's treatment programme:

a) Patient versus therapist.
b) Patient versus patient in a one-to-one capacity.
c) Patient versus several other patients in a group situation.

REHABILITATION CENTRES

'A REHABILITATION CENTRE IS FOR A MAN WHO IS RUN DOWN TO GO TO BE WOUND UP'.

Throughout the United Kingdom there are specialised units where traumatic cases are admitted for concentrated treatment. Some centres are for patients requiring 24-hours-a-day, seven days a week attention e.g. The Spinal Injuries Unit at Stoke Mandeville, Bucks.

A few operate as residential centres from Monday to Friday for ambulant patients only, e.g. The Hermitage, County Durham.

A number accommodate both residential and day patients from Monday to Friday, e.g. Hartford Hall, Northumberland.

Many are day centres only, e.g. The Medical Rehabilitation Centre, Camden Road, London NW1.

In these centres the patient learns to be a 'little fish in a big pond' instead of being the 'only pebble on the beach'. In his own home he may be surrounded by a doting family, waited on hand and foot, until such time as the ambulance transports him two or three times per week to a hospital out-patient department. The conscientious, non-compensationitis fellow will practise his basic home exercises between hospital visits but the awareness of his injured limb is heightened when there is no other traumatised person present. He has no one with whom to share the experience of trauma, nobody similarly afflicted with whom to discuss the subsequent pain or discomfort and the obvious limitation of movement in normal activity. He may well become introspective.

'THE MAN WHO GETS WRAPPED UP IN HIMSELF MAKES A VERY SMALL PARCEL'.

A Rehabilitation Centre/Unit provides a varied daily programme which covers most activities over the period of a full working week.

TREATMENT VARIATIONS

Group Exercise Classes	a. Competitive
	b. Non-Competitive

Individual treatment sessions (as required)

Hydrotherapy	A.	Passive – Aeration baths
		1. One limb
		2. Whole body immersed
	B.	Active
		1. Organised group exercise (in treatment pool excluding swimming)
		2. Swimming and diving in standard size swimming pool.

Circuit Training (Variations)		a. Non weight-bearing
		b. Weight-bearing
		c. For general activity
	or	d. To work specific area only competing against other members of the group
	or	e. Working to improve an individual score

Weight Lifting		a. For correction of lifting techniques *only*
	or	b. To develop strength and endurance – brick-layers etc.

Weight and Pulley Work:	a. To encourage joint mobility and/or
	b. Increase muscle power

Functional tests	1. In a specially devised area, e.g. scaffold climbing, rough ground walking and crawling – pushing and pulling a) 'free' (wheelbarrow loaded or empty) b) vehicle on rails containing variable weights 2. In a workshop situation a) woodwork b) car maintenance
'Outdoor' Work	1. Walks – various 2. Gardening 3. Logging 4. Leaf sweeping, snow clearing etc.
Games	1. Indoor ⎱ both in teams, or with a partner 2. Outdoor ⎰ and individually against an opponent

The rules for 99 per cent of all games can be adjusted to suit a specific need. The patient with normal intelligence is usually able to adapt his thought processes rapidly and easily to the altered situation and gain added enjoyment from the 'new' approach to an 'old' game.

The rehabilitation centre provides many advantages whether residential or not. The patient may see the medical staff in situ instead of making a tedious journey to a hospital to wait in a frustratingly long queue. He may contact the administration staff concerning sick notes or benefits without travelling to some distant ministerial building there to wait in another long queue, at the end of which is an unfamiliar face.

The unit administrator is available to discuss alternative employment using the patient's existing skills or to arrange re-training for more suitable work developing some latent or new dexterity. All these points assist the patient to regain his equilibrium mentally as well as physically, especially if his injury is likely to render him permanently disabled to some degree. There are at least two sides to everything and conflict between one therapist and another as to the correct approach to rehabilitation is inevitable. Provided the ultimate aim of 'restoring the patient' is achieved, then 'let variety be the spice of life!'

DEBATABLE POINTS

The following 'debatable points' are designed deliberately to provoke controversy. As well as a standard comment, the author's own point of view is expressed and openly invites criticism!

STANDARD COMMENT

AUTHOR'S VIEWPOINT

A1 The same exercises should be repeated at each session so that the patient achieves a high standard of performance in one particular movement before progressing to another.

A2 Different exercises should be given at each session so that boredom is avoided (for both the patient *and* the therapist) and, with a wider range of general activities, a greater variety of joint movement is obtainable.

B1 The patient should have individual gait training to prevent a limp-pattern forming and no attempt should be made to progress to a trot until a limp-free walk is established. This prevents the formation of bad postural habits.

B2 The patient should be encouraged to trot, run and jump, swerve and possibly fall over; laugh, get up off the floor and try again regardless of a limp or any other irregular pattern of movement. By this means he will prove to himself that he is ambulant once more and only *then* should formal correction of gait be introduced into his treatment programme.

C1 The patient's clothing should be reduced to the minimum to allow for freedom of movement and so enable the therapist to observe the precise working of muscles and joints.

C2 The patient should be allowed considerable freedom in the choice of clothing worn during treatment sessions. This prevents embarrassment or other mental discomfort which could inhibit natural movement. Muscle groups contract and relax whether or not they are visible to the therapist!

D1 All exercises and activities in group therapy should be non-competitive thus preventing over-strain of the injured limb. This ensures that the less competent patient never feels inferior to his fellow patients.

D2 A high proportion of exercises and activities in group therapy should be competitive so that the patient exerts himself to the fullest extent as soon as possible. This aim of competition prepares him for a return to the 'outside world' and the inevitable rat race. Learning to laugh at himself when he fails dismally in some minor game or contest will

E1 When patients are required to work in pairs during a treatment session always ensure that
a) the injuries of each are at the same stage of recovery
b) the two patients are of the same sex and within the same age group and
c) that both are of similar build to one another.

E2 Make sure that everyone partners everyone else regardless of injury, sex, age or size. Life in the world outside the hospital walls is not designed to accommodate people in neat pigeon holes! 'The wind blows as hard on the weak as it does on the strong'.

F1 The patient should be treated two or three times each week in a hospital outpatient department. This enables him to continue a normal life at home with his family and friends thus aiding his recovery in a familiar environment. Good training in basic home exercises is sufficient to guarantee development of mobility and muscle power both in the affected limb and in the body generally.

F2 The patient gains most benefit when he is outside his home environment and may learn to become independent more rapidly when he is living and working with others similarly disabled. Very few patients work their muscles and joints to full capacity when performing formal exercises solo at home!

G1 A man's hobby is his own concern and no time should be allotted to this during a treatment session. His ability to perform leisure-time activities will return naturally with time. All effort should be concentrated on the work situation.

G2 The average man works one third of a 24 hour span in order to play for the second eight hour period and sleep, to recover from both types of exertion, commandeers the remaining one third! To promote full rehabilitation, time should be allowed for the patient to discover whether or not his leisure activities – be they boisterous football, peaceful fishing or relatively strenuous gardening – are again possible.

DO'S AND DON'TS

The follow 'do's' and 'don'ts' are not 'laws' so much as comments. They are designed to stimulate discussion and provoke argument out of which may arise a new approach or a treatment scheme ideal for the particular unit or department.

DO'S

1. DO believe in what you are doing!
2. DO keep the final aim in view, i.e. to rehabilitate the patient back to a 24-hours-a-day life.
3. DO remember rehabilitation is a team effort with the patient as the focal point.
4. DO work to restore confidence, stamina and co-ordination; a sense of community living and, above all, a sense of humour.
5. DO use 'contact exercises' wherever possible. So many jobs these days are computerised, mechanised and 'conveyor belted' and person to person contact is often absent. Advanced rehabilitation can help to restore this deficiency.
6. DO remember that 'the injured man is stronger than the average woman' and female therapists should not underestimate the ability of patients – severely injured or not. So much time is wasted by giving 'feeble' exercises.
7. DO remember full and correct use of the voice is vital if success is to be maximal. 'ENTHUSIASM AND LAUGHTER ARE LIKE THE MEASLES – INFECTIOUS!'
   Let the patient laugh at *you* so that you are then entitled to laugh at him too . . . Develop the power of repartee which can be used to great advantage in class work.
8. DO use the patient's name! This is a 'personal touch' and reduces his feeling of being merely a number on a filing card. Introduce yourself to your class whenever a new patient is injected into it.
9. DO offer the patient a challenge and the latent CAVEMAN INSTINCT will rise to the occasion!
   a) Let them cheat a little – but catch them at it!
   b) Let them make a noise whenever it is feasible to do so – a 'cathedral atmosphere' is not conducive to merriment – but make sure there is silence when you wish to give a command or correction.
   c) Always remember to announce the winners of a race or competition – a little praise goes a long way!
   d) Devise a 'penalty or prize plan' – a press-up is an excellent

exercise in itself and may be utilised as a 'penalty' for anything from being late for a class to 'cheating' in a game. Most male patients *delight* in the opportunity to display their prowess in this direction! The therapist also must be prepared to pay the same penalty for a misdemeanour. It is not 'one rule for them and another one for us'. The 'prize' need not be an enormous one. Sometimes a mere reduction in the number of penalty press-ups which may have accrued is sufficient reward! Some rehabilitation units provide a 'Personalised Prize', in the shape of a keyring, a coaster or a bookmark with suitable words inscribed, and the effort expended by the majority of patients in the attempt to win these 'favours' is well worth any initial financial outlay involved. A simple inexpensive item stamped 'Super Star of the Year Award' becomes tantamount to the World Cup in value. Try it!

10. DO 'trick' him into using his injured limb during group therapy. During individual treatments it is more advantageous to allow the patient to demonstrate a movement with his unaffected limb which will then 'teach' the injured limb what is required of it.

11. DO remember to have enough apparatus for everyone in the class to work simultaneously.
    a) This equipment should be basic, inexpensive and easily obtainable for use in the home situation so that activity can be continued outside the hospital or centre environment. Many children would delight in the opportunity to 'play' with 'Daddy' or 'Grandpa' when he returns from hospital and teaches the family the exercises and activities he has been doing.
    b) Use a piece of apparatus if it
       i) makes the exercise more interesting (Fig. 14/2) or
       ii) distracts the patient's attention from the injured area (Fig. 14/3)

12. DO try to keep the number of patients down to a maximum of twelve for class work.
    This allows for:
    a) Greater use of available space and reduces the risk of collision etc. and
    b) With a small number there is a better chance that the individual patient can be seen and praised – or corrected – and the personal level is maintained.

13. DO remember to keep the patient 'on the move', especially in an outpatient situation where time is limited. 'Waiting for one's turn' in a game or activity is a time waster.

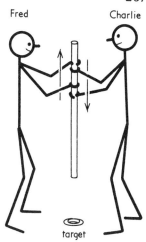

Fig. 14/2 Challenge for patients with painful hands, arms or shoulders. Charlie attempts to pull the pole downwards towards the target while Fred prevents him. The challenge offered to both men is sufficient to overcome a 'normal' pain; at any point either man can concede victory to his opponent by merely 'giving in' to the superior opposition and so prevent overstrain of a joint or muscle group

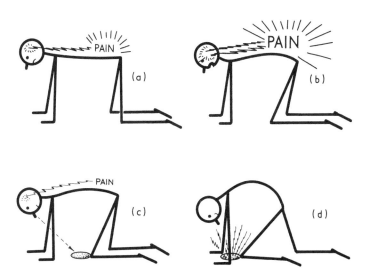

Fig. 14/3 a) Patient in prone kneeling in preparation for a hip and spine flexion exercise (to mobilise joints following removal of plaster jacket or the equivalent). b) Increase in awareness of pain on movement of one hip. c) Add a piece of apparatus e.g. a rubber quoit or bean bag (*not* a ball). The 'awareness' is now divided between pain and the piece of apparatus. d) Flexion of same hip pushing the bean bag with knee toward the thumb. *Target* – to propel the bean bag beyond the thumb and double the range of movement is achieved. 'Pain' is now in the bean bag as the thought processes concentrate on knee and thumb regions

14. DO teach lifting techniques as part of any class activity regardless of injury. 'Prevention is better than cure.' Hopefully, the correct lifting of stools, forms, medicine balls etc. will become automatic eventually.

DON'TS

1. DON'T give 'lethal' exercises:
   a) where one patient is 'fixed' to another and, therefore, unable to free himself when he so wishes.
   Examples: i) arms linked (Fig. 14/4) and
                ii) 'wheelbarrows' (Fig. 14/5)
   b) i) leapfrog over a partner's back (Fig. 14/6)
      ii) somersaults (Fig. 14/7) and even
     iii) double leg raising (Fig. 14/8)
   These are all potential 'hazard exercises'. AVOID THEM!
2. DON'T stop the class following a minor incident, e.g. a grazed knee, a 'jumped' finger or a nose bleed. Send the patient to the nearest 'first aid' department, in company with a volunteer from the same class, and carry on as before. School children, sportsmen and housewives in particular are prone to minor accidents and are used to 'just getting on with it'.

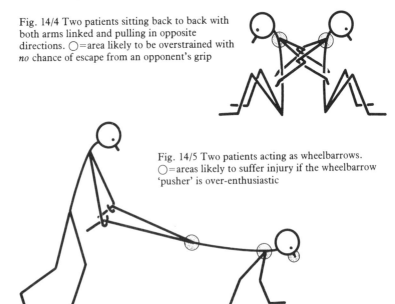

Fig. 14/4 Two patients sitting back to back with both arms linked and pulling in opposite directions. ○=area likely to be overstrained with *no* chance of escape from an opponent's grip

Fig. 14/5 Two patients acting as wheelbarrows. ○=areas likely to suffer injury if the wheelbarrow 'pusher' is over-enthusiastic

Fig. 14/6 Leap frog. ◯=area which could succumb to forced flexion especially in the patient who is not expecting his partner to 'land' on his back

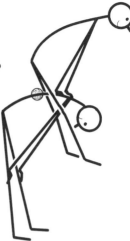

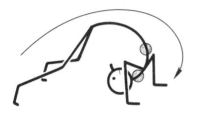

Fig. 14/7 Somersaults. ◯=areas most vulnerable to damage when the weight of the body, travelling at speed, hits the ground

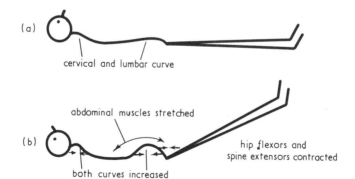

Fig. 14/8 Double leg raising. a) Body in normal back-lying position; b) Double leg raising. The patient usually holds his breath, thereby increasing his abdominal pressure to abnormal heights

3. DON'T demonstrate an exercise badly or half-heartedly. If you can *do* the exercise – do it well. If not – don't do it at all! Instead, declare your inability to do a press-up or touch your toes, or whatever, to your class and the patients will gleefully attempt to succeed where you have failed.

4. DON'T sit down or lean against the wallbars with arms folded or hands resting on the hips (teapot!) when taking a class. The VOICE gives the command and the hands and arms should be used to emphasise the order 'make a circle right round the room' or 'Jump up' etc.

5. DON'T join in as a fully participating member of the group activity. You will see more of the work your class is doing if you are an active spectator, involved without being embroiled.

After all these DON'TS, the final declaration is a DO:

Make your patient work *so* hard that it is easier for him to return to his work than it is to continue on an Advanced Rehabilitation programme! He will have proved to himself that he is able to cope with the unexpected as well as with routine requirements in his daily life and the therapist will have the satisfaction of knowing that it has been human endeavour and not a machine-wrought treatment that has brought the patient to 'the end of the beginning'.

ACKNOWLEDGEMENT

The author acknowledges the co-operation, inspiration and toil of all the patients, staff and students at the Hermitage; without it this chapter would not have been written.

Chapter 15

Cranial Surgery

revised by P. A. DAWE, M.A.P.A.

Brain lesions may cause motor and sensory defects but may be accompanied by other severe disorders, for example, of sight, hearing, intellect, speech and personality. Psychological disturbance, requiring full understanding and suitable management, may accompany both brain and spinal cord lesions. Early diagnosis of brain lesions and early admission to a neurosurgical unit is essential to ensure maximum benefit as delay may cause irreparable damage and permanent disability.

Research continues to increase understanding of the central nervous system in terms of anatomy, physiology and function, although much still remains to be discovered. Increasing knowledge of brain areas, pathways, connections, spinal cord tracts and functions has opened up new fields in surgical neurology. Improved investigative and operative equipment and techniques, anaesthetics, antibiotics and other drugs continue to reduce operating time and minimise postoperative complications and morbidity.

Team work is essential to rehabilitate the patient for normal living. The team includes surgeons with their medical teams, nursing staff, physiotherapists, occupational therapists, speech therapists, psychologists, social workers and chaplain, and the patient and his relatives who should have an important contributory role. Interchange of knowledge between members of the team allows a full understanding of the particular problems of each patient. Encouragement, patience, and perseverance are of paramount importance during the rehabilitation period, which can be said to begin immediately the patient enters hospital. As rehabilitation proceeds, other support services may be required, e.g. the disablement resettlement officer (D.R.O.), to arrange job retraining.

TABLE I. THE ANATOMICAL SUBDIVISIONS OF THE BRAIN

				Cavity Enclosed
Prosencephalon (forebrain)	Telencephalon	Cerebral hemispheres — Cerebrum — Cerebral cortex	Frontal / Parietal / Temporal / Occipital / Insula / Rhinencephalon } lobes	Lateral ventricles
		Connections between = corpus callosum the hemispheres		
		Anterior part of the hypothalamus		
		Nuclei of the basal ganglia		
	Diencephalon	Thalamus, geniculate bodies, epithalamus / Subthalamus / Part of hypothalamus		Third ventricle
Mesencephalon (midbrain)	Cerebral peduncles	Crus cerebri / Substantia nigra / Tegmentum		Cerebral aqueduct
Rhombencephalon (hindbrain)	Pons (mentencephalon) / Medulla oblongata (myelencephalon) / Cerebellum	Cerebellar hemispheres connected by vermis / 3 peduncles connecting cerebellum to brainstem*		Fourth ventricle

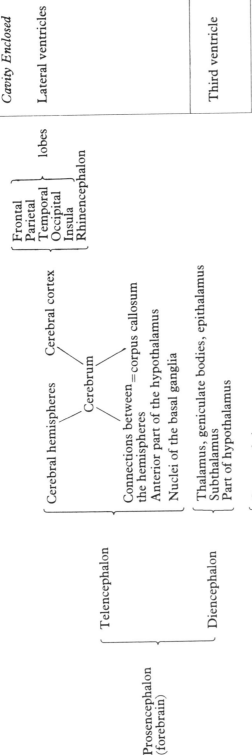

* The midbrain, pons, and medulla oblongata connect the prosencephalon to the spinal cord, and together are called the brainstem

ANATOMY AND PHYSIOLOGY

For the purposes of description, the brain can be divided into the forebrain or prosencephalon, the midbrain or mesencephalon and the hindbrain or rhombencephalon. Table 1 shows further subdivisions which are required for clarity and accuracy. It must be remembered that the entire mechanism is extremely complex; no one part works as a separate entity, and the response of the brain is the result of the integrated action of its various systems. The anatomical units are not necessarily the functional units. For example, the extra-pyramidal system and the reticular formation appear to have specific functions and yet are comprised of widely spread grey and white matter; the distribution of the blood supply divides the brain into areas different from the anatomical lobes.

The effects of lesions at some strategic sites throughout the brain are given in the following brief guide.

Cerebrum (Figs. 15/1 and 15/2)

The cerebrum is the largest part of the brain, and consists of two hemispheres connected by bundles of nerve fibres, the corpus callosum. The surface of each hemisphere covered by layers of cells constitutes the cerebral cortex. This represents the highest centre of function and can be roughly mapped into areas, each concerned with a specific function. To facilitate reference each hemisphere is divided into four lobes, frontal, temporal, parietal and occipital. The right hemisphere controls the left side of the body, and the left hemisphere controls the right side of the body and usually speech function.

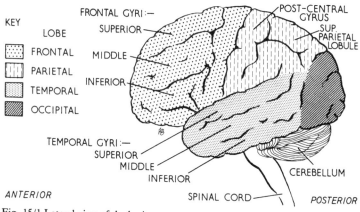

Fig. 15/1 Lateral view of the brain

KEY

LOBE

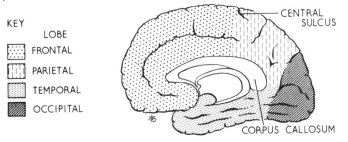

CENTRAL SULCUS

CORPUS CALLOSUM

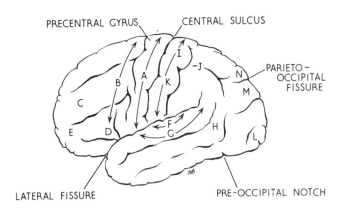

PRECENTRAL GYRUS   CENTRAL SULCUS

PARIETO-OCCIPITAL FISSURE

LATERAL FISSURE   PRE-OCCIPITAL NOTCH

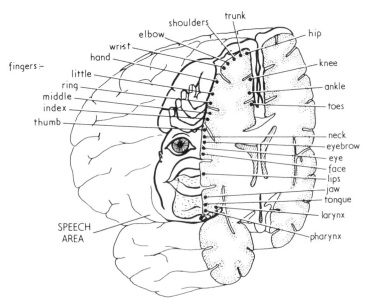

FRONTAL LOBE (Figs. 15/1 and 15/3)

Area	Function	Effect of a lesion
(A) Motor area (which gives rise to the cerebro-spinal tracts)	Controls voluntary movement of the opposite half of the body which is represented on the cortex in an upside down position (Fig. 15/4)	Flaccid paralysis. A lesion between the hemispheres produces paraplegia
(B) Pre-motor area	Localisation of motor function	*Spastic paralysis. Psychological changes
(C)	Controls movements of the eyes	The eyes turn to the side of the lesion and cannot be moved to the opposite side
(D)	Motor control of larynx, tongue, and lips to enable movements of articulation	Inability to articulate
(E) 'Silent area'	Believed to control abstract thinking, foresight, mature judgement, tactfulness	Lack of a sense of responsibility in personal affairs

*The effects of a lesion in the pre-motor area vary with the rate of onset; a lesion which occurs suddenly, such as a head injury or a haemorrhage, will result in a flaccid paralysis initially, spasm gradually developing over a variable period of time. A lesion which has a slow mode of onset, such as a slowly growing neoplasm, will produce spasm in the early stages.

Fig. 15/2 (*top left*) Sagittal section of the brain

Fig. 15/3 (*centre left*) Diagrammatic representation of some of the cortical areas of the brain

Fig. 15/4 (*bottom left*) The motor homunculus superimposed on the pre-central gyrus illustrates the proportions and positions of body representation in the motor cortex. In the post-central gyrus there is a similar representation for sensation

TEMPORAL LOBE (Figs. 15/1 and 15/3)

Area	Function	Effect of a lesion
(F and G)	Hearing and associ- ation of sound	Inability to localise the direction of sound
(H) Auditory speech area	Understanding of the spoken word	Inability to understand what is said

Other areas on the medial aspect of the temporal lobe are associated with the sense of smell and taste. The optic radiations sweep through the temporal lobe to reach the occipital lobe and these may also be damaged by a lesion of the temporal lobe giving rise to a homonymous hemianopia. (See Fig. 15/5)

PARIETAL LOBE (Figs. 15/1 and 15/3)

Area	Function	Effect of a lesion
(I, J and K)	Sensory receptive areas for light touch, two- point discrimination, joint position sense and pressure	Corresponding sensory loss giving rise to a 'neglect phenomenon'. 'Body image' loss is associated with lesions of the non-dominant hemisphere

Visual defects arising from lesions in the parietal area may be highly complex and the patient unaware of them. Sensory loss gives a severe disability, which is out of proportion to any associated voluntary power loss.

OCCIPITAL LOBE (Figs. 15/1 and 15/3)

Area	Function	Effect of a lesion
(L)	Receptive area for visual impressions	Loss of vision in some areas of the visual fields. (See Fig. 15/5)
(M and N)	Recognition and interpretation of visual stimuli	Inability to recognise things visually

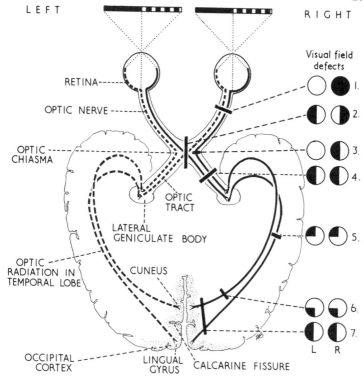

Fig. 15/5 Diagram to show the effects of injury on the visual pathway. 1. Complete blindness in one eye. 2. Bi-temporal hemianopia. 3. Complete nasal hemianopia, right eye. 4. Left homonymous hemianopia. 5 & 6. Quadrantic defects. 7. Complete left homonymous hemianopia

Brainstem

All nerve fibres to and from the cerebral cortex converge towards the brainstem forming the corona radiata, and on entering the diencephalon they become the internal capsule (Fig. 15/6). When the cerebral cortex is removed the remainder, or central core, is termed the brainstem. Its components from above downwards are: the diencephalon; the basal ganglia; the mesencephalon or midbrain; the pons; and the medulla oblongata.

The nuclei of the cranial nerves are scattered throughout this area.

DIENCEPHALON (Fig. 15/6)

Components	Function	Effects of a lesion
(A) Hypothalamus lies in the grey matter near the floor and lower walls of the third ventricle	1. Influences respiration, heart rate and blood pressure 2. Due to its connection with the reticular formation, it influences the conscious level 3. Influences the pituitary gland 4. Influences appetite 5. Has some influence over emotional behaviour 6. Regulation of body temperature 7. Fluid balance	1. Alterations in respiratory and heart rate and blood pressure 2. Pathological sleep 3. Refer to pituitary gland dysfunction 4. Appetite may be increased or decreased 5. Effects on emotional behaviour are very variable 6. Increase in body temperature 7. Diabetes insipidus
(B) The thalamus. To date over 150 areas have been defined	1. Relays impulses of all types to the cerebral cortex 2. Incomplete but conscious awareness of peripheral sensory stimuli 3. Focussing attention	A postero-lateral lesion causes hemiparesis, sensory loss and intractable pain, loss of co-ordination and vasomotor changes. Anterior lesions may cause involuntary movements and impaired sensation. Lesion of the mid-portion may cause mental changes

Basal Ganglia and Extra-pyramidal System

Broadly speaking the basal ganglia include the corpus striatum, amygdala, claustrum, substantia nigra and subthalamic nuclei. The corpus striatum consists of the caudate nucleus and the lenticular nucleus, the latter being composed of the putamen and the globus pallidus.

The extra-pyramidal system includes parts of the cerebral cortex, thalamic nuclei connected with the striatum, corpus striatum, subthalamus, rubral and reticular systems and its functions are concerned with associated movements, postural adjustments and autonomic

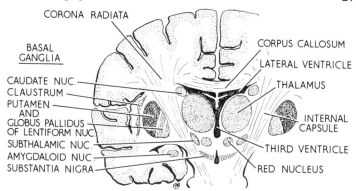

Fig. 15/6 The brain in cross-section shown diagrammatically

integration. Lesions may result in voluntary movement being obscured or abolished and replaced with involuntary movements.

Lesions of the extra-pyramidal system can produce either hyperkinetic or hypokinetic disorders.

HYPERKINESIS

Examples of hyperkinetic lesions are: chorea, characterised by quick, jerky, purposeless movements; athetosis, which gives slow, writhing movements of the limbs; hemiballismus, causing continual wild, flail-like movements usually confined to one arm; and torsion dystonia with involuntary movements causing torsion of the limbs and trunk. Frequently the lesions are in the caudate nucleus and the putamen of the striate bodies, and in the midbrain nuclei.

HYPOKINESIS

The rigidity of the Parkinsonian syndrome is an example of hypokinesis and may result from destruction of the globus pallidus, its cortical projections, the substantia nigra or reticular substance of the midbrain.

Midbrain, Pons and Medulla Oblongata

The midbrain, pons and medulla oblongata also act as a funnel for tracts passing from higher levels downwards to the spinal cord and for sensory tracts from the spinal cord passing upwards to higher centres. In view of it being a relatively small area, any lesion can give rise to widespread effects. Involvement of any of the following are likely.

Cerebellar function may be affected due to interference of the efferent and afferent pathways·passing through the brainstem.

Sensation of all types may be affected as the fasciculi gracilis and cuneatus terminate in nuclei in the medulla oblongata. Nerve fibres then arise from these nuclei, cross the mid-line and continue upwards to the thalamus in the medial lemniscus. The spinothalamic tracts which cross in the spinal cord pass directly upwards through the brainstem.

Loss of motor function occurs if the cerebrospinal tracts are damaged. These pass downwards from the internal capsule to decussate at the lower end of the medulla oblongata.

The conscious level can be depressed if there is damage to the reticular formation which is scattered throughout the brainstem.

Vomiting and disturbed respiratory rate can occur with pressure on the vomiting and respiratory centres in the medulla oblongata.

Cranial nerve nuclear lesions may result with characteristic palsies.

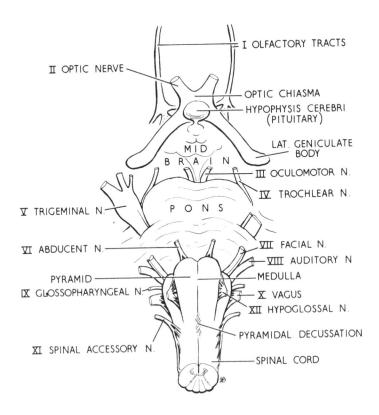

Fig. 15/7 The brainstem and cranial nerves from the front

CRANIAL NERVES (Fig. 15/7)

Cranial nerve	Function	Effect of a lesion
1. Olfactory	Sense of smell	Loss of sense of smell
2. Optic	Vision	Various visual field defects (see Fig. 15/5). Visual acuity affected
3. Oculo-motor	Innervates medial, superior, inferior recti and inferior oblique muscle and voluntary fibres of levator palpebrae superioris. Carries autonomic fibres to pupil	Outward deviation of the eye, ptosis, dilation of the pupil
4. Trochlear	Motor supply to the superior oblique eye muscle	Inability to turn the eye downwards and outwards
5. Trigeminal	(a) Motor division to temporalis, masseter, internal and external pterygoid muscles (b) Sensory division: touch, pain and temperature sensation of the face including the cornea on the same side of the body	(a) Deviation of the chin towards the paralysed side when the mouth is open (b) Loss of touch, pain and temperature sensation and of the corneal reflex
6. Abducent	Innervates the external rectus muscle	Internal squint and therefore diplopia
7. Facial	Motor supply to facial muscles on the same side of the body	Paralysis of facial muscles
8. Acoustic	Sensory supply to semicircular canals. Hearing	Vertigo. Nystagmus. Deafness
9. Glosso-pharyngeal	Motor to the pharynx. Taste: posterior one-third of the tongue	Loss of gag reflex. Loss of taste in the appropriate area

Cranial nerve	Function	Effect of a lesion
10. Vagus	Motor to pharynx. Sympathetic and parasympathetic to heart and viscera	Difficulty with swallowing. Regurgitation of food and fluids
11. Accessory	The cranial part of the nerve joins the vagus nerve	
12. Hypoglossal	Motor nerve of the tongue	Paralysis of the side of the tongue corresponding to the lesion, thus it deviates to the paralysed side when protruded

Cerebellum (Fig. 15/8)

The cerebellum lies in the posterior cranial fossa of the skull connected to the pons and medulla oblongata by the cerebellar peduncles. The surface is corrugated and consists of cells forming the cerebellar cortex. It is divided into two cerebellar hemispheres which join near the mid-line with a narrow middle portion called the vermis. Each hemisphere can be divided into the archicerebellum and the corpus cerebelli, of which the latter is composed of the paleocerebellum and the neocerebellum.

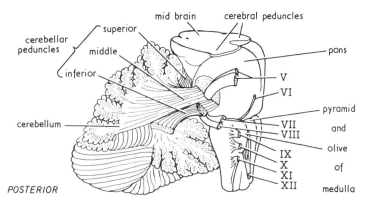

Fig. 15/8 Right antero-lateral view of the dissected cerebellar hemisphere and peduncles showing the lower cranial nerves

Although the whole of the cerebellum is highly integrated, and disease often results in diffuse damage, Lance and McLeod (1975) summarise the signs and symptoms of cerebellar syndromes as follows:

Archicerebellar syndrome: a) ataxia of gait, b) vertigo and c) nystagmus.

Paleocerebellar syndrome (anterior or mid-line cerebellar syndrome): ataxia of gait and inco-ordination of the lower limb.

Neocerebellar syndrome: a) hypotonia, b) dyssynergia, c) dysmetria, d) static or postural tremor, e) intention tremor, f) ataxia of gait and falling to the side of the lesion, and g) nystagmus.

ATAXIA

Where the equilibrium is disturbed and there is poor orientation in space, truncal ataxia is seen as a swaying and staggering gait. A unilateral lesion causes the patient to overbalance towards the side of the lesion.

When performing a movement which involves several joints, the joints tend to move asynchronously instead of in the normal rhythm of movement.

When reaching out to pick up an object the hand either stops before the object is reached or overshoots it. There is an inability to stop one movement and follow it immediately by a movement in the opposite direction.

When speaking, the spacing of sounds is irregular with pauses in the wrong places, termed dysarthria.

HYPOTONIA

Diminution of tonic reflexes is demonstrated by reduced resistance to passive movements and palpable flaccidity of muscle.

Tendon reflexes remain brisk, but are undamped so a characteristic change is seen, illustrated by a 'pendular' knee jerk.

DYSMETRIA

The sensorimotor system misjudges the distance for a particular movement, and thus a limb may over- or undershoot the target, or deviate to either side.

TREMOR

A static or postural tremor may be present, but more commonly a tremor is seen on attempted controlled movement which increases as the limb approaches the target. This is sometimes known as an intention tremor.

TABLE II.   BRAIN STRUCTURES AND THEIR MAIN BLOOD SUPPLY

Areas of structure	Blood supply
Cerebral Hemispheres: lateral surface	Middle cerebral artery
anterior and supero-medial surface	Anterior cerebral artery
occipital lobe and most of the inferior temporal gyrus	Posterior cerebral artery
Corpus striatum and the internal capsule	Mostly by the medial and lateral striate rami of the central branches of the middle cerebral artery, with a little supply from the anterior cerebral artery.
Choroid plexus of the third and lateral ventricles	Internal carotid and posterior cerebral arteries
Thalamus	Posterior communicating, posterior cerebral and basilar arteries
Midbrain	Posterior cerebral, superior cerebellar and basilar arteries
Pons	Basilar artery, and anterior, inferior and superior cerebellar arteries
Medulla	Vertebral arteries, and the anterior and posterior spinal arteries
Cerebellum	All the cerebellar arteries
Choroid plexus of the fourth ventricle	Posterior inferior cerebellar artery
Optic chiasm	Anterior cerebral artery
Optic tract	Anterior choroidal and posterior communicating arteries
Optic radiations	Deep branches of the middle cerebral and posterior cerebral arteries.

NYSTAGMUS

Jerking movements of the eyes – an oculomotor inco-ordination – may be seen, and this may be due to irritation of vestibular fibres in the cerebellum, or to pressure on the vestibular nuclei of the brainstem.

Thus, smoothly performed, accurate and skilled movements are the responsibility of the cerebellum, and the speed with which it can correlate the information it receives and effect controlled actions is phenomenal.

Circulation of the Brain

The four major vessels which supply the brain, the right and left vertebral and internal carotid arteries, form an anastomosis at the base of the brain, called the Circle of Willis (see Fig. 15/15c, p. 303). From this arterial complex many branches are given off, to be distributed to the brainstem, cerebellum and cerebrum. Interference with the circulation in any of these branches will cause characteristic deficits, depending on the parts of the brain deprived of blood supply. Table II shows the main blood supply to the key areas of the brain.

The Ventricular System

The ventricular system consists of four fluid-filled cavities within the brain (see Table I, p. 272). There is a right and left lateral ventricle, and a third and fourth ventricle in the mid-line (Fig. 15/9). Cerebro-spinal fluid (C.S.F.) is produced in the choroid plexuses of the ventricles and circulates within the system to the fourth ventricle where it escapes through the foramina of Luschka and Magendie, into the subarachnoid space. C.S.F. flows all around the brain and spinal cord, bathing it and cushioning it against jarring forces.

Obstruction of the system leads to hydrocephalus, raised intracranial pressure and eventually neurological deficits as the underlying structures are compressed or distorted.

EXAMINATIONS AND INVESTIGATIONS

Before surgery can be considered, extensive examinations and investigations may need to be carried out to localise the lesion and decide upon its nature and likely prognosis.

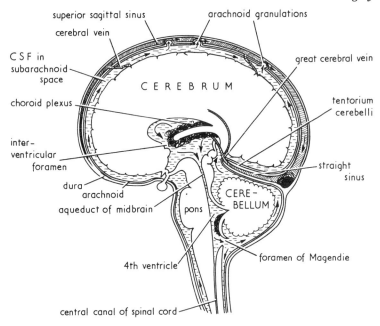

Fig. 15/9 The circulation of the cerebrospinal fluid

Examinations

A history of the patient's present illness, previous illnesses and any relevant family illness is noted; social circumstances, occupation, drinking and smoking habits are taken into account. This information is obtained directly from the patient whenever possible, but if the patient's conscious level or language function is disturbed the family history and relevant details will probably have to be obtained from other convenient sources, such as a wife or parents. If the patient has a history of unconscious episodes, such as epileptic attacks, a description of these attacks from an observer may provide useful information.

The patient undergoes a general examination but special attention is devoted to the central nervous system; each cranial nerve is tested, reflexes, motor power and all types of sensation are carefully checked. Full assessment of the central nervous system may be complicated by lack of co-operation, but adequate information is usually obtained to establish a diagnosis.

Assessment by the Physiotherapist

Detailed and precise pre-operative assessment is ideal but this may be difficult if the patient requires immediate surgery, or if the conscious level affects co-operation.

The assessment will give a base line from which further improvement or deterioration can be measured. A postoperative deterioration may be the result of removal of brain tissue during the course of surgery, but more important it may be one of the signs of onset of postoperative complications, such as haemorrhage or thrombosis.

The assessment by the physiotherapist requires an accurate evaluation of:

1. Voluntary movement and muscle power, as this is useful both for diagnosis and future treatment. This should be recorded carefully, perhaps using a numerical scale, although this is not always appropriate in the presence of spasticity.
2. The range of movement which may be correlated with any incidental findings of importance, for example previous underlying orthopaedic pathology.
3. Muscle tone, which may be either hypo-, normo-, or hyper-tonic. Changes in muscle tonus may be subtle but they are important indications of the patient's progress. Awareness of the state of muscle tone is an integral part of treatment. Muscle tone may be described as the resistance to stretch, and can be judged by palpation of the muscle belly, the resistance felt to velocity sensitive passive movements, tendon responses, observation of active movements and posture.
4. Equilibrium and righting reactions.
5. The sensorium and mental status of the patient.
6. Sensory modalities particularly cutaneous, deep and proprioceptive responses.
7. The functional ability of the patient to determine the level and quality of his independence. Full details of the assessment of neurological patients will be found in Chapter 4 of the companion volume *Neurology for Physiotherapists*.
8. The early assessment of the patient's respiratory function is desirable but will depend upon his physical state and the degree of urgency for operation.

Special Investigations

These procedures may be carried out while the patient is having physiotherapy treatment, and this in consequence may need to be modified for a few days.

LUMBAR PUNCTURE

A needle is inserted in the subarachnoid space between the third and fourth lumbar spinous processes; the pressure of the cerebrospinal fluid is determined and a sample of fluid taken for diagnostic purposes. Following lumbar puncture the patient is nursed lying flat in bed for 24 hours, and active physiotherapy can be given in any of the lying positions. A severe headache may develop after a lumbar puncture. This can be relieved by elevating the foot of the bed for several hours during which time no physiotherapy treatment is given.

X-RAY

Plain films of the skull are usually necessary and can be supplemented by special views of various areas. A note is made of any intracranial calcification and possible displacement of a calcified pineal body. General X-ray examination may be indicated and chest X-rays are always taken.

COMPUTERISED AXIAL TOMOGRAPHY (C.A.T. SCAN)

This is a relatively recent technique which has revolutionised the field of investigation. A large series of X-rays are taken from different angles in one plane, and the densities computed. A photograph is produced as part of the computer output.

ECHO-ENCEPHALOGRAPHY

By means of ultrasonic waves echoes from mid-line supratentorial structures can be obtained and mass lesions causing displacements can be detected easily and safely and may serve to indicate the need for further appropriate investigations.

LUMBAR AIR ENCEPHALOGRAPHY

Small quantities of air are injected after lumbar puncture with the patient seated erect. Films are taken with the patient successively erect, supine and prone. The whole ventricular system, the basal cisterns and the subarachnoid spaces are displayed showing any displacements or deformities, thus accurately indicating the site of any lesions. Improved X-ray tubes and television screening have allowed better detail to be produced and the use of tomography allows a more detailed study. Tomography is more extensively practised with particular reference to the petrous bones. Nursing care and physiotherapy treatment are the same as following lumbar puncture.

CEREBRAL ANGIOGRAPHY

This is an extremely important procedure, which is usually carried out under a general anaesthetic. Injections of radio-opaque solutions into the carotid or vertebral arteries are followed by taking films of the arterial, capillary and venous phases of the circulation. Displacement of the blood vessels shows the site of intracranial masses such as clots, tumours, abscesses or cysts. In a proportion of tumour cases, the circulation of the tumour itself may also be seen and may give an accurate assessment of its pathological type.

Angiography is of great value in cerebrovascular disease. The site of arterial stenosis or occlusion is easily seen. In spontaneous intracranial haemorrhage the site of an aneurysm or arteriovenous anomaly can only be determined by angiography. Postoperative angiography is a useful means of checking the efficiency of surgical treatment of aneurysms and anomalies.

Indirect methods of angiography are now more frequently used. A catheter is inserted into the femoral or axillary artery and its tip passed into the aortic arch. Large quantities of contrast medium injected under pressure allow the display of all major cerebral arteries.

Following angiography the patient is nursed flat for 24 hours, then allowed to sit up and get out of bed if no headache is present. Physiotherapy treatment consists of breathing exercises and maintenance exercises. If the femoral or axillary artery has been used, care must be taken to ensure that the patient maintains full range of hip or shoulder joint movement.

VENTRICULOGRAPHY

A burr hole is drilled in the skull allowing insertion of a needle into a lateral ventricle. A positive contrast medium, either a radio-opaque solution, or air, is then introduced and manoeuvred into the third and fourth ventricles. This procedure is often used to demonstrate lesions in the posterior fossa, and is a routine measure during stereotaxic surgery, when it is used to outline appropriate cerebral landmarks. This allows accurate measurements to be made, which are necessary for the introduction of electrodes into chosen positions. The procedure is carried out under general anaesthesia and the nursing care and physiotherapy will be similar to that following angiography.

RADIO-ISOTOPE SCANNING

The use of radio-active isotopes in investigation of cerebral disorders may take the form of one of the following:

1. Intravenously in order to delineate masses such as tumours.
2. Introduced into the cerebral circulation to investigate the blood supply.
3. Introduced into the C.S.F. for the study of obstruction to the circulation of the C.S.F. This helps to distinguish between atrophy and hydrocephalus with gross increase in intracranial pressure.

ELECTRO-ENCEPHALOGRAPHY

The electro-encephalograph (E.E.G.) amplifies and records the electrical activity of the brain, but it can only give a measure of the extent of the disorder of brain function. No abnormal E.E.G. pattern is specific to the disease which produces it, thus interpretation of records requires an appreciation of the clinical problems involved and close liaison between the interpreter and the clinician. An E.E.G. can be recorded within 45 minutes, with no danger or discomfort to the patient.

In surgical neurology, in the light of the patient's history and clinical signs, the E.E.G. may be used to help distinguish between cerebral tumours and cerebrovascular accidents; psychiatric symptoms with a suspected organic cause; and in localising the site of abnormal electrical activity in intractable epilepsy.

Electro-corticography, the recording from the exposed brain at operation, is also particularly helpful when dealing surgically with epilepsy.

MONITORING INTRACRANIAL PRESSURE

A monitoring device can be used to measure intracranial pressure over a period of approximately 48 hours. The information gained allows fuller assessment of the patient's condition and his further management. (This means of measuring intracranial pressure over a period of time has been extremely useful in the management of certain head injury patients whose condition has remained static for no apparent reason. The monitoring can show up huge variations in pressure over a long period, which could go undetected with random measurements, and can indicate the need for a 'shunt' to reduce intracranial pressure, with a resultant improvement in the patient's condition.)

Because the patient is connected to a delicate piece of apparatus, he is necessarily kept lying quietly in bed for the duration of the monitoring. However, physiotherapy will probably need to continue, particularly chest care. It is important to note that moving or turning the patient, and coughing or straining, will dramatically alter the C.S.F. pressure, and hence the recording needle may swing violently. It is necessary to note both type and time of physiotherapy treatment, so that when the results are analysed these changes in pressure are interpreted correctly.

GENERAL SIGNS AND SYMPTOMS OF CEREBRAL LESIONS

Raised Intracranial Pressure

Intracranial pressure depends on the volume of the skull contents. In a child under the age of 18 months, any slow abnormal increase in volume will result in a disproportionate increase in the size of the head. In individuals over the age of 18 months there is no increase in the size of the head, thus the effects of raised intracranial pressure will produce a disturbance of cerebral function more rapidly. Increased volume may be caused by a space-occupying lesion, such as a tumour or abscess, a blockage in the cerebrospinal fluid pathways or by haemorrhage from an aneurysm. With raised intracranial pressure the soft-walled veins become compressed, giving rise to oedema and subsequent lack of oxygen to the brain tissue, and although the symptoms vary in degree, the classical picture of raised pressure is a combination of the following features.

HEADACHE

In the early stages of raised intracranial pressure, headache may be paroxysmal occurring during the night and early morning. With continued increase in pressure it becomes continuous and is intensified by exertion, coughing or stooping. The pressure headache is usually bilateral and becomes worse when the patient is lying down and is relieved when sitting up. Other causes of head pain are irritation of parts of the meninges, involvement of the fifth, ninth and tenth cranial nerve trunks, referred pain from disorders of the eyes, sinuses, teeth and upper cervical spine, and tension headaches due to muscle spasm.

PAPILLOEDEMA

This is oedema of the optic discs which can cause enlargement of the blind spot and subsequent deterioration of visual acuity and complete blindness.

VOMITING

This occurs when the headache is most severe and tends to be projectile in nature.

PULSE AND BLOOD PRESSURE

Acute and sub-acute rises in pressure cause a slowing of the pulse rate, but if pressure continues to rise the pulse rate becomes very rapid. A rapid increase in intracranial pressure causes a rise in the blood pressure, but a chronic rise does not affect it, and in some lesions below the tentorium cerebelli the blood pressure is below normal.

RESPIRATORY RATE

This is not affected by a slow rise in pressure but a sufficiently rapid increase in pressure, which produces a loss of consciousness, usually results in slow deep respirations. This may change after a period and become irregular, of the Cheyne-Stokes type.

MENTAL SYMPTOMS

These can vary from confusion and disorientation to complete loss of consciousness.

EPILEPTIC CONVULSIONS

Generalised fits may occur but it is not clear whether these are caused by the raised intracranial pressure or by the actual lesion itself.

Eye Symptoms

It is essential to realise that eye symptoms are often present with a brain lesion and they can directly affect a patient's capabilities during his rehabilitation. Among those most commonly found are:

Damage to the optic nerve, optic chiasm or optic tracts will cause field defects. (See Fig. 15/5.)

Damage to the third cranial nerve can cause a ptosis, an inability to open the eye.

Nystagmus. This is frequently present in cerebellar or brainstem lesions and is an involuntary jerky movement of the eyes.

Diplopia or double vision. This is present if there is any imbalance of the eye muscles and may be overcome by covering alternate eyes on alternate days until the imbalance adjusts itself.

Ear Symptoms

Deafness may be caused by tumours of the eighth cranial nerve such as acoustic neurinomas; these tumours may give rise to vertigo.

Speech Disorders

These have already been briefly mentioned and are mainly associated with lesions of the temporal lobe on the dominant side.

The Level of Consciousness

Numerous factors can be responsible for alteration in the level of consciousness:

haemorrhage which can be either extradural, subdural or sub-arachnoid;
infection as in the case of encephalitis;
certain types of trauma producing a craniocerebral injury;
space-occupying masses causing increased intracranial pressure and compression of the brainstem;
operational trauma;
postoperative complications such as oedema or haemorrhage.

Any known disturbance of hearing, vision or speech function must always be taken into account, and the patient given every opportunity to be able to respond. Sometimes a scale denoting the stages of coma, stupor, confusion, and normality may be used, but this is not always a reliable guide.

General attitudes of the patient should be noted also:

1. A patient who lies curled up, turned away from the light, and does not like being interfered with, who is irritable to varying degrees and who may be confused or even delirious might be showing signs of cerebral irritation.
2. When the neck is held stiffly into extension, and the patient resists flexion sometimes accompanied by retraction of the head, it may be due to irritation from subarachnoid haemorrhage, meningitis or raised intracranial pressure (Fig. 15/10).
3. Trunk and limb rigidity or tiffness may be signs of involvement of the base of the brain. The spine and lower limbs are held in total extension, the forearms pronated and the wrists and fingers flexed. The elbows may be either flexed or extended. This posture is usually described as decerebrate rigidity, and one or both sides may be affected (Fio. 15/11).

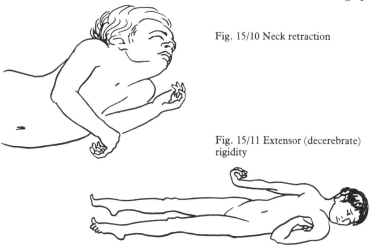

Fig. 15/10 Neck retraction

Fig. 15/11 Extensor (decerebrate) rigidity

Other localising signs may include:

a) ataxia
b) cranial nerve palsies
c) reflex changes.

ASSESSMENT OF CONSCIOUSNESS

A convenient guide for the physiotherapist assessing the patient's conscious level is to note the motor activity, verbal performance and eye opening responses, as suggested in the Glasgow Coma Scale (Teasedale and Jennett, 1974).

Motor activity, if not in response to commands, can be assessed by the response to painful stimuli. The response may be either 'localising' e.g. if the hand moves towards the stimuli, or 'flexor' or 'extensor' to indicate the direction of the movement. There may be no response. If one limb or one side is clearly worse than the other side, this is regarded as evidence of focal damage. The physiotherapist may be able to use these techniques, together with passive movement, to establish for example the presence of a hemiplegia.

Verbal responses can indicate either full orientation and awareness of self and surroundings or confusion, inappropriate speech or incomprehensible speech.

Eye opening responses indicate whether the arousal mechanisms in the brainstem are active. The eyes may open in response to speech, to pain, or spontaneously.

CRANIAL SURGERY

TABLE III.   NEUROLOGICAL CONDITIONS FOR WHICH SURGERY
MAY BE APPLIED

Condition	Adult	Paediatric and juvenile
Cerebral trauma	Head injuries	Head injuries

Neoplastic lesions	Cerebral – primary
	         – metastatic
	Tumours from related structures e.g.:
	  meninges
	  cranial nerves
	  pituitary fossa
	Cerebellar
		Cerebral – primary
		
		Tumours from related structures e.g.:
		  choroid plexus of ventricle
		
		Cerebellar

Cerebrovascular disease Haemorrhage Ischaemic lesions	Intracranial aneurysms Spontaneous subdural or extradural haemorrhage Angiomatous malformations Carotid stenosis	 Angiomatous malformations

Hydrocephalus	Secondary (e.g. with space-occupying lesions)
	Aqueduct stenosis
		Congenital
		Secondary – tumours
		            – spina
		               bifida

Spina bifida		Spina bifida cystica
		  meningocele
		  myelomeningocele
		Encephalocele

Dyskinesia	Parkinsonism	Cerebral palsy
		  spastic hemiplegia
		  choreoathetosis

Epilepsy	Intractable Primary focus	Primary focus, associated with e.g. Sturge-Weber syndrome
Cerebral infections	Abscess	Abscess
Repair of skull defects	Cranioplasty	Craniosynostosis

Psychiatric conditions	Psychosurgery e.g.
	  stereotactic
	  amygdalotomy	

Miscellaneous	Intractable pain, e.g. trigeminal neuralgia	

PHYSIOTHERAPY IN CRANIAL SURGERY

The general principles of physiotherapy in cranial surgery are virtually the same as for other surgical procedures.

1. To prevent respiratory complications.
2. To maintain circulation of the lower limbs.
3. To help prevent pressure sores occurring.
4. To help prevent the development of soft tissue contractures, particularly in the unconscious or paralysed patient.
5. To make any necessary assessment of the patient and where appropriate to treat any neurological deficit.

Specific physiotherapy will be indicated in the succeeding sections relating to the different types of surgery.

General Methods

Rather special anaesthetic conditions are required for neurosurgery (Greenbaum, 1976) and although techniques are continually improving, the operation may still take many hours and the patient be subjected to long periods of anaesthesia. It is a frequently stated fallacy that anaesthesia produces excess secretions. It is far more likely that some degree of dehydration will occur and thus secretions will become thick and stickier and therefore more difficult to clear. General anaesthesia also apparently reduces muco-ciliary activity and therefore slows down the velocity of mucus along the broncho-tracheal tree (Landa, Hirsch and Lebeax, 1976). Breathing exercises are taught and the patient is asked to practise them hourly before operation and as soon as he is sufficiently awake afterwards. A check must be made that the patient can cough and he should demonstrate that he is able to cough effectively, as a shallow throat cough is quite ineffective in clearing secretions. Patients who are known smokers should be advised to stop doing so prior to operation.

The patient should also be instructed to keep moving his legs (particularly feet and ankles) after operation to prevent venous stasis which reduces the risk of deep vein thrombosis. Passive movements are substituted when the patient is unable to do them voluntarily, and the use of anti-embolitic stockings may be helpful.

Postoperative assessment of voluntary movement, power, muscle tone, sensation, degree of ataxia, balance and gait is carried out appropriately when the patient's condition allows.

The preparation of a patient for a cranial operation is extremely important. In the majority of operations involving the brain, the hair

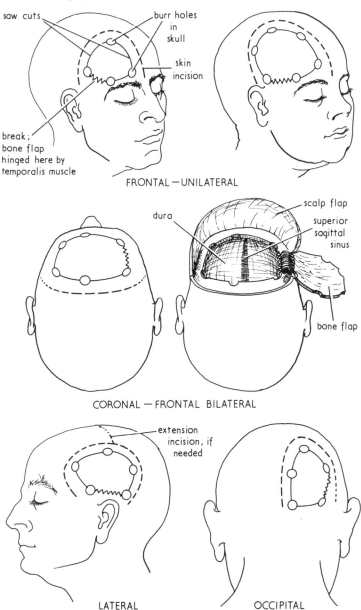

Fig. 15/12 Some supratentorial surgical approaches

must be totally removed and the scalp carefully prepared. The female patient may require reassurance if she becomes distressed at the prospect. Most operations are performed under general anaesthesia and take a considerable period of time to complete. During the course of surgery a bone flap may be turned back, but this is usually replaced at the end of the operation. Figures 15/12 and 15/13 illustrate some of the surgical approaches.

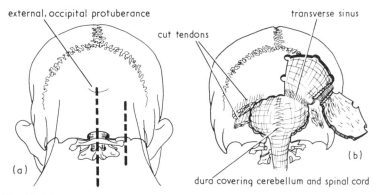

Fig. 15/13 Surgical approaches to the posterior fossa. a) Midline or paramedian incision. b) Craniectomy with an additional occipital bone flap when more exposure is necessary. The posterior arches of C 1 and C 2 are also gone

Postoperative Treatment

On return from the operating theatre the patient will have a pressure bandage on the head to control swelling; this may be extended to include the eye on the side corresponding to the operational site, for the same purpose. Eyes are very vulnerable to swelling and do so as a result of operational trauma. The position of the patient on the operating table may also be a contributory factor, hence for the first two or three postoperative days the patient may be unable to open either eye.

Intravenous infusion begun during the operation may be continued for one or two days; then, if the ability to swallow is affected, the patient is artificially fed via a nasogastric or naso-oesophageal tube.

Patients are generally nursed naked initially, to ensure accurate observations of limb responses, and to facilitate skin care. A urinary catheter is usually in situ.

Care must be taken to restrain a restless, confused patient, as he may attempt to remove head dressings, which will allow easy access of infection and meningitis may result. Padding and bandages on the hands, which may need to be tied down, reduce this danger. Cot sides should be attached to the bed in the early postoperative phase. It is important to replace hand bandages and cot sides after any treatment.

During the first few postoperative days intensive nursing care is required, the patient's condition being carefully observed and charted. Deterioration can occur very rapidly due to postoperative complications, thus any change must be reported immediately as it can be a matter of life and death. Surgical resection of brain tissue may account for neurological deficits.

BONE FLAP

This may be removed if the brain is very swollen during operation, or if the skull is splintered as a result of a head injury. When bone has been removed the patient is not nursed on the affected side until he shows signs of recovery of his conscious level. Replacement of this flap is advisable once oedema has subsided, as the patient tends to suffer from headache, dizziness when stooping and is afraid of damage from a bump to the area. Following head injury the bone may be so badly damaged it has to be discarded, and the defect is then filled with plastic material.

The young active male who is once more ambulant may be provided with a protective metal plate inside a cap, or a crash helmet to prevent further trauma, until the defect is repaired.

VENTRICULAR DRAINAGE

The patient may return from theatre with ventricular drainage if there are signs of inadequate cerebrospinal fluid circulation at operation. A catheter is introduced into a lateral ventricle by means of a burr hole in the skull and the cerebrospinal fluid drained into a flask; the height of the flask is dependent upon the pressure of the cerebrospinal fluid. Care should be taken when treating the patient to ensure that the level of the head is not altered in relation to the flask as this alters the drainage pressure.

If the doctor's permission has been given for postural drainage, the height of the flask must be adjusted as the bed is tipped and readjusted on its return to the horizontal, this being done under medical supervision.

LUMBAR DRAINAGE

This may be set up several days postoperatively if there are signs of continued raised intracranial pressure. The needle is placed as for a lumbar puncture and rubber tubing connects it to a drainage flask, the height of which is dependent upon the cerebrospinal fluid pressure. If the drainage is to be continuous the patient is nursed in side lying, well supported by pillows. Turning is done by lifting the patient from side to front, to his other side.

Complications

Apart from the complications arising from brain damage the following may also arise:

Cerebrospinal fluid may leak following the original operation, which may require further surgical repair.

Postoperative oedema, thrombosis or haemorrhage from cerebral blood vessels, or arterial spasm occurs in a small number of patients.

Thrombosis may occur elsewhere and pulmonary embolus.

Epilepsy may develop after a variable period of time.

Infection at the operation site is serious, particularly if the dura has been opened, as it can lead to meningitis and encephalitis.

Respiratory complications are fairly common.

Respiratory Complications

Postoperative oedema can cause pressure on the respiratory centre and the vagus nerves in the medulla oblongata, causing alteration in the respiratory rate and loss of the cough reflex. The ability to swallow may also be lost, thus there is a constant danger of aspiration of mucus and vomit. Until the ability to swallow returns the patient is artificially fed by means of a Ryle's tube passed down the nose into the stomach to prevent aspiration of food or fluids.

Involvement of the lower cranial nerves (ninth, tenth, eleventh and twelfth) may increase the difficulties of maintaining an open airway.

The physiotherapist is obviously concerned with the possibility of respiratory complications, and she must be always on the alert for these. Treatment and prevention of chest complications following cranial surgery may have to be carried out within the limitations imposed as follows:

1. Postural drainage may be contra-indicated immediately after operation as it will cause an increase in intracranial pressure.
2. Change in blood pressure may govern the position in which the patient must remain, for example a patient may have his head elevated to about 30 degrees, in an attempt to control raised blood pressure. It is therefore imperative to check the patient's charts prior to treatment, and permission to begin postural drainage should be obtained from the surgeon.

3. The patient may not be allowed to lie on one side if there is no bone flap in situ.
4. The patient may have a diminished cough reflex or weakness of oro-facial musculature, and therefore have difficulty expectorating.
5. When the conscious level is disturbed it is necessary to constantly try to gain the patient's co-operation. Deep breathing must be encouraged, and manual pressure on the sides of the chest when the patient breathes out is helpful. Clear instructions to cough should be given accompanied by pressure of the hands on the sides of the chest as the patient attempts this. A demonstration of a cough by the physiotherapist can also be helpful to the dysphasic patient.

SUCTION

When a patient's conscious level is depressed, or he is conscious but incapable of coughing, suction may be necessary to remove secretions. Vibrations, shakings and clapping may help to loosen secretions. A patient who requires suction is most successfully treated by two people, either a physiotherapist and a nurse or two physiotherapists, one using the suction apparatus while the other assists the patient with breathing and attempts to cough.

It is recommended that one of the 'atraumatic' varieties of suction catheter now widely available should be used. The multiple side-holes create an air cushion around the tip. This dramatically reduces the invagination of mucosa and resulting trauma which occurs with conventionally designed catheters (Pincus, 1975). Two such catheters are the Aero-flo and Tri-flo (Fig. 15/14).

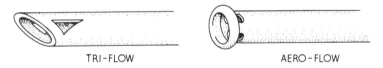

TRI-FLOW   AERO-FLOW

Fig. 15/14 Diagram of atraumatic suction catheters

TRACHEOSTOMY

This may be necessary if the patient has carbon dioxide retention due to respiratory insufficiency, or a clear airway cannot be maintained by use of a mouth airway and suction. Tracheostomy is also required to deal with the hypersecretions associated with midbrain damage following a head injury.

The removal of secretions from a patient with a tracheostomy should be regarded as an aseptic technique, the physiotherapist masked and gowned and the hands well scrubbed before touching the suction catheters.

Chest work with a patient who has respiratory complications can be very time-consuming and it may take almost constant attention throughout the day, but it is well worth the time and effort. An 'on call' system for physiotherapists is necessary when a patient has respiratory complications, which allows the patient to have chest care at any time throughout the 24-hour period.

FACILITATION TECHNIQUES

Some respiratory facilitation techniques suitable for the unconscious adult patient have been described by Bethune (1975). These include stimulating a co-contraction of the abdominal muscles, pressure on upper and lower thoracic vertebrae, stretch of isolated intercostal muscles, moderate manual pressure on the ribs, stretch of the anterior chest wall by lifting the posterior basal area of the supine patient, and peri-oral stimulation by firm pressure applied on the top lip.

INTRACRANIAL ANEURYSMS

Intracranial aneurysms are balloon-like dilatations occurring at the bifurcation of vessels in the Circle of Willis (Fig. 15/15). The precipitating cause is thought to be a defect in the wall of the blood vessel of congenital origin. Aneurysms are also associated with arteriosclerosis and hypertension. The size varies from a pea to a plum and multiple aneurysms may be present. Age-groups most affected are individuals between 30 and 50 years old.

Rupture of an aneurysm is the most common cause of spontaneous subarachnoid haemorrhage. Signs and symptoms from such a haemorrhage naturally depend on the severity and site of the bleeding. A minor leak from an aneurysm gives sudden severe neck pain, the pain then radiates up over the head and settles to a generalised headache and stiffness of the neck. Severe haemorrhage will cause increased intracranial pressure and loss of consciousness with various neurological deficiencies, depending on the degree of damage from the haemorrhage.

INVESTIGATIONS

The investigations to establish the diagnosis are: *lumbar puncture*, to establish the presence of blood in the cerebrospinal fluid, *a C.A.T. scan* to estimate the position of haematoma formation and *angio-*

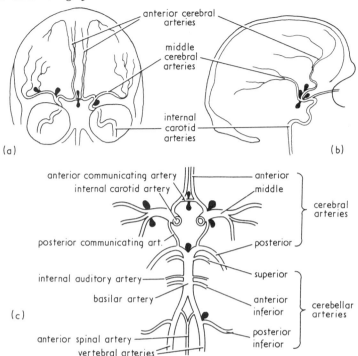

anterior cerebral arteries

middle cerebral arteries

internal carotid arteries

(a)

(b)

anterior communicating artery

internal carotid artery

posterior communicating art.

internal auditory artery

basilar artery

(c)

anterior spinal artery

vertebral arteries

anterior
middle
posterior
} cerebral arteries

superior
anterior inferior
posterior inferior
} cerebellar arteries

Fig. 15/15 Common sites for aneurysms. a) Antero-posterior view.
b) Lateral view. c) Vessels of the Circle of Willis

graphy, to determine the exact site of the aneurysm. As soon as a subarachnoid haemorrhage is suggested precautionary measures are taken. The patient is generally on strict bed rest, and kept as flat as possible but recently some neurosurgeons have been suggesting that patients should be allowed to sit up or get up for toilet purposes, as this actually raises the intracranial pressure less than straining hard when lying down.

Surgical Treatment

Unless an attempt is made surgically to deal with the aneurysm there is a constant danger of further haemorrhage which can be fatal.

To obtain a satisfactory result, operative procedure is undertaken only if the patient is conscious and showing improvement from any neurological deficits arising from the initial bleeding. All procedures are directed towards occluding the aneurysm by one of the following methods: by use of clips; by a clip and wrapping the aneurysm in muslin gauze or muscle; or by clipping the feeding vessel intra-cranially to reduce the force of blood entering the aneurysm.

Physiotherapy

The patient is taught breathing exercises and how to cough. If the level of consciousness is depressed suction may be necessary to remove secretions.

Passive movements may be given if there are motor deficiencies.

All muscles which are active will be strengthened and maintained and facilitation techniques used to re-educate weak muscles.

If no complications occur as a result of operation the patient will be allowed to get out of bed on about the fifth day. Prior to getting up, the head of the bed is slowly elevated until the patient can tolerate sitting up.

Balance re-education begins with the patient sitting on the edge of the bed and paying particular attention to check the righting and equilibrium reactions. His blood pressure may require checking. A significant rise or fall will necessitate his return to bed, otherwise he can progress to balance in standing, a short walk, then return to bed.

Walking re-education will require minimum attention if no motor deficiencies were present after surgery. If a hemiparesis does exist re-education will be necessary.

PROGRESSION OF TREATMENT

The patient is allowed up for progressively longer periods and gradually takes over his own personal care such as bathing, dressing and going to the toilet.

His rehabilitation programme in both physiotherapy and occupational therapy departments is increased until he can cope with a full programme without undue fatigue, and demonstrate his ability to live independently.

These patients do tend to become tired very easily in the early days following operation; it is well known that intensive care nursing is an exhausting experience as sleep must be regularly disturbed in order that the patient's conscious level and vital signs can be checked. Physiotherapists must remember this and not overtax these patients at the beginning.

Complications

Further bleeding from the aneurysm may occur while the surgeon is attempting to obliterate it. This may lead to further damage to the brain with a resultant increase in neurological defects.

Traction upon blood vessels in the field of surgery can cause ischaemia of the brain area they supply, which may be severe enough to give rise to defects.

Oedema and thrombosis may follow surgery, and may be severe enough to disturb the conscious level. These postoperative complications manifest themselves 48 hours after surgery and can completely alter the patient's prognosis.

The rehabilitation of a patient suffering from these complications may be either as for the unconscious patient, or as for the patient with hemiplegia or hemiparesis and is fully described in the companion volume *Neurology for Physiotherapists*.

LIGATION OF THE COMMON CAROTID ARTERY

This is carried out when certain aneurysms are difficult to approach by a direct method e.g. those arising directly from the internal carotid artery and those in the cavernous sinus, and only if the patient is neurologically intact, or nearly so. If there is an adequate cross-circulation in the brain, the vessel is ligated in the neck under local anaesthetic. If cross-circulation is not adequate a clamp is put on the vessel and the vessel occluded over a period of 48 hours, then finally ligated.

POSTOPERATIVE TREATMENT

The patient is nursed lying flat on the back with a thin pillow under the head; foam wedges can be used to prevent head movements (see Fig. 16/9, p. 349). A constant check is kept on the blood pressure, pulse rate, conscious level, motor power and the reaction of the pupils to light, in case the patient's condition shows signs of deterioration.

Forty-eight hours after occlusion of the artery the patient can be gradually elevated in bed. Side lying is allowed on approximately the third day. To minimise the risk of any thrombus formation (at the site of the ligation) breaking off during turning, the patient holds his head in his hands, so effectively reducing neck movement.

The patient is allowed to get out of bed on about the seventh day. Prior to getting up he must be able to tolerate sitting erect in bed. His blood pressure must be checked before he is allowed to sit over the edge of the bed, when he achieves this position and when he returns to bed after being up. Any significant drop in blood pressure necessitates return to bed.

Physiotherapy

The patient must be treated gently, and disturbed as little as possible. Exercises in bed are kept to a minimum: foot and ankle movements, and static muscle contractions of the leg, abdominal and back muscles. When the patient is ready to get up, balance re-education may be required in sitting and standing, before walking.

PROGRESSION OF TREATMENT

Progression of treatment must be slow and careful to allow the cross-circulation to compensate adequately. It should start with gradual increase in sitting tolerance. Then walking is introduced with increasing distances and eventually he is allowed to go up and down stairs.

Rapid changes in position may cause dizziness. The patient is therefore warned to move slowly when getting out of bed, standing up or turning around.

His stay in hospital is usually short and on discharge home he is instructed to continue with the slow, gradual resumption of normal activities.

INTRACRANIAL ANGIOMATOUS MALFORMATIONS (ARTERIOVENOUS ANOMALIES)

These malformations are congenital abnormalities of vascular development and occur on the surface of the brain or within the brain tissue, deriving a blood supply from one or both hemispheres, usually found in the younger age-groups including children. Most of the lesions are arteriovenous malformations. The blood vessels of the malformation show degeneration of their walls, and direct communication between arteries and veins in some areas. If the malformation is small no diversion of blood from the capillary bed occurs, but a large one robs the brain of its blood supply.

Signs and Symptoms

These are variable but the following may occur: headaches of a migrainous character; focal epilepsy; subarachnoid haemorrhage; spastic monoparesis or hemiparesis together with a sensory or visual loss.

INVESTIGATIONS

Electro-encephalography may be used for diagnosing the cause of headaches and epilepsy. *Angiography* will serve to display the malformation.

Surgical Treatment

A direct intracranial approach is made and the lesion excised if it lies on the surface. Sometimes very complex lesions may be treated by occlusion of the feeding vessels.

PHYSIOTHERAPY

This follows the same course as previously described for aneurysms (p. 304).

CAROTID ARTERY STENOSIS

Discussion of occlusive cerebrovascular disease can be confusing because of the terminology used. Jennett (1977) has described it as follows: 'Stenosis implies narrowing only, occlusion a complete block, while thrombosis describes a pathological state which may sometimes be the cause of an occlusion but is more often a consequence of obstruction. Ischaemia refers to inadequate perfusion of an area of brain with functional failure; only if it is sufficiently severe and prolonged, does infarction develop. Carotico-vertebral insufficiency is a useful term for symptomatic extra-cranial obstructive vascular disease.'

Atheroma is the most usual cause of stenosis of the common and internal carotid arteries, and thrombus formation may complete the occlusion. The site of the narrowing is most frequently at the origin of the internal carotid artery, and the severity variable.

The deprived hemisphere is dependent upon the collateral circulation derived through the Circle of Willis for its blood supply.

If the major problem is caused by multiple emboli shooting off from the site of the thrombus, then anti-coagulants may be used but with great care.

Signs and Symptoms

A wide variety of symptoms and modes of onset can be produced by carotid artery occlusion.

Hemiplegia. This may be profound and occurs suddenly, with loss of consciousness usually accompanying this type of onset. There may be hemiparesis progressing to hemiplegia. There may be transient motor weakness ('stuttering') usually affecting one extremity.

Dysphasia, *sensory loss* and various *eye symptoms* are associated in some degree with the loss of voluntary power.

Headache behind the eye is often present.

INVESTIGATIONS

A C.A.T. scan will differentiate between infarct and haemorrhage and angiography will reveal any stenosis or occlusion.

Surgical Treatment

In carefully selected cases surgery is of great value. Contra-indications are gross arteriosclerotic involvement of other cerebral vessels, and loss of consciousness with the onset of symptoms, which carries a poor prognosis.

Surgical measures aim to restore the normal blood flow and prevent further progression of the disease. Carotid endarterectomy is often performed by vascular surgeons as opposed to neurosurgeons.

ENDARTERECTOMY

The atheromatous portion of the artery and any thrombus is removed. If the atheromatous area is too extensive, a bypass arterial graft is carried out.

Physiotherapy

Immediate measures are required for the re-education of the hemiplegic limbs. Bearing in mind the likely sensory loss and field defects of the eyes, the patient must be constantly reminded of the affected limbs. The position of the affected limbs should be checked regularly to reduce the danger of damage to joints, and circulatory obstruction. Passive movements and facilitation techniques should be used to re-educate the affected muscles and the patient must be able to watch his limbs.

Balance and re-education in sitting aided by use of a mirror can begin when the patient is allowed to get up, approximately between the fifth and seventh day.

Walking re-education is also aided by use of a mirror.

During mat work the patient must first be taught to adjust the position of his affected arm and leg before rolling and similar activities.

When sitting in a chair he must constantly be reminded to check the position of his limbs. When walking unaided he must also be taught constantly to check that his foot is not catching on objects in his path, and that he allows ample clearance going through doorways and when walking near a wall.

INTRACRANIAL TUMOURS

Tumours found in and around the brain can be classified into:

PRIMARY TUMOURS

These are either *malignant*, of the glioma type (the malignancy of a tumour is judged upon its rate of growth and its tendency to infiltrate the brain tissue), or *benign*, such as the meningiomas.

SECONDARY TUMOURS

These are blood-borne metastases from primary tumours mainly in the lung and breast.

The rate of growth of a tumour is very variable depending on whether it is malignant or benign. Tumours of the glioma type invade the brain substance making complete removal difficult. Types like the meningioma do not invade the brain, but present problems in view of their size and extreme vascularity.

The location of a tumour is the most important factor irrespective of its pathology, because it may involve the vital centres, thus directly threatening the patient's life, or limiting surgical accessibility.

SIGNS AND SYMPTOMS

Some degree of raised intracranial pressure usually exists. Focal signs develop pointing to the site of the tumour.

INVESTIGATIONS

These will include C.A.T. scan, radio-isotope scanning, angiography and a lumbar puncture. Skull and chest radiographs will always be taken.

Surgical Treatment

A craniotomy is necessary and where possible the tumour is removed either in toto or as much as is surgically feasible. If it is not possible to remove the tumour a biopsy will be taken to enable a diagnosis to be established. Following an incomplete removal the tumour may recur.

If the tumour is known to be radio-sensitive i.e. it will respond to radiotherapy treatment, a course may be given. Alternatively cytotoxic (anti-tumour) drugs may be given either alone or combined with radiotherapy. Occasionally a bone flap may be removed to effect a decompression.

Intrinsic tumours of the dominant temporo-parietal area are not usually removed surgically as severe defects would result, namely dysphasia and hemiplegia. Tumours of the brainstem are rare but surgical intervention is often contra-indicated in view of the fatal damage which could result.

Physiotherapy

A patient without complications is allowed to get up on about the fifth day.

The patient with a hemiparesis or hemiplegia will be treated as described in *Neurology for Physiotherapists*.

Where the prognosis is known to be poor, all steps must be taken to ensure maximum independence without recourse to sophisticated techniques (Downie, 1978).

Cerebellar Tumours

The majority of cerebellar tumours arise in or near the mid-line and may extend into one or both hemispheres, such as the medullo-blastomas and astrocytomas, and are commoner in young people.

SIGNS AND SYMPTOMS

These differ considerably depending on the site of the tumour. The following occur in varying degrees:

Raised intracranial pressure.
Hypotonia.
Ataxia; this is probably most marked when the patient is walking. Ataxia is the result of the inability to stabilise the background activity essential for co-ordinated movement. Repeated movement tends to increase ataxia.
Giddiness.
Nystagmus.
Disturbance of function of some cranial nerves.
Sensory loss may occur but it is the exception, not the rule.

Surgical Treatment

To excise this type of tumour a different approach is necessary. Generally a mid-line incision is followed with a craniectomy of the occipital bone and laminectomy of C1. For a particularly extensive procedure a small occipital bone flap may be turned as well (see Fig. 15/13b, p. 298).

POSTOPERATIVE TREATMENT

Due to operative trauma and postoperative oedema, the ninth, tenth, eleventh and twelfth cranial nerves may be temporarily out of action, causing loss of the cough reflex and inability to swallow.

Nursing care is of importance. The patient must be nursed in side lying to prevent possible aspiration of vomit and mucus, and he is artificially fed by a nasogastric tube until he is able to swallow. This further reduces the risk of aspiration of food or fluids.

Physiotherapy

Breathing exercises must be practised by the patient. Suction may be necessary to remove secretions until the cough reflex returns. Even after return of the cough reflex, suction may still be required, as the patient becomes quickly exhausted.

Other aims of treatment are to strengthen the general musculature with particular attention to the neck muscles, and to re-educate balance and co-ordination.

Methods. As the patient's condition improves postoperatively exercises can be given to strengthen the general musculature, particularly the back extensor muscles. Re-education of the neck muscles begins with static contractions on about the seventh day and active exercises when sutures are removed about the tenth day.

Re-education of co-ordination begins in bed. The patient will find it easier to produce a co-ordinate movement against resistance, thus re-education can begin with resisted isotonic exercises for the ataxic limbs; and isometric holding against resistance from varying directions (this is termed stabilising).

Balance re-education begins when the patient is allowed to get up, usually between the fifth and seventh days. Balance is re-educated in sitting on the edge of the bed using techniques to facilitate postural holding and co-contraction around the joints, particularly the proximal and vertebral joints. Equilibrium reactions should also be reinforced at this stage.

PROGRESSION OF TREATMENT

It must be emphasised that a patient with a cerebellar lesion fatigues quickly. He will probably have a history of vomiting for a variable period of time before operation, leading to debility and dehydration.

His programme of treatment in the physiotherapy and occupational therapy departments must be carefully graded to guard against exhaustion.

As his condition improves the following progressions will be made:

Mat work. Resisted exercises are more accurately carried out than free exercises, thus mat work begins with resisted activities such as rolling, hip raising. Stabilising is done in each new position.

Activities are progressed to rolling from side to front to the other side. Sitting up from lying down and moving up and down and from side to side on the mat, using the arms to lift the buttocks off the mat. From prone lying practice in getting to the hands and knees position, sitting over from side to side and practice in crawling in all directions. From the hands and knees attaining the kneeling position, then half kneeling, then standing. Resisted crawling in all directions greatly helps balance and co-ordination.

Walking. Parallel bars and a mirror are of great value in the early stages. Stabilising in standing and resisted walking, walking forwards, backwards and sideways helps to regain the patient's self-confidence. Resistance against the head helps to steady a grossly ataxic patient.

If a walking aid is necessary to gain the patient's independence, elbow crutches or a reciprocal walking aid are more easily managed by the more ataxic patient. A stick may be adequate to support a less severely handicapped person.

Tumours of the Cerebello-Pontine Angle

A sub-section of the cerebellar tumours worthy of special mention are those conditions affecting the cerebello-pontine angle (Fig. 15/16). These surgically difficult procedures require a more lateral approach. Several types of tumour occur in this confined and critical area, and any space-occupying lesion will gradually compress the nearby structures, and result in deficits related to the appropriate cranial nerves, as well as producing a rise in intracranial pressure.

SIGNS AND SYMPTOMS

These will include:

Tinnitus, progressing to deafness if the eighth cranial nerve is involved.

Vertigo.

Facial weakness resulting from compression of the seventh cranial nerve.

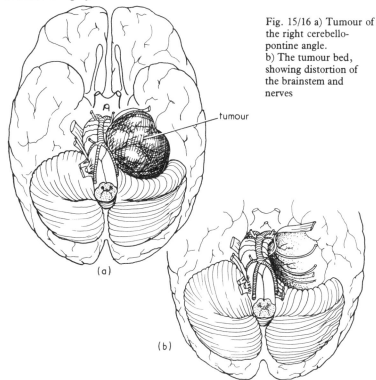

Fig. 15/16 a) Tumour of the right cerebello-pontine angle.
b) The tumour bed, showing distortion of the brainstem and nerves

tumour

(a)

(b)

Loss of the corneal reflex, and loss of sensations of pain and temperature occur with compression of the fifth cranial nerve.

Ataxia of the limbs on the side of the tumour occurs with compression of the cerebellar hemisphere and cerebellar peduncles.

The most common lesion to occur here is the acoustic neurinoma, which arises from the sheath of the eighth cranial nerve.

Surgical Treatment

Some tumours in this area can be completely removed but large tumours which are adherent to nearby related structures may prove more difficult to excise and lower cranial nerves may have to be sacrificed.

POSTOPERATIVE TREATMENT

The patient may have swallowing difficulties and loss of the cough reflex; this requires the same nursing care as for a cerebellar tumour.

If there is a facial nerve palsy the patient will be unable to close his eye, and an eye-glass will be provided to prevent damage to the cornea, and to prevent infection. The nurse devotes special care to the eye until the patient's condition allows a tarsorrhaphy (this is a partial suturing together of the upper and lower lid). Vision of the eye is thus reduced, which must be remembered during rehabilitation.

Physiotherapy

Physiotherapy is as for cerebellar tumours, but special attention is frequently required to retrain oro-facial dysfunction. This is best done by a co-ordinated programme arranged between the speech therapist, the physiotherapist and the nursing staff. It can be a most frustrating and humiliating experience for a patient to find he is unable to feed himself, that he dribbles and drools, and that he is unable to manipulate the food in his mouth. If he cannot control liquids adequately, and hence coughs and splutters, he feels he is choking with every mouthful. Some of these difficulties can be overcome by ensuring correct head position, by facilitating a co-contraction of the tongue and cheeks, by encouraging mental practice, and by carefully selecting a food of appropriate consistency. Water, although safest to attempt, is very difficult because it is so runny, and the patient is unable to control it with his slower and inaccurate movements. Clearly lumpy or chunky foodstuffs are equally inappropriate to begin with, and generally the most satisfactory consistency is that of ice-cream, purée, custard or yoghurt. Slowly and carefully the patient progresses to both more-liquid and more-solid foods as he learns to cope with the difficulty.

PARKINSONIAN SYNDROME

Parkinsonism is described in *Neurology for Physiotherapists*, and only points relating to the surgical management of the condition will be discussed.

Stereotaxic surgery is used mainly for the treatment of tremor, and careful selection of patients is essential, with an upper age limit usually of 65 years. A patient older than this is only considered if he is essentially unilaterally affected and has no physical or mental deterioration. The best results are obtained from the under-60 age-group with a slowly progressive form of the disease.

INVESTIGATIONS AND ASSESSMENTS

Plain X-ray films of the skull are taken. Electro-encephalography is performed and neuro-physiological measurements of the tremor are recorded. The patient is fully assessed by the psychologist, the speech therapist, the occupational therapist and the physiotherapist.

Surgery

Before describing the surgical procedure for treating Parkinsonism it is proposed to discuss the technique of stereotaxy.

STEREOTAXY

This surgical technique aims to obliterate a small amount of brain tissue, and is becoming widely used for the treatment of quite diverse conditions, for instance certain movement disorders, epilepsy, intractable pain, and some psychiatric conditions.

The general procedure requires fixing a special frame containing the lesion-making apparatus to the skull. Water soluble contrast medium is introduced into the ventricles via a burr hole, and X-rays are taken. Measurements on the X-rays are taken relating the outlined structures to the target area. The target point is then related to the stereotactic frame, and an electrode introduced to the target point.

The trajectory of the electrode is checked by recording from the nervous tissue during advancement of the electrode. At the target point a radio-frequency current is passed and the lesion made at the electrode tip. The size of the lesion is adjusted by the electrode size, or by moving it slightly. Usually the lesion is only about 5mm×3mm (Hitchcock, 1978).

Specific lesions may be made into the thalamic or dentate nuclei of the brain, and are sometimes indicated for the abolition or reduction of involuntary movements such as dystonias, dyskinesias (for example choreo-athetosis and hemiballismus) and spasticity. The classic example is in the treatment of Parkinsonian tremor. Some psychiatric conditions benefit from discrete surgical lesions, and occasionally leucotomy, amygdalotomy, cingulectomy, and partial fronto-thalamic lesions are made. These latter procedures are usually carried out through a burr hole, and complications are rare.

Stereotaxic surgery for Parkinsonism is carried out under local anaesthetic in two stages, occasionally completed within the same day, but usually with a day of rest between.

The first stage consists of placing markers in the skull as a guide to the mid-sagittal plane of the brain.

The second stage consists of performing contrast ventriculography to outline the anterior and posterior commissures. An electrode is passed through an occipital burr hole to the thalamus (Fig. 15/17).

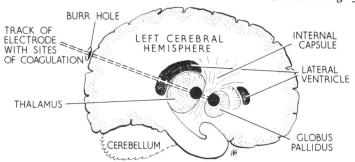

Fig. 15/17 Diagram showing the position of the burr hole in stereotaxic surgery for Parkinsonism

Coagulation is carried out in the ventro-lateral nucleus of the thalamus to reduce tremor and in the globus pallidus to reduce rigidity.

Stereotaxy is now being used mainly for the relief of tremor. Rigidity is being treated by the use of drugs, L-dopa being widely used.

Physiotherapy

Breathing exercises must be practised hourly by the patient to reduce the risk of bronchopneumonia. Coughing may be difficult for the patient whose main symptom is rigidity.

The limbs freed from rigidity and tremor may require functional re-education. After loss of severe tremor the type of stabilising exercises described for cerebellar ataxia (p. 311) help the patient to regain functional use of his limbs, particularly the upper limb. Full range joint mobility is rapidly regained when symptoms have been relieved.

The patient is allowed to sit up in bed the day after operation and to get up on the second postoperative day. Balance re-education is important for a patient with rigidity as the main symptom, and stabilisation in sitting and standing is useful, the patient watching himself in a mirror. A patient with mainly tremor has little or no problem in regaining balance. Re-education of standing up and sitting down, walking, walking with arm swinging and turning round require patience and perseverance.

Standing up and sitting down, especially if a low chair is being used, is difficult for a Parkinsonian patient. He must be taught to tuck his feet well underneath him, then use his hands on the edge of the chair to push his weight forward over his feet, then to straighten up. When sitting down he must be taught to feel for the chair and lower himself down gently.

Walking. To re-educate walking it must be impressed upon the patient to lift his feet and take a big step. Lifting the feet is over-emphasised at the outset; marking time on the spot prior to walking can be a useful preliminary followed by stepping over lines on the floor.

To re-educate arm-swinging while walking, poles are used, the patient holding one end of the pole in each hand, and the physiotherapist walking behind holding the other ends. Arm-swinging is done at first by the physiotherapist pushing the appropriate pole with the patient gradually taking over.

Turning. The great tendency is for the patient to jerk round suddenly when turning. He must be taught to do this slowly and lift his feet up. Re-education can begin with marking time on the spot, then turning round slowly still marking time.

Stairs. Apart from any difficulty with balance, the Parkinsonian patient rarely has difficulty in going up or down stairs.

PROGRESSION OF TREATMENT

Progress can be made rapidly in the physiotherapy and occupational therapy departments once the patient is allowed up. About the third day he will be able to participate in some class work to music to assist re-education of balance and mobility. The class work can be increased on successive days to a full programme which includes exercises in sitting, standing and on the mat. Mat work to retrain rolling, sitting up, standing up to lying down and vice versa, and exercises on the mat to strengthen back extensor muscles are useful in that they help the patient regain his independence. He can then begin to move about in bed and get in and out of bed, activities which he will previously have found difficult.

EPILEPSY

Epilepsy can be described as a paroxysmal transitory disturbance of the functions of the brain which develops suddenly, ceases spontaneously, with a strong tendency to recurrence. Many varieties of epileptic attack exist, depending upon the site of origin, extent of spread and the nature of the disturbance of function.

Causes

Epilepsy may be caused by:

A local lesion in the brain, such as tumour or abscess, where epilepsy is the presenting feature.

Complication of a head injury due to a post-traumatic scar.
Hereditary predisposition.
Unknown causes.

INVESTIGATIONS

Electro-encephalography. Recordings of the electrical activity of the brain can help to pinpoint the cause of epilepsy. If a focus can be determined, its nature can be investigated by other means.

Further appropriate measures will be selected according to the particular history of the patient.

Surgical Treatment

Until recently surgery has only been indicated for certain selected cases and has been of value to a patient who has epilepsy as the presenting feature of a brain lesion, or a definite focus which gives rise to his epileptic attacks.

Surgical procedures vary with the type of lesion to be excised. Temporal lobe epilepsy may be treated by lobectomy. Increasingly stereotaxic procedures are being employed to treat certain forms of epilepsy, particularly a diffuse type which cannot be treated by drugs or cortical excision.

Physiotherapy

A general programme of rehabilitation is carried out; defects are treated according to the symptoms.

INTRACTABLE PAIN

In conditions where pain is unable to be controlled pharmacologically, or where other surgical procedures which are potentially less hazardous have failed, it is sometimes necessary to attempt to control pain at higher neurological centres (Fig. 15/18). Chapter 16 also discusses procedures for relief of pain (p. 351).

INVESTIGATIONS

In all cases a thorough assessment of the pain is essential; skull and chest X-rays are a usual preliminary to stereotactic surgery.

Thalamotomy

Sometimes small lesions of the ventro-postero-medial part of the

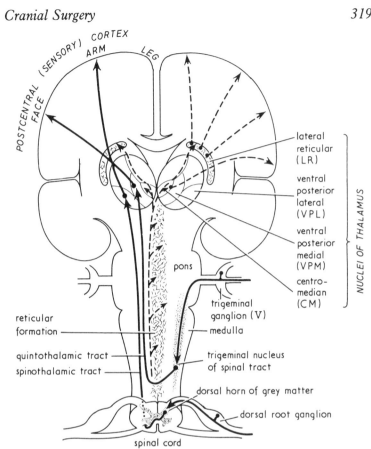

Fig. 15/18 Projections of some pain pathways. The centromedian nucleus (CM) and the ventro-postero-medial nucleus (VPM) of the thalamus are sites for stereotaxic interruption of central pain pathways. Interruption of the trigeminal nerve tract at spinal or pontine levels or at the trigeminal ganglion are possible sites for treating facial pain

thalamus or para-fascicular nuclei are made stereotactically to relieve pain, without causing significant sensory loss.

REFERENCES

Bethune, D. D. (1975). 'Neurophysiological facilitation of respiration in the unconscious adult patient'. *Physiotherapy, Canada*, 27 (5), 241.

Downie, Patricia A. (1978). *Cancer Rehabilitation: an Introduction for Physiotherapists and the Allied Professions*. Faber and Faber.

Greenbaum, R. (1976). 'General anaesthesia for neurosurgery'. *British Journal of Anaesthetics*, **48**, 773.

Hitchcock, E. R. (1978). 'Stereotactic surgery for cerebral palsy'. *Nursing Times*, **74,** 50, 2064.

Jennett, B. (1977). *An Introduction to Neurosurgery.* 3rd edition. William Heinemann Medical Books Ltd.

Lance, J. W. and McLeod, J. G. (1975). *A Physiological Approach to Clinical Neurology.* 2nd edition. Butterworths.

Landa, J. F., Hirsch, J. A. and Lebeax, M. I. (1975). 'Effects of topical and general anaesthetic agents on tracheal mucus velocity of sheep'. *Journal of Applied Physiology*, **38** (5), 946.

Pincus, S. (1975). *Respiratory Therapist Manual.* The Bobbs-Merrill Co. Inc.

Teasedale, G. and Jennett, B. (1974). 'An assessment of coma and impaired consciousness. A practical side'. *Lancet*, July 13.

BIBLIOGRAPHY

See end of Chapter 16.

Chapter 16

Spinal Cord Surgery

revised by P. A. DAWE, M.A.P.A.

ANATOMY AND PHYSIOLOGY

The spinal cord lies within the vertebral canal and extends from the foramen magnum to the lower border of the first lumbar vertebra. It is surrounded by three fibrous coverings known as the meninges, as is the brain, and the cerebrospinal fluid circulates in the subarachnoid space between the pia mater and the arachnoid mater (Fig. 16/1). This space descends as far as the second sacral vertebra.

The blood supply is rich but complex and mainly derived from the posterior spinal arteries, the anterior spinal artery and segmental arteries which enter by the intervertebral foramina (Fig. 16/2).

Thirty-one pairs of nerves are given off symmetrically from the cord, thus dividing the cord into segments (Fig. 16/3). As the cord is

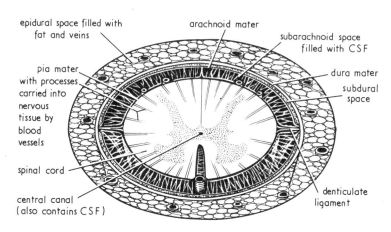

epidural space filled with
fat and veins

arachnoid mater

subarachnoid space
filled with CSF

pia mater
with processes
carried into
nervous
tissue by
blood
vessels

dura mater

subdural
space

spinal cord

central canal
(also contains CSF)

denticulate
ligament

Fig. 16/1 The meninges of the spinal cord in the spinal canal

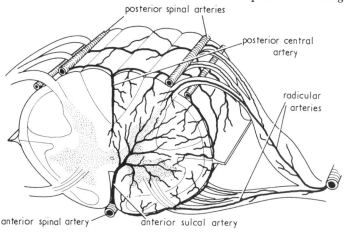

Fig. 16/2 Cross-section of the cervical spinal cord showing the distribution of blood supply from the anterior spinal and posterior spinal arteries

shorter than the vertebral canal the segments are not aligned with the numerically corresponding vertebrae. In the cervical region the segments lie one vertebra higher, while in the lumbar region the fifth lumbar nerve root is given off at the level of the twelfth thoracic vertebra. The mass of lumbar and sacral nerve roots given off at the lower end of the spinal cord is termed the cauda equina (Fig. 16/3).

Each nerve root consists of an anterior motor root and a posterior sensory root, which pass separately through the dura mater, then unite. They then descend to the appropriate intervertebral foramen through which they issue. The course of these nerves is almost horizontal in the cervical region, but the lumbar nerves have a long vertical course before reaching their appropriate point of exit (Fig. 16/3).

EFFECTS OF COMPRESSION ON THE SPINAL CORD

Any lesion in the region of the spinal cord which causes pressure affects the spinal cord and nerve roots in several ways:

Direct pressure interferes with conduction in the nerve roots and the spinal cord. Myelin is more vulnerable to both mechanical pressure and minor degrees of anoxia than nerve cells or axons and therefore the effects of compression are usually greatest in the myelinated fibres of the white columns (Blackwood and Corsellis, 1976).

Pressure on the veins leads to oedema.

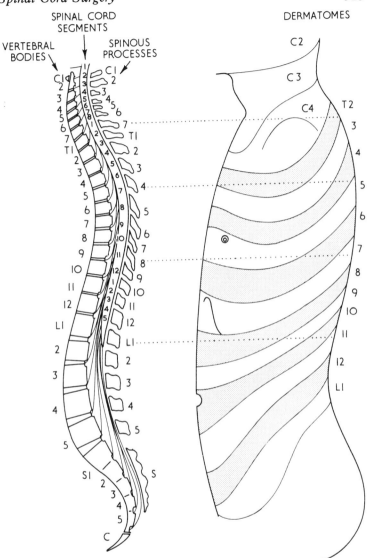

Fig. 16/3 Spinal cord segments and spinal nerves

Spinal Cord Surgery

Pressure on the arteries leads to ischaemia and degeneration of nerve cells and fibres then takes place in the area (Fig. 16/2).

The subarachnoid space becomes obstructed.

Compression of the cord can occur anywhere throughout its length and affects one or several segments. The pressure may affect both sides if the lesion is central, or one side more than the other if the lesion is lateral. Pressure on one side of the cord can gradually displace the cord and the nerve roots towards the opposite side of the vertebral canal, thus involving the healthy side. Motor and sensory symptoms can arise on both sides of the body if the lesion is central but can give a Brown-Séquard type of syndrome if the lesion is confined to one side of the cord.

Brown-Séquard Syndrome

Complete hemi-section of the spinal cord (the Brown-Séquard Syndrome) rarely occurs clinically. It is generally a matter of degree. Ipsilaterally, i.e. on the side of the lesion, the following occurs:

1. There is ipsilateral loss of voluntary power, since the cerebrospinal tracts cross mainly in the medulla oblongata which lies above the area of compression. There is lower motor neurone paralysis in the segments of the lesion, and upper motor neurone paralysis below the level of the lesion.
2. There is ipsilateral loss of muscle and joint sense, vibratory sense and tactile discrimination due to involvement of the posterior column.
3. Fibres of the lateral spinothalamic tract entering the cord just below the level of the lesion are caught before they cross, causing a narrow zone of pain and temperature loss immediately below the lesion.
4. There is an ipsilateral zone of cutaneous anaesthesia in the segment of the lesion (Fig. 16/4).

On the contralateral side i.e. opposite to the side of the lesion, the findings are as follows:

1. There is loss of pain and temperature sensations due to destruction of the lateral spinothalamic tract, fibres of which enter the cord and ascend for several segments, then cross. The upper level of the sensory loss is therefore a few segments below the level of the lesion.
2. Fibres carrying light touch and tactile localisation are partly crossed and partly uncrossed, thus there is rarely loss of these sensibilities in a unilateral lesion.

MOTOR TRACTS
(DESCENDING — EFFERENT)

SENSORY TRACTS
(ASCENDING – AFFERENT)

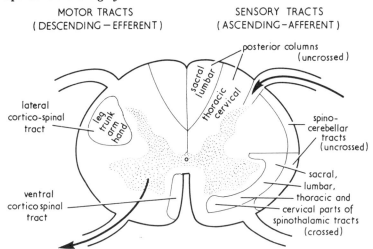

Fig. 16/4 Ascending and descending spinal cord tracts

Pressure may be localised and affect only one nerve root, resulting in pain, sensory loss and motor weakness in the distribution of this particular nerve root. In this case the sensory loss will be incomplete as structures are rarely supplied by one nerve, but hyperaesthesia can be present as an early feature.

Onset of Cord Compression

Acute compression usually occurs with either malignant disease or sudden vertebral collapse or abscess formation. It may be accompanied by severe pain and rapidly progressing motor and sensory disturbances.

Chronic compression which develops slowly, may produce symptoms of pain first, due either to bone erosion, root pain or spinal mechanics.

Cord compression is considered a matter of surgical urgency, and clinical examination and special investigations are made to establish the exact site, extent and nature of the lesion.

PAIN

Pain is a perceived response to noxious stimuli, so there are physiological as well as psychological connotations. It is the experience of 'pain' for which the patient seeks help; and in relation to the spine, there are a number of structures which appear to produce a pain response.

Lesions of the spine and spinal cord may also involve the related structures: joints, muscles and skin. Irritation or swelling of these structures causes deformity of the pain receptors; impulses are discharged and pain is experienced. Dilatation and oedema of the local blood vessels is commonly present, producing a throbbing quality to the pain, caused by pulsation of the capillaries.

Root pain is the result of the irritant effect of a lesion on the nerve fibres, and is a prominent feature in extramedullary lesions, such as neurinoma and extradural neoplasms, and when nerve roots are involved in cauda equina or disc lesions. Pain is usually the earliest symptom and has a specific distribution relating to the involved nerve (Figs. 16/5 and 16/6). Kellgren (1939) showed that inflammation or compression of a posterior root produced pain referred to the sclerotome and paraesthesia to the appropriate dermatome.

Continuing and severe pressure results in decreased conductivity of the nerves and pain then diminishes.

Movements which stretch a tethered or trapped nerve root will cause sharp pain, radiating along the course of the nerve.

Pressure over the spinous processes may elicit pain. Vertebrae receive their nerve supply from several segments above.

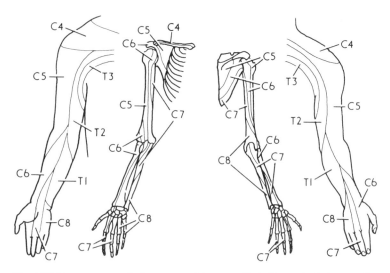

Fig. 16/5 Dermatomes and sclerotomes of the upper limb. Paraesthesia is generally referred to the dermatome and pain to the sclerotome

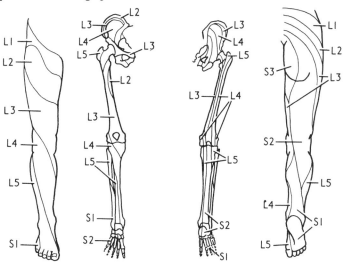

Fig. 16/6 Dermatomes and sclerotomes of the lower limb

A sudden increase of the pressure in the intraspinal canal, caused by coughing, sneezing and straining, causes increased root pain.

Involvement of the spinothalamic tracts at any part of their course may initiate a burning pain in the opposite half of the body below the point at which the tracts are affected.

LOSS OF MOTOR POWER

This usually follows the sensory disturbance and takes the form of a progressive weakness. The muscles affected are those supplied by the segments of the cord which are being compressed and those supplied by the segments below the lesion. If the lesion is unilateral the weakness is present on the same side of the body; with a central lesion both sides are involved, but one side is usually more affected than the other.

MUSCLE TONE

At the level of the lesion tone will be diminished or lost, as this constitutes a lower motor neurone lesion. Below the level of the lesion there is an upper motor neurone lesion and tone will be increased as the pyramidal and extrapyramidal tracts are interrupted and the reflex arc is no longer inhibited by higher centres. In a cauda equina lesion, which is essentially a 'root' problem, only a lower motor neurone lesion exists.

It soon becomes apparent to the physiotherapist who treats patients with spinal cord lesions and those with lesions originating from a higher neurological level, that while both may have spasticity, there are different characteristics in the behaviour of such spasticity, depending on the degree of control, or lack of it, from higher centres.

REFLEXES

A summary of the reflexes usually tested is given in Table I.

As with muscle tone, reflexes are diminished at the level of the lesion and increased below the lesion. For example, a cord lesion at the 5th cervical level, causes a lower motor neurone lesion of C5 and an upper motor neurone lesion of muscles innervated below this level. At this particular level it can be demonstrated by the so-called 'inverted supinator jerk', where, when testing the 'supinator' jerk, there is diminished or absent activity of the brachioradialis (C5, C6) and elbow flexors, and exaggeration of finger flexion (C7, C8, T1) and triceps (C6, C7, C8) activity (Bickerstaff, 1976).

SENSATION

This is diminished or lost below the lesion. Types of sensation involved will depend on which ascending tracts are affected (Fig. 16/4). Involvement of the posterior column will affect kinaesthetic sensation, while the antero-lateral column will affect pain and temperature. In cauda equina lesions sensory loss of all types is likely in the root distribution.

SPHINCTERS

These are not involved in the early stages but later precipitancy or difficulty with micturition develops and this may progress to retention of urine. Constipation is most usual with spinal neoplasms. Rectal incontinence rarely occurs.

Impotence may occur with cauda equina lesions.

AUTONOMIC DISTURBANCES

Since the whole of the sympathetic output leaves the spinal cord between the first thoracic and the second lumbar segments, spinal cord lesions will show discrepancies between the distributions of the somatic and sympathetic disturbances. Lesions at or above C8 may cause disturbances of sympathetic function over the whole body, and lesions below L2 have no sympathetic effects.

Lesions at T1 or T2 may involve the ascending sympathetic fibres which supply the orbit (the back of the eye, the dilator muscle of the pupil and the smooth muscle of the upper lid). Interruption of these

TABLE I. REFLEXES

Superficial reflexes	Deep (muscle) reflexes	Visceral reflexes	Segmental level	Peripheral nerve
		Pupillary light response }	Midbrain	Cranial 2 and 3
Corneal			Pons	Cranial 5 and 7
Gag (pharyngeal and uvular)			Medulla	Cranial 9 and 10
	Jaw		Pons	Cranial 5
	Biceps		C5, C6	Musculo-cutaneous
	Brachio-radialis (Supinator)		C5, C6	Radial
	Triceps		C6, C7	Radial
	Wrist flexion		C6, C8	Median
	Wrist extension		C7, C8	Radial
	Finger flexion		C8	Median
Upper abdominal			T7, T8, T9, T10	T7, T8, T9, T10
Lower abdominal			T10, T11, T12	T10, T11, T12
	Knee (patella)		L3, T4	Femoral
	Hamstrings		L5, S1 S2	Sciatic (trunk)
	Ankle (Achilles)		S1, S2	Tibial

fibres may then produce Horner's syndrome (de Palma and Rothman, 1970).

If there is considerable disruption of conduction the control from higher centres is impaired, and with complete transection of the cord, excessive sweating frequently occurs over the parts thus isolated. Vasomotor disturbances may occur, with impaired body temperature and blood pressure regulation resulting in impaired circulation.

CEREBROSPINAL FLUID

If there is an obstruction of the subarachnoid space the chemical composition of this fluid changes. Its protein content is increased, which provides useful diagnostic information.

Special Investigations

After careful clinical examination special investigations are carried out to establish the exact site, extent and nature of the lesion.

X-rays. Plain films are usually necessary.

Lumbar puncture is carried out to obtain specimens of cerebrospinal fluid for diagnostic purposes and to establish if there is a block of the subarachnoid space (see p. 286).

Myelography. Myodil, or air, usually the former, is introduced via a lumbar puncture needle and guided to the appropriate region. Where a complete spinal block is present, the contrast medium may be introduced via a cisternal puncture into the cisterna magna and allowed to flow down to outline the upper level of the lesion. Myodil is removed at the end of the examination as it tends to act as an irritant.

Lumbar radiculography. A water-soluble contrast medium such as Conray 280 or Dimer X is now being used to investigate lumbar nerve roots. Following this examination the patient has to remain erect (seated or propped up in bed) for six hours in order to prevent the contrast medium reaching the spinal cord, as it is very irritating.

Assessment

A full neurological investigation will be carried out by the medical staff. Physiotherapists who would like to know more about the rationale of these are referred to the bibliography at the end of the chapter.

The physiotherapy assessment for a spinal cord or nerve root condition will include:

1. Carefully reading the patient's notes.
2. Enquiring from the patient how the condition has developed.
3. Examination which will include defining the site and type of pain; muscle power; muscle tone; reflexes; sensation; range of movement of limbs and cautious examination of vertebral movements; palpation of spine and paravertebral muscles; standing posture and balance; gait (unless paralysed); functional activities; special tests e.g. Lasègue's straight leg raising test for sciatic nerve stretch; femoral nerve stretch test; Kernig's bent-knee stretch test.
4. Pre-operative chest assessment and care if necessary.

GENERAL CLASSIFICATION OF CONDITIONS IN WHICH SURGERY HAS A ROLE

NEOPLASMS

1. Primary neoplasms may arise from the cord or its central canal, the meninges and the sheaths of the spinal nerves.
2. Secondary neoplasms usually involve the vertebral bodies and may cause compression of the spinal cord and nerve roots.

INFECTIONS

These are either intradural, e.g. staphylococcal infection or extradural, e.g. epidural abscess from tracking infection, tuberculosis.

DEGENERATIVE LESIONS

These will include protruded intervertebral discs, cervical spondylosis and lumbar stenosis.

CONGENITAL CONDITIONS

These will include spina bifida, diastematomyelia, syringomyelia, cervical rib and vascular anomalies e.g. angiomas.

These conditions will not be discussed in this chapter and physiotherapists who wish to know more about them should consult the bibliography.

SPINAL CORD INJURY

Physiotherapists are referred to *Neurology for Physiotherapists* for full details of the care required for these patients.

INTRACTABLE PAIN

NEOPLASMS

Neoplasms of the Spinal Cord

Spinal neoplasms occur in any age-group, but are rather more common between the ages of 20 and 60. The sexes are affected equally.

They are classified as extradural (those which lie outside the membranes surrounding the cord), and intradural (those which lie inside the membranes). The intradural type is further classified into extramedullary tumours, which do not enter the spinal cord (such as the meningiomas) and intramedullary tumours which arise in the substance of the cord (such as gliomas and meningiomas) (Fig. 16/7).

The onset of symptoms is variable depending on the specific tumour.

SURGICAL TREATMENT

To relieve compression of the spinal cord caused by neoplasms, a laminectomy is usually carried out at the appropriate level. For fairly extensive lesions, adequate exposure is needed, so several vertebral segments may be included. Although it is argued that multiple laminectomy may leave the spine unstable, this appears to be unfounded provided the intervertebral discs are healthy and left intact.

Laminectomy

A fairly long mid-line incision is made and the back muscles stripped from the spinous processes and the laminae, which are then removed; the number removed depends on the extent of the lesion. Neoplasms of the extramedullary type are removed entirely or as far as possible. The intramedullary type which invade the cord substance may not be removed entirely. The cord will be incised and as much material as possible removed, the dura being left open to effect a further decompression.

POSTOPERATIVE TREATMENT

On return from theatre the patient is nursed in side lying with a pillow supporting his back, his underneath leg straight and the top leg flexed at hip and knee and supported by two pillows, one under the thigh and one under the leg. To prevent pressure sores two-hourly turns are essential, the patient going from side to front, from front to his other side. If there are signs of bladder involvement prior to operation, a catheter will be draining the bladder, which is maintained until bladder function returns or an automatic bladder trained.

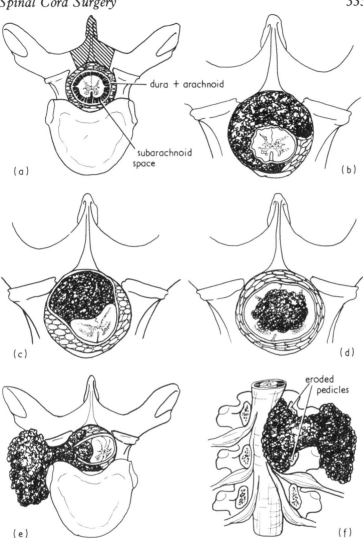

Fig. 16/7 Sites and types of spinal tumour. a) Normal appearance. b) Extradural. c) Intradural (extramedullary). d) Intramedullary. e) Intraspinal – partially intradural and also outside the vertebral column. f) Coronal section

If there is loss of sensation the patient will be nursed on pillow packs to prevent the development of pressure sores. Great care must be taken to ensure that the coverings on the packs are kept unwrinkled. Positioning and turning procedures are as previously described. A bed cage is used to keep the weight of the bedclothes off the feet and a firm support placed at the bottom of the bed to maintain the feet at right angles, thus preventing a foot drop.

For a lesion of the cervical spine, with loss of power and sensation in the upper limbs, careful positioning of the arms is necessary to ensure that the elbows do not develop flexion contractures. A roll of Sorbo rubber in the hand keeps the fingers in a functional position and the wrist in slight extension. If necessary a pillow can be used to keep the upper arm away from the chest wall.

With an extensive laminectomy the patient may find lying on the back uncomfortable until the tenth day, when sutures will be removed, or partly so, and the wound feels less tender. The patient is generally only allowed to sit out of bed after the wound is well healed and frequently requires analgesics. As these lesions frequently occur in the dorsal region, respiratory movements may be responsible for some of the pain. The physiotherapist will need to be guided in the extent of her treatments by the progress of the patient and by the preferred wishes of the surgeon.

Neoplasms of the Vertebral Column

The most common type of neoplasm is a secondary deposit which develops in a vertebral body. The primary lesion is often in the breast in women and the prostate gland or the lung in men. Metastatic lesions may progress very rapidly, be extremely painful and give rise to acute spinal cord compression which requires emergency treatment. Primary neoplasm, such as sarcoma, is very uncommon.

SURGICAL MANAGEMENT

Laminectomy and decompression are generally required, and the postoperative care is as for spinal neoplasms. Occasionally where there is gross bony destruction, it may be necessary to stabilise the spine, e.g. by fusion or posterior wiring, and then the postoperative treatment is much more conservative, frequently with several weeks of bed rest. This procedure would only be undertaken either where the prognosis in the case of disseminated malignant disease was considered reasonable or if the presenting condition was caused by a benign lesion.

When these patients are finally allowed to get out of bed, it is usually necessary to use a spinal brace for extra support and protection. When measuring for and fitting such braces, great care must be taken to ensure that the patient's spine is not moved unnecessarily.

Some types of spinal and vertebral neoplasms are sensitive to irradiation and decompression procedures may be followed by a course of radiotherapy. During such time, physiotherapy treatment may have to be modified because of side-effects.

INFECTIONS OF THE SPINE

Epidural Abscess

This can result from the spread of infection from the vertebral column, e.g. osteomyelitis; it may be blood-borne from the lungs, peritoneal cavity, or from a skin infection; or be introduced from without, e.g. at lumbar puncture. The mid-thoracic level is the most commonly affected, and pus is usually posterior to the cord. The onset of the symptoms may be acute, sub-acute or chronic. Once pressure on the spinal cord has been relieved, antibiotics are introduced by means of a drain to control the infection.

Tuberculosis (Pott's Disease)

This condition, now relatively uncommon in Western Countries, occurs predominantly in children and young adults, although no age-group is exempt. The infective process usually begins in the body of a vertebra and spreads to adjacent vertebral bodies which leads to their collapse. An angular deformity of the spine is thus produced. This deformity, associated tuberculous abscess, or interference with the vascular supply of subjacent segments, can disturb spinal cord function and result in paraplegia.

SURGICAL TREATMENT

Laminectomy and decompression, excision of the abscess cavity, and sometimes spinal fixation is carried out.

On return to the ward, the patient is 'barrier nursed' to prevent spread of infection, and the physiotherapist must be meticulous in carrying out the procedures advocated by the ward sister. Post-operative physiotherapy is appropriate for the level of the lesion, but similar to that after spinal cord and vertebral neoplasms.

Physiotherapy

BREATHING EXERCISES AND COUGHING

When a lesion involves the intercostal and abdominal muscles, the diaphragm is the only remaining muscle of respiration. The patient must be encouraged to practise breathing exercises regularly to reduce the danger of bronchopneumonia. Coughing will be reduced in force and can be assisted by pushing up under the diaphragm with the hand. Where voluntary power allows, the patient is taught to do this for himself, and if he is unable to do so the nurses are taught how to assist him.

MAINTENANCE EXERCISES

These are carried out where possible to maintain circulation. If no voluntary power is present, passive movements are carried out twice daily.

CAREFUL POSITIONING AND PASSIVE MOVEMENTS

These are necessary to prevent contractures. When the arms are involved it is important to retain full range shoulder movements, full extension of the elbow and prevent tightening of the wrist and finger flexors. Flexion and extension of the metacarpophalangeal joints and a full stretch on the web of the thumb are important. In the lower limb it is important to retain full extension of the hip and knee and the ability to get the feet to a right angle. Hamstring muscles should not be allowed to become tight. During the first few postoperative days no hamstring stretching should be given as it might produce pain due to stretching of the nerve roots and a pull on the meninges. After approximately one week gentle hamstring stretching can be commenced in a small range, gradually increasing until the leg, with the foot at 90° to the leg, can be raised to a right angle to the body.

RETURN OF FUNCTION

This is encouraged by means of facilitation techniques.

STATIC CONTRACTIONS

Static abdominal and back muscle contractions can begin on the first day. Active abdominal work can begin when the sutures are removed and active back extension is begun gently on approximately the third day.

SHOULDER GIRDLE STRENGTHENING

This may be started immediately with arm exercises. If the incision is a high one care must be taken that there is no pull on the wound. Spring resistance can be given if there is no danger of pulling on the wound, and can be commenced when the patient's back is comfortable. When there is gross loss of voluntary power in the lower limbs it is most important to develop the muscles of the shoulder girdle and latissimus dorsi as they will be required for lifting and when walking with crutches.

BALANCE RE-EDUCATION

This begins when the patient is allowed to get up approximately after the fourth day. It is advisable to get him to tolerate an upright position in bed before he gets up. Balance re-education can begin by sitting the patient over the edge of the bed with the feet supported on the floor or on a stool, then in a wheelchair. In the early stages a mirror is useful to help the patient regain his balance, especially if he has sensory loss. When he has gained balance in a wheelchair and on the edge of the bed, mat work can be started and balance in long sitting.

Mat work. The patient must practise sitting up, rolling from side to side and rolling on to his front, getting into a kneeling position and balancing in this position. He must practise moving across and up and down the mat using his arms to lift his buttocks. Hip raising and balancing in this position helps to regain stability. Back extension, hip extension and hamstring exercises can be given in prone lying. Crawling in all directions, free and against resistance, helps to strengthen hip muscles. Further balance re-education is done in kneeling and half kneeling and practise in getting from this position on and off a chair or stool is the next progression.

Wheelchair. If the patient has a gross or permanent disability a wheelchair will be necessary to enable him to become independent. Each patient is measured and a chair and Sorbo cushion ordered to his specific requirements. The patient must be taught to control and manoeuvre his chair. When his balance and arm power are adequate the patient is taught to transfer himself from bed to wheelchair and from wheelchair to bed. Later he is taught to get from his chair to the mat and vice versa.

RE-EDUCATION OF WALKING

Re-education of walking commences with balance in standing. This usually begins with the patient between parallel bars with a mirror in front of him. When the patient can balance satisfactorily, walking re-education is commenced. The ability to progress along these lines depends on the degree of voluntary power loss. When the patient is ready to stand, various aids may be necessary. As a temporary measure plaster back slabs to keep the knees straight may be used. If gross muscle weakness persists calipers will be needed. The calipers are made to measure with a corset top, jointed at the knee, and a toe-raising device if necessary. If weakness is only in the anterior tibial muscles below-knee calipers may be needed.

The type of gait taught depends upon the level of the lesion. This may be four-point if the lesion is at or below the tenth thoracic segment, or swing-to, for lesions above this level. Once walking has become controlled in the parallel bars the patient can progress to using elbow crutches, beginning with one bar and one crutch, then balancing on both crutches, then to walking. A mirror can be used at the beginning of each progression until the patient gains the correct idea of balance and gait. If the patient uses a wheelchair he must be taught how to stand up and sit down using his crutches.

Stairs. The patient can be re-educated to use the stairs by using a banister rail and one elbow crutch. Going up the stairs the patient puts his crutch up on the step first then jumps his feet up. Coming down he swings his legs down one step then brings his crutch down.

When a patient has voluntary control of his hips and knees, elbow crutches are not necessary. He can walk with the aid of quadruped or tripod sticks in initial stages, and may be progressed to walking sticks when his balance and confidence improve. When going upstairs he uses the banister rail and one stick. He puts his stick up first, then his right foot, the stick goes up to the next step, followed by his left foot. Coming down he puts his stick down first, then his right foot to the same step, his stick down to the next step followed by his left foot.

A patient with sensory loss. Measures taken to prevent pressure sores developing in the early stages of postoperative care have already been mentioned (p. 332) and nursing care has been directed to this end. If beds become wet they are immediately changed and the patient sponged and dried. Time must be taken to explain to the patient what this sensory loss means to him and he must be taught to look after his skin to prevent any sores developing. He should be instructed in the following points:

He must examine his skin carefully each day, using a mirror where necessary.

A hot-water bottle must never be used.

Special care must be taken when cutting toe and fingernails. If there is a tendency to ingrowing toenails the skin should be massaged away from the nail. If the nail does grow into the skin, suppuration may occur and the nail may need to be removed.

If thick hard skin develops on hands and feet it should be softened with cream or olive oil and removed.

Bath water must be checked for temperature before the patient gets into the bath. A piece of sponge rubber in the bottom of the bath prevents the patient getting bruised. Cold water should be run into the bath first in case the heat of the bath itself causes a burn.

Warning should be given with regard to sitting near fires and radiators and in direct sunlight.

In cold weather the feet must be kept warm to prevent chilblains developing.

For patients with loss of sensation in the hands, cups should have a protective covering or holder and a cigarette holder must be used if the patient smokes.

When sitting in a chair he must frequently lift his buttocks off the cushion to relieve pressure. This is taught immediately he starts using his wheelchair. If arm power is inadequate a physiotherapist, or nurse, must lift the patient regularly until his balance will allow him to move sufficiently from hip to hip to relieve pressure.

If the patient wishes to sit in an ordinary armchair he must make sure it has a soft seat.

Shoes must be chosen carefully to ensure they do not produce sores; it is advisable for them to be of soft leather with no toecaps and a half-size larger and wider fitting than previously worn.

If a pressure sore develops the quickest way to heal this is to keep the patient in bed and nurse him in a position which will keep all pressure from the area. He should not be allowed to get up again until the sore is adequately healed.

INTERVERTEBRAL DISCS

Intervertebral discs are found between the bodies of the movable vertebrae and extend from the second cervical vertebra to the lumbo-sacral junction. In the lumbar region they are much thicker and shaped to the lumbar curve. Each vertebral body is covered with hyaline cartilage and the disc, consisting of an outer fibrocartilaginous annulus fibrosus and an inner gelatinous nucleus pulposus, is sandwiched between. The annulus fibrosus is weakest posterolaterally where it is inadequately supported by the spinous ligaments. This is where it becomes thinned as a result of trauma and may rupture completely if the initial trauma is sufficiently severe.

When the annulus fibrosus becomes thinned the results are as follows (Fig. 16/8):

The nucleus pulposus bulges at the weakened point. The nerve root passing down the vertebral canal to emerge through the appropriate intervertebral foramen becomes stretched over this bulge. This causes

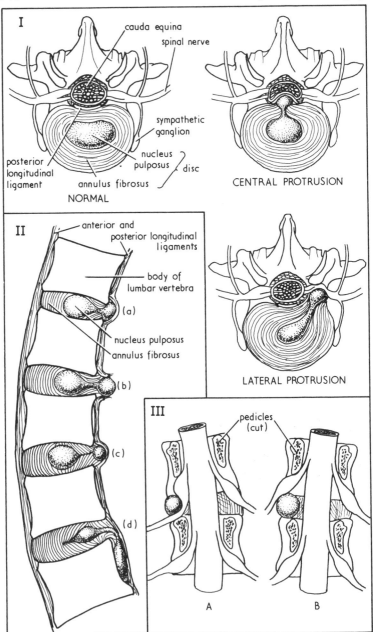

Fig. 16/8 Lumbar intervertebral disc herniations. I. Normal disc and nerve roots. Central protrusion. Lateral protrusion (Lumbar 3 seen from above). II. Lateral view of central disc herniations. III. Inclination of the spine to relieve compression of the nerve root pain due to irritation with subsequent compression, causing loss of sensation and motor power.

The annulus fibrosus may rupture and allow the nucleus to pass through the opening in the spinous ligaments to lie in the vertebral canal.

Occasionally the nucleus pulposus may herniate in the mid-line giving rise to symptoms similar to a spinal cord neoplasm in the cervical region and a cauda equina lesion in the lumbar region.

LUMBAR DISC HERNIATIONS

The lumbar region is the commonest site of a disc herniation. The highest incidence is between the fourth and fifth lumbar vertebrae and the fifth lumbar and the first sacral vertebrae.

General Signs and Symptoms of a Lumbar Disc Herniation

Pain. Backache may be the presenting feature, but the patient usually complains of pain in the distribution of the sciatic nerve. Bending and straining will increase the pain.

The lumbar curve is obliterated and the paravertebral muscles are in spasm.

Scoliosis. Some degree of scoliosis may occur, usually away from the side of the lesion, which relieves pressure on the nerve root.

Straight leg raising is decreased.

Sensory changes. These are usually found over the lateral aspect of the calf and heel.

Depressed tendon reflexes. The ankle jerk is diminished or lost if the first sacral nerve root is compressed. The knee jerk is diminished or lost if the fourth lumbar nerve root is compressed. These signs and symptoms are intermittent and will recur with any fresh trauma.

SYNDROME OF A DISC PROTRUSION BETWEEN THE FOURTH AND FIFTH LUMBAR VERTEBRAE

Pain, down the postero-lateral aspect of the thigh and lateral aspect of the leg, to the ankle.

Sensory changes, usually pins and needles, over the lateral aspect of the leg.

Motor weakness, involving extensor hallucis longus first, but may eventually involve all the other dorsiflexors.

SYNDROME OF A DISC PROTRUSION BETWEEN THE FIFTH
LUMBAR AND FIRST SACRAL VERTEBRAE

Pain, down the postero-lateral aspect of the thigh and lateral aspect of
the leg extending to the outer border of the foot.

Sensory changes, usually over the outer border of the foot and little
toe, which may extend over the foot and involve the other toes.

The ankle jerk is depressed.

Motor weakness, involving the plantar-flexors.

Conservative Treatment

The patient should rest in bed until the symptoms abate. He must lie
on a firm mattress or have fracture boards under the mattress to ensure
that his spine is adequately supported.

Continuous lumbar traction can be used to separate the vertebral
bodies in the hope that the nucleus pulposus will return to its normal
position.

A plaster jacket may be used.

Physiotherapy may be given.

Indications for Surgical Treatment

The relief of symptoms by surgical means becomes necessary when
conservative treatment no longer affords relief, when progressive
nerve root involvement appears, namely weakness and sensory loss,
and/or when there are signs of cauda equina compression and bladder
involvement. Emergency surgery is required in this instance to prevent irreparable damage to the spinal cord.

SPECIAL INVESTIGATIONS

Lumbar radiculography. This is now being used as a routine measure.
X-rays. These are always taken in order to exclude other pathology.

Surgical Treatment

This treatment is aimed at the removal of the protruding part of the
nucleus pulposus, or the ruptured part of the annulus fibrosus. The
method of approach depends on the site and size of the protrusion.

Several operative techniques can be used to remove a lumbar disc
herniation, all requiring a fairly long mid-line incision, to expose the
spinous processes and laminae. The following procedures can then be
carried out:

Fenestration. At the site of the disc protrusion the ligament is removed between the laminae, then a small portion of the lamina of the vertebrae above and below the protrusion is removed and the nerve root retracted. The exposed protrusion is then incised and as much as possible of the nucleus pulposus gouged out.

Laminectomy. This procedure is used when both sides of the disc space require exploration, usually in the case of a centrally protruded disc. The spinous process and both laminae are removed at the appropriate level and the disc protrusion dealt with as before.

POSTOPERATIVE TREATMENT

Nursing care is of paramount importance during the first few post-operative days. The patient is nursed in the side-lying position previously described and turned two-hourly, going from side to front to his other side, all pillows being removed to facilitate turning. By about the second postoperative day the patient will probably be able to turn unaided.

Physiotherapy

A wide variety of postoperative routines exists, each surgeon having his own ideas as to how the patient should be progressed. Each patient presents an individual problem and any routine must be adjusted to suit his capabilities. Early postoperative ambulation is being increasingly widely employed, ranging from the first to about the third postoperative day, and it is rare that a patient needs to be kept in bed for more than one week before ambulation begins. However, all ambulation is initially strictly limited, particularly with the patient who, now being pain-free, is so enthusiastic that he wants to be up and doing too much, too soon.

Some surgeons consider that formal exercises are unnecessary, as the natural use of the back and limbs is just as effective (Pennybacker, 1968). They also maintain that no formal exercise reduces the degree of over-reaction by the patient to his symptoms. Where exercises are given, the general principles which always apply are 1) limit all exercises to the pain-free range of movement, and 2) when giving mobilising exercises, never force a movement.

METHODS

Breathing exercises and coughing. The patient may require encouragement if his wound is painful. Firm pressure over the wound from the physiotherapist's hand and instructions to tighten his abdominal muscles as he coughs are helpful measures. Breathing exercises should be practised regularly.

Maintenance exercises confined to foot and knee movements are practised hourly by the patient. Hip movements in a small range of flexion and extension to mid-line can begin on the first day, together with static abdominal work. Abduction of the hip and increased range of flexion with extension beyond the mid-line and straight leg raising follow as progressions of hip movement.

Static contractions of back extensor muscles are usually commenced on the third day. At this stage the patient can begin lying on his back for short periods. Care must be taken with his posture so he is taught to appreciate when he is lying in a straight line. Active extension usually follows on the fourth day and the number of times the exercises are repeated and the strength of the exercises are gradually increased.

Any specific muscle weakness is re-educated by means of facilitation techniques.

The re-education of posture in lying is progressed to re-education of posture in standing. The surgeon decides when the patient should be allowed to get up, which will be between the first and fifth day. Before the patient gets up it is advisable to elevate the bed to allow him to adjust to a more upright position. It must be noted that the entire bed is elevated: the patient is not placed in a sitting position. The patient is taught to lie on his side at the edge of the bed, put his feet over the edge and sit up keeping his back straight. His posture is corrected as soon as he stands up and he is re-educated in walking when necessary. On returning to bed he sits on the edge of the bed and with his back straight lies down on his side, bringing his legs into bed as he does so. Some patients may find it easier to get out of bed from a prone lying position. To do this he moves himself into a diagonal position across the bed; when his feet touch the floor he then pushes himself into an upright position keeping his back straight. Getting into bed, he keeps his back straight and lowers the top of his body by bending from the hips, then lifts his legs into bed. The patient is encouraged to get up for short periods and walk about.

The following instructions should be given:

A hard upright chair must be used and he must keep his back straight when sitting down and standing up. The sitting position should only be used at mealtimes and for short periods as it is usually an uncomfortable one.

When picking objects up from the floor he should be taught to go down on one knee keeping his back straight.

No lifting should be attempted.

If his back becomes uncomfortable he should lie down and rest.

Mobilisation of the spine begins after the sutures are removed, usually the tenth day. Side flexion, rotation and forward flexion are all encouraged. Hydrotherapy is a useful means by which mobility can be encouraged.

When the patient is ready for discharge home he should be given a scheme of exercises to practise daily and instructed to continue these exercises for an indefinite period. The surgeon will decide when the patient is able to assume his normal activities and if any change of employment is necessary.

Cervical Disc Herniations

Herniation of the nucleus pulposus in the cervical region is less common than in the lumbar region. The usual sites of herniation are between the fifth and sixth, and sixth and seventh cervical vertebrae. This is probably due to the greater stress at these levels, as they lie at the point where the free mobility of the cervical spine is changing to the relative immobility of the thoracic spine. Herniation can occur spontaneously or as a result of trauma. The protrusion is usually in a postero-lateral direction, but a central herniation can occur giving symptoms of spinal cord compression.

Signs and Symptoms

Pain occurs in the neck on movement and may be severe. Referred pain in the distribution of the compressed nerve root is also present.

There is rigidity of the neck muscles.

The head may be slightly flexed to the side of the lesion.

Muscle wasting occurs in the motor distribution of the compressed nerve root, but severe loss of muscle power is not usual.

Sensory changes may occur over the appropriate dermatome.

Tendon reflexes innervated by the compressed nerve are diminished or lost.

CONSERVATIVE TREATMENT

Neck traction may be given to relieve pressure on the nerve root, and the neck immobilised by use of a collar.

SURGICAL TREATMENT

When conservative measures fail to relieve the symptoms, surgical intervention is indicated (p. 348).

Cervical Spondylosis

Degeneration of the intervertebral discs with the formation of osteophytes, especially at the intervertebral joints, are the pathological changes giving rise to cervical spondylosis. These intervertebral joints are the articulations between the bodies of the cervical vertebrae; they lie at the lateral margins of the intervertebral discs and are sometimes known as the joints of Lushka.

Individuals most affected are those in the middle and older age-groups. The most common site of the lesion is between the fifth and sixth and sixth and seventh vertebrae. Compression of the nerve roots can occur on one or both sides, at one or several levels.

The disease presents in two main patterns: cervical spondylosis with brachialgia, when the nerve roots are involved, and cervical myelopathy when there is spinal cord involvement.

Cervical Spondylosis with Brachialgia

The history of symptoms is very variable and onset of radicular symptoms may be acute, sub-acute or insidious. An acute onset of symptoms which involves one nerve root closely resembles an acute cervical disc herniation. An insidious onset is characterised by burning and tingling sensations down the arm.

SIGNS AND SYMPTOMS

A general picture of the signs and symptoms is as follows:

Burning and tingling sensations are often accompanied by pain radiating down the arm and into the fingers, the little and ring finger usually being involved. It has been suggested that the distribution of pain is widespread and conforms to the scleratomes (segmental distribution of muscles and bones) rather than to dermatomes, although there may be some dermatomal hyperaesthesiae. These symptoms tend to be worse at night.

The ability to appreciate light touch and pinprick is diminished in the dermatomes supplied by the compressed nerve roots.

There is localised tenderness of muscles supplied by the affected nerves.

Kinaesthetic sensation is impaired.

Slight muscle wasting and hypotonia are present in the muscles supplied by the compressed nerve roots.

Tendon reflexes are diminished or lost.

Neck movements are limited but relatively pain-free.

Local tenderness in the neck is elicited on pressure.

CONSERVATIVE TREATMENT

This is by immobilisation by use of a collar, and physiotherapy including traction, heat, massage and exercises.

Cervical Myelopathy

SIGNS AND SYMPTOMS

The patient usually presents with insidious onset of difficulty with walking and clumsiness and weakness of the hands. It is the picture of progressive spastic tetraparesis, with variable sensory loss, and which is difficult to diagnose unless the syndrome is well developed. Clinically it cannot be differentiated from the signs and symptoms of a spinal cord neoplasm, which have already been described, and similar special investigations would be done.

SURGICAL MANAGEMENT

This is designed to relieve nerve roots and spinal cord compression by the degenerated disc and osteophyte formation. The anterior approach is superseding the posterior approach but both will be mentioned.

If the lesion is lateral and the nerve root only is involved, a posterior approach with a hemilaminectomy is usually undertaken.

If myelopathy is present two alternative approaches are possible: a wide decompression of the spinal cord by means of a laminectomy, or an anterior cervical decompression and fusion which is discussed fully on p. 348.

POSTOPERATIVE TREATMENT FOLLOWING HEMILAMINECTOMY
OR LAMINECTOMY

The patient is nursed in side lying, until his neck wound becomes less tender and he can tolerate back lying.

Physiotherapy

FOLLOWING HEMILAMINECTOMY

If this involves one level only, the patient will be allowed to get up three or four days postoperatively, and usually the neck is immobilised in a collar, partly for protection and partly as a reminder to the nursing staff to be gentle with it. Static neck exercises, particularly for the neck extensor muscles, may begin about the same time. Active neck and shoulder girdle exercises follow when the sutures are removed on approximately the tenth day. Any specific muscle weakness is treated with appropriate strengthening exercises.

FOLLOWING LAMINECTOMY

If several laminae have been removed, the patient's treatment is more conservative. He generally remains in bed, nursed in a collar, for about one week. Static exercises can begin when the patient can tolerate them. The surgeon will decide how long the collar has to be worn, but usually once the sutures have been removed gentle neck and shoulder exercises may be performed without the collar. Particular attention must be paid to the patient's head and shoulder posture.

Anterior Cervical Decompression and Fusion

This operation has been found to be more effective than a laminectomy.

The anatomy of the cervical region is such that a posterior approach by means of a laminectomy requires retraction of the spinal cord in order to reach the disc protrusion and the osteophytes. Manipulation of the spinal cord may upset its blood supply with disastrous results. The posterior approach can also weaken the neck muscles and subluxation may occur as a postoperative complication.

The anterior approach is a much safer procedure. Discs and osteophytes can be completely excised and the spine fused to prevent further osteophyte formation. Indications for operation are:

1. Disease of the cervical discs when conservative measures have failed to relieve the symptoms.
2. Certain types of injury to the cervical spine due to hyperextension and hyperflexion of the neck.
3. Certain neoplasms and infective processes such as tuberculosis of the cervical spine.

Surgical Procedure

The patient lies supine with 25 pounds (11·3kg) head traction. An incision is made in a skin crease in the right carotid triangle, exposing the anterior aspect of the spinal column from the second cervical to the first thoracic vertebral body. At the appropriate level a hole, half an inch (13mm) in diameter is drilled through the disc and adjacent vertebral bodies until the posterior longitudinal ligament is reached. The debris of disc material and osteophytes is removed and a plug of bone, usually from the left iliac crest, inserted in the hole.

POSTOPERATIVE TREATMENT

The patient returns from theatre in a supine position with the head and neck positioned in a specially fashioned foam-rubber support (Fig. 16/9), which maintains the head in a mid-line position, allowing no lateral movement or rotation. A check X-ray is done early on the first day and if this is satisfactory the patient is then allowed to get up wearing a cervical collar.

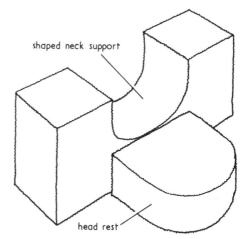

Fig. 16/9 A shaped foam neck and head support suitable for use after cervical surgery

Although the operation site is inherently stable a collar is usually worn as a protective measure and as a reminder to both the patient and the staff to be careful when moving. The collar is worn for variable lengths of time, depending on the opinion of the surgeon, the severity of the condition and on the number of bony segments fused. It may be worn for up to six weeks. A further X-ray is done before the decision is made to discard the collar altogether. A great advantage of this method of treatment is that it allows early ambulation and early return to normal duties.

Postoperative Physiotherapy

Breathing exercises and coughing. The patient practises his breathing exercises hourly. He may require particular encouragement to cough as the neck and throat are sore.

Maintenance exercises. Particular attention is given to the left lower limb, especially hip movements. The patient needs encouragement to begin hip movements and quadriceps contractions, as the hip area is stiff and painful following the removal of bone from the ilium. Gentle full range movements of the shoulder joints must be encouraged. Maintenance exercises must be practised hourly.

Re-education of any muscle weakness is carried out by means of facilitation techniques.

Walking re-education is often necessary, especially if the lower limbs were spastic due to spinal cord compression. Walking between parallel bars with the aid of a mirror helps the patient to appreciate where to place his feet. Later some type of walking aid may be necessary to make him independent.

CARE OF THE PATIENT'S NECK

The aims are to strengthen neck and shoulder muscles, and to regain mobility.

Methods. Static contractions of the neck and shoulder muscles are begun approximately on the third day with the patient in a supine position. When he is out of bed wearing a collar he is encouraged to practise these static contractions at regular intervals.

When the collar is removed between three to six weeks from the date of operation, active neck and shoulder exercises are given.

Lumbar Stenosis

Stenosis means 'narrowing' and lumbar stenosis is characterised by narrowing of the spinal canal, nerve root canal (or 'tunnel') and/or the intervertebral foramen. Occasionally a congenitally trefoil-shaped spinal canal contributes to the narrowing but the symptomatology is generally found in association with other degenerative changes. It is fairly common at the higher lumbar levels, unlike disc lesions. As well as nerve root entrapment in any of the structures, there is also pressure on the arteries, capillaries and veins in the same regions, and venous hypertension in the vertebrae.

The patient may complain of weakness and pain in a root distribution similar to that associated with disc disease, but may also have pain at rest which is probably a feature resulting from the vascular involvement. Spinal movements may be little affected, but pain is often bilateral and the straight leg raising test symmetrical. Long-standing cases at the highest lumbar levels may eventually result in spastic paraparesis if left untreated.

SURGICAL TREATMENT

For effective decompression, the spinous process has to be removed and a bilateral laminectomy performed. The articular processes are saved if possible. The intervertebral foramen may also be widened.

Physiotherapy

The patient is nursed on his side, turning regularly, via prone. Generally this activity requires some help for the first couple of days until the wound pain settles.

Special exercises in bed consist of active hip, knee and foot exercises, begun in side lying and progressing to supine and prone. Isometric abdominal and back extension exercises are necessary to ensure adequate muscular support. Re-education of any weak muscles begins immediately, and the patient is got up to walk as early as possible, usually about the fourth postoperative day. Help is required in the same way as after disc surgery. Posture and gait may need retraining, particularly where there has been long-standing pain, and an antalgic posture adopted.

As with all spinal surgery, the patient is urged to progress his activities slowly and gently, interspersing short exercise periods with frequent rests lying down, and occasional periods of sitting in a suitable chair. Sitting tolerance must be carefully increased to avoid back pain. Sutures are removed about the tenth day. Home exercises should be continued and the patient instructed in 'back-care' i.e. correct bending and lifting, sitting and sleeping positions.

INTRACTABLE PAIN

Intractable pain describes a chronic severe pain which persists after the primary lesion has been treated. Figure 15/18, p. 319, shows some of the pain pathways. This type of pain serves no useful purpose and the patient's suffering can be relieved only by constant narcotic therapy. This becomes progressively less effective and there is constant danger of addiction to the drugs used.

Pain cannot be measured and has different characteristics depending on its origin. Innumerable factors can influence it; among the most important are the patient's personality, intelligence and emotional maturity. A careful assessment is thus essential before surgical measures are undertaken to relieve pain. When surgery is used for this purpose it is an indication that no further treatment is possible for the original disease. Figure 16/10 shows some of the surgical procedures used in pain alleviation.

Lesions giving rise to intractable pain are largely carcinomas outside the central nervous system. Herpes zoster, operational scars, amputation stump neuromas, phantom limb pain, and some cord lesions are non-malignant causes.

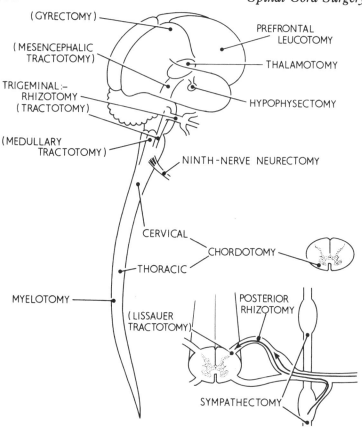

Fig. 16/10 Various surgical procedures designed to alleviate pain

Surgical Treatment

POSTERIOR RHIZOTOMY

The appropriate posterior spinal nerve roots are sectioned between the spinal cord and the posterior spinal ganglion, on the same side of the body as the intractable pain is appreciated. Due to the overlap of the sensory supply from one dermatome to another, it is necessary to section at least two sensory roots above and below the area in which pain is localised by the patient. This operation is carried out for post-herpetic pain and painful scars, but after a period of time the intractable pain tends to recur. It is of no use for limb pain, as it destroys muscle and joint sensation, which would give rise to a severe disability.

SPINOTHALAMIC CORDOTOMY

Fibres of the lateral spinothalamic tract are divided on the opposite side of the body to that on which the pain is appreciated. To achieve a permanent result this procedure must be done several segments higher than the localisation of pain, to allow for the fact that fibres carrying sensations of pain and temperature enter the spinal cord and ascend for several segments before crossing the mid-line to join the lateral spinothalamic tract, and that no matter how deep the incision made at operation, the level of sensory loss always descends during the first postoperative week.

The patient is so anaesthetised during this type of operation that he can be roused when the surgeon is ready to divide the lateral spinothalamic tract. The patient co-operates by telling the surgeon the level of his sensory loss and when an adequate level is reached he is re-anaesthetised and the operation completed.

Spinothalamic cordotomies are used to relieve pain from malignant disease, especially affecting the pelvic region. A bilateral cordotomy may be necessary for a patient who suffers from bilateral symptoms, but this procedure can produce motor weakness below the level of the surgical lesion. Bladder and bowel function are often permanently disturbed, accompanied by the loss of sexual function in the male. High cervical cordotomy may damage the respiratory pathway, innervating the diaphragm and intercostal muscles, producing an ipsilateral paralysis.

Physiotherapy

Following cordotomy in the thoracic region static contractions of the back extensor muscles can begin about the fifth postoperative day, and active extension exercises when sutures are removed, on approximately the tenth day.

Following a high cervical cordotomy, neck extensor muscles require retraining; static contractions can begin about the seventh postoperative day, and gentle neck mobilisation when sutures are removed, on approximately the tenth day. Chest care is most important if there is a diaphragmatic and intercostal muscle paralysis.

The patient should be allowed to get up between the seventh and tenth day if his general condition is satisfactory. It is important to teach him how to look after the area of pain and temperature loss. A patient with a unilateral loss should be reminded to use his normal side for testing the temperature of bath water. He must look after his affected side in the manner previously described for the paraplegic patient (p. 308).

Further Advances

Percutaneous cordotomy is gradually replacing open procedures, while stereotaxic cordotomy is now being developed to bring greater accuracy in lesion making. Obvious advantages of percutaneous procedures are that the patient only requires a local anaesthetic, there is no longer a painful wound and earlier mobilisation is therefore possible.

If for any reason a high cervical cordotomy is contra-indicated a stereotaxic lesion can be made in a portion of the thalamic nucleus, and is often successful in relieving pain. Certain patients whose pain may not have been adequately relieved by a surgical lesion at a lower level may derive greater benefit from thalamotomy.

REFERENCES

Bickerstaff, E. R. (1976). *Neurological Examination in Clinical Practice*. 3rd edition. Blackwell Scientific Publications.

Blackwood, W. and Corsellis, J. A. N. (Eds.) (1976). *Greenfield's Neuropathology*. 3rd edition. Edward Arnold.

Kellgren, J. H. (1939). 'On the distribution of pain arising from deep somatic structures with charts of segmental pain areas'. *Clinical Science*, **4**, 35.

de Palma, A. F. and Rothman, R. H. (1975). *The Intervertebral Disc*. W. B. Saunders Co.

Pennybacker, J. (1968). 'Lumbar disc protrusion'. *Hospital Medicine*, June, 1088–1095.

BIBLIOGRAPHY

This list comprises only a selection of further reading on this specialised subject of neurosurgery. It is compiled by both the author of Chapters 15 and 16 and the overall editor of the book.

Arnoldi, C. C. et al (1976). 'Lumbar spinal stenosis and nerve root entrapment syndrome. Definition and classification'. *Clinical Orthopaedics and Related Research*, **115**, March to April.

Bickerstaff, E. R. (1972). *Neurology for Nurses*. English Universities Press.

Bobath, B. (1978). *Adult Hemiplegia: Evaluation and Treatment*. 2nd edition. William Heinemann Medical Books Ltd.

Brain's Clinical Neurology. (Ed. Bannister, R.) (1978). 5th edition. Oxford University Press.

Brain's Diseases of the Nervous System. (Ed. Walton, J. N.) (1977). 8th edition. Oxford University Press.

Carr, J. and Shepherd, R. (1978). *Physiotherapy in Disorders of the Brain.* William Heinemann Medical Books Ltd.

Cash, J. E. (Ed.) (1977). *Neurology for Physiotherapists.* 2nd edition. Faber and Faber.

Chusid, J. G. (1976). *Correlative Neuroanatomy and Functional Neurology.* 16th edition. Lange Medical Publications.

Downie, P. A. (Ed.) (1979). *Cash's Textbook of Chest, Heart and Vascular Disorders for Physiotherapists.* 2nd edition. Faber and Faber.

Jennett, B. (1977). *An Introduction to Neurosurgery.* 3rd edition. William Heinemann Medical Books Ltd.

Lance, J. W. and McLeod, J. G. (1975). *A Physiological Approach to Clinical Neurology.* 2nd edition. Butterworths.

Matson, D. (1969). *Neurosurgery of Infancy and Childhood.* 2nd edition. Chapter 2: *'Diastematomyelia'.* Charles C. Thomas.

Naylor, A. (1977). 'Surgical treatment in lumbar disc protrusion'. *British Medical Journal*, **1**, 567.

Northfield, D. W. C. (1973). *The Surgery of the Central Nervous System – A Textbook for Post-graduate Students.* Blackwell Scientific Publications.

Purchese, G. (1977). *Neuromedical and Neurosurgical Nursing.* Baillière Tindall.

Walsh, K. W. (1978). *Neuropsychology – A Clinical Approach.* Churchill Livingstone.

van Zwanenberg, Dinah and Adams, C. B. T. (1979). *Neurosurgical Nursing Care.* Faber and Faber.

Glossary

SUFFIXES

-ectomy From a Greek word meaning 'a cutting out'. Removal of the whole or part of an organ

-gram From the Greek, *gramma*, meaning a mark. Usually used to describe the radiograph obtained following the outlining of organs or vessels by a radio-opaque substance

-ography The examination of a particular organ or system of the body, and the methods used to do so

-oscopy From the Greek word 'to look'. An inspection of a hollow organ or body cavity by means of instruments specially made for this purpose

-ostomy From the Latin, *ostium*, meaning a mouth. The formation of an artificial opening on to the surface of the body, e.g. colostomy

-otomy From the Greek word meaning 'incision'. A surgical incision

-plasty From the Greek word 'to mould'. A surgical procedure for repair of a defect and restoration of a part

resection From the Latin *re*, 'again' and *secare*, 'to cut'. It indicates the operation of cutting out e.g. rib resection

SURGICAL TERMS

ablation The removal of a part by surgery, drugs or radio-active means

amputation The surgical removal of part of the body, e.g. a limb, breast, penis

arthrodesis The surgical fixation of a joint

arthroplasty The making of an artificial joint by the surgical introduction of a suitable prosthesis; e.g. total hip arthroplasty where both the acetabulum and head of femur are replaced by metal or plastic prostheses

caecostomy An opening into the caecum through the abdominal wall for drainage; it is never permanent

cholecystogram The radiograph (X-ray) of the gall bladder obtained following the outlining of the gall bladder with a radio-opaque substance

colectomy The excision of part of the colon, e.g. hemicolectomy

colostomy The surgical formation of an artificial anus, either temporary or permanent, by making an opening into the colon, from the skin

gastrectomy The excision of the whole or part of the stomach

gastrostomy The establishment of an opening into the stomach from the skin, for the purpose of feeding

haematoma A collection of extravasated blood in the body causing swelling and bruising

ileostomy The surgical formation of a passage through the abdominal wall into the ileum; it is usually permanent and is performed in cases of ulcerative colitis

laparotomy An incision through the abdominal wall to allow an exploratory examination

laryngectomy The surgical removal of the larynx

lymphogram A radiograph of lymph vessels or nodes

lymphography The radiographic examination of lymph vessels or nodes which are rendered radio-opaque by the injection of dye

mammaplasty A plastic surgery procedure for the breasts; either augmentation or reduction

mastectomy The surgical removal of the breast

mediastinoscopy The examination of the mediastinum by the use of a mediastinoscope

pancreatectomy The excision of the pancreas

prosthesis The replacement for a limb or organ which has been either removed or is missing, e.g. an artificial limb, breast form or eye

pyloroplasty An operation to widen a contracted pylorus. The fibres of the pyloric canal are divided longitudinally and closed transversely

splenectomy The surgical removal of the spleen

thoracoscopy The examination of the pleural cavity by the use of a thorascope

tracheostomy The surgical formation of an opening into the windpipe (trachea) through the neck

tracheotomy The operation of incising the trachea

List of Useful Organisations

Cancer Information Association
2nd Floor, Marygold House
Carfax, Oxford

0865 46654

Colostomy Welfare Group
38/9 Eccleston Square (2nd Floor)
London SW1V 1PB

01–828 5175

Ileostomy Association of Great Britain and Ireland
First Floor, 23 Winchester Road
Basingstoke RG21 1UE

Basingstoke 21288

Marie Curie Memorial Foundation
124 Sloane Street
London SW1X 9BP

01–730 9157

Mastectomy Association of Great Britain
1 Colworth Road
Croydon CRO 7AD

National Association of Laryngectomee Clubs
38 Eccleston Square
London SW1V 1PB

01–834 2704

Women's National Cancer Control Campaign
1 South Audley Street
London W1Y 5DQ

01–499 7532

Index

abdominal lipectomy 130
abdominal pain due to nerve
    entrapment 70–1
accidents, causes of 257
Achilles tendon, rupture of 187–8
acoustic neurinoma 293
acromioclavicular lesions 165
adrenalectomy 38
amputations 133–60
    bilateral 152–4
    lower limb 134–57
        early ambulation 148
        physiotherapy 138–57
        prosthesis 149–52
    upper limb 157–60
        physiotherapy 157–8
        prosthesis 158
ankle, inversion injury 190–1
annulus fibrosus 197, 339–41
anterior cervical decompression
    fusion 348–50
    physiotherapy 349–50
A.O. technique 218, 221, 224
apronectomy 130
ataxia 283
atelectasis following surgery 47
athletic and sports injuries,
    physiotherapist's approach
    202–5
avascular necrosis of femoral head
    242–3

bandaging after amputation
    above-knee and through-knee
    145–6
    below-knee 146–7
Bartholin's abscess, incision 72
    cyst, excision 72
basal ganglia 278–9

bat (prominent) ears 130
Bell's palsy 95
below-knee amputation 137
Bennett's fracture 238–9
biceps tendon, rupture 186–7
bicipital tendonitis 164
bilateral amputee 152–4
bladder 64–7
    gold grains inserted 43
    nerve supply 67
    operations 42–3
bone flap 299
bone repair following fracture
    213–15, 221
Boutonnière deformity 122
brain
    anatomy and physiology 272–
    85
    blood supply 284, 285
    examinations and investigations
    285–91
    functional assessment by
    physiotherapist 287
    subdivisions 272
brainstem 277–8
Braun's splints 218, 223
breast surgery 38–40
Brown-Séquard syndrome 324–5
buried dermal flap 126
burns 209
bursae 180
bursitis 180–2
    subacromial 164, 181

caecostomy 36
calcaneum, fracture 250–1
callus formation 215
capsulitis, acute 164–5
carcinoma of larynx 100–1

cardiac arrest and resuscitation 46,
    57–61
carotid artery stenosis 307–9
catalogue
    dictionary 21
    library 20–1
    periodical 23–5
    subject 21–3
catarrhal endocervicitis chronic,
    treated by short wave
    diathermy 91
catheter 37
C.A.T. scan 288
causalgia, following fracture of
    wrist and hand 240
cerebello-pontine angle, tumours
    312–14
cerebellum 282–3
    tumours 310–11
cerebral angiography 289
cerebral lesions, signs and
    symptoms 291–4
cerebrospinal fluid 285
    in spinal cord compression
    330
cerebrum 273–6
cervical disc herniation 345
cervical lymph node, block
    dissection 93–4
cervical myelopathy 347
cervical spondylosis 346
    with brachialgia 346–7
cervix uteri, cautery 72
C.E.T. 156–7
Charles operation 127
chest injury 206–8
cholecystectomy 37
circle of Willis 285, 302,
    307
circuit training 204–5
clavicle, fracture 230–1
cleft lip and palate 117
Colles' fracture 238–41
colonic and rectal surgery,
    physiotherapy 40–1
colostomy 40–1
colpoperineorraphy 72
colporrhaphy, anterior 72
colpotomy 74

common carotid artery, ligation
    305–6
    physiotherapy after 306
common peroneal nerve damage
    246
complications of cranial surgery 300
    of surgery 45–56
compound fractures 128–9
compression plating of fracture 218,
    221, 224–5
computerised axial tomography 288
cone biopsy 71
consciousness, levels in cerebral
    lesions 293
    assessment of 294
contractures, prevention after
    amputation 140
contra-planar short wave diathermy
    89–90
controlled environment treatment
    (C.E.T.) 156–7
cosmetic surgery 129–30
coughing 31–3, 85
    effective 48–9
    following Pfannenstiel approach
    76
cranial nerves 281–2, 292, 293
cranial surgery 271–320
    complications 300–1
    physiotherapy 296
    postoperative treatment 298–9
cross-fire short wave diathermy
    89
cross-leg flaps 112–13
cruciate ligament damage 170–1,
    246
cystectomy 42–3
cystocele 80

deafness in cerebral lesions 293
deep breathing exercises 48
deep vein thrombosis 50–1
    physiotherapy 51, 75–6
De Quervain's disease 179–80
dermabrasion 129
dilatation and curettage (D & C) 71
diplopia 292
direct flaps 112
dislocations 195–7

double vision 292
drains, surgical 36
drop foot 250
Dupuytren's contracture 121
dysmetria 283

ear symptoms in cerebral lesions 293
echo-encephalography 288
ectopic pregnancy 69
elbow region, fractures 232–5
electro-corticography 290
electro-encephalography (E.E.G.) 290, 318
endarterectomy 308
epidural abscess 335
epilepsy 292, 317–18
Excerpta Medica 25
extensor pollicis longus, rupture of 240
extra-pyramidal system 278–9
eye symptoms in cerebral lesions 292

face lifting 129
facial fractures 115–17
   physiotherapy 116–17
facial palsy 94–8
   idiopathic 95
   nerve conductivity tests 96
   physiotherapy 96–8
   strength-duration curves 96
   surgical treatment 117
facilitation techniques for unconscious patient 302
Fajersztajn's sign 175
Fallopian tubes 63–4
   inflammation 69
   insufflation 72
   plastic operation 74
faradism, for pelvic floor conditions 87–8
femur fractures:
   shaft 240–3
   supracondylar 244–5
   upper end 240–3
fenestration 343
fibula fractures:
   malleolus 248–50

neck 248–50
   shaft 248–50
fibular collateral ligament damage 170
flail chest 207–8
foot amputations 138
forearm, fractures 234–7
fractures 210–55
   causes 210–12
   charts of common 228–55
   internal fixation 218–21
   march 212
   pathological 212
   physiotherapy 222–6
   repair 213–15
   signs and symptoms 212–13
   supports 216–21
   treatment, general principles 215–16
      lower limbs 216
      upper limbs 215–16
   see also individual bones and regions
free flaps 113
free skin grafts 109
frequency of micturition 83
frontal lobe 275
frozen shoulder 167–8
full thickness skin grafts 110
functional activities after amputation 143

gastrectomy 37
general surgical care, introduction to 29–44
gold grains insertion in bladder 43
graduated exercises 76
Gritti-Stokes amputation 136–7
group therapy in pelvic floor exercises 86
gynaecological conditions 62–92
   infra-radiation 77
   operations using vaginal route 71–2
   in outpatient department 78–83
   physiotherapy 75–7, 83–92
   short wave diathermy 77, 88–91

haematoma, in fracture repair 214
haemorrhage, postoperative 46, 54
hands, crush injuries 118
surgery 117–25
headache 291
head and neck surgery 93–107, 114–17
physiotherapy 114–15
head injury 208–9
hemilaminectomy, physiotherapy 347–8
hemi-mandibulectomy 99
hemiplegia 307–8
physiotherapy 308–9
herniae, repair 43–4
hindquarter amputation 135
hip and thigh, fracture 240–3
hip disarticulation 135
Homan's sign 50
humerus fractures:
great tuberosity 230–1
shaft 230–1
supracondylar 232–3
surgical neck 230–1
hyperkinesis 279
hypokinesis 279
hypophysectomy 98–9
physiotherapy 98–9
hypospadias 130–1
hypotonia 283
hysterectomy, total 73
vaginal 72
Wertheim's 73–4
hysterotomy 73

ileal conduit 42–3
ileostomy 41
incisions, surgical 35–6
for gynaecological diseases 72–5
incontinence, urinary 78–80
Index Medicus 24–5
infertility, treatment by short wave diathermy 91
infra-red radiation for gynaecological conditions 77
inter-lending library systems 26–7
internal fixation of fracture 218–21, 223–4

intervertebral disc lesions 197–201, 339–42, 345
treatment 200–1, 342–5
intra-aortic balloon counterpulsation 60–1
intracranial aneurysms 302–5
physiotherapy 304
intracranial angiomatous malformations 306–7
intracranial pressure 290–1
intracranial tumours 309–14
physiotherapy 310, 311–12, 314
intractable pain 318–19, 351–4

jaw surgery 99
osteotomies 117

knee, examination 168–72
fluid in 171–2
fractures in region 244–7
history 168–9
ligamentous damage 170–1
locking 168–9, 194
meniscus damage 171, 192–4
movement 169–70
provocative exercises 194
springing 171
knee joint level amputation 136

lacerations with skin necrosis 128
lamellar bone 215
laminectomy 200–1, 332–4, 343
physiotherapy 348
laparoscopy 75
laryngectomy 100–1
physiotherapy 101
larynx, carcinoma of 100–1
Lasègue's sign 174–5
ligament, damage 189–92
complete rupture 191–2
in knee 170–1
mild sprain 190
severe sprain 190–1
stretched 189–90
ligamentum patellae damage 171
Limb Fitting Centre 134–5, 149, 150, 151, 158

locking of knee 168–9, 193
low back, examination 172–6
  history 172
  movements 173–4
  muscle power 176
  nerve root lesions 175–6
  observation 172
  posture 173
  reflexes 176, 328
  sensory loss 176
low cardiac output 59–60
lumbar air encephalography 288–9
lumbar disc herniation 341–5
  physiotherapy 343–5
lumbar drainage 299–300
lumbar nerve root lesions 175–6
lumbar puncture 288, 330
lumbar radiculography 330, 342
lumbar stenosis 350–1
  physiotherapy 351
lymphoedema 39–40, 126–7

malignant melanoma 125–6
mallet finger 120–1
mammaplasty 130
mammary hyperplasia 130
mammary hypoplasia 130
mandible, fracture 115
march fracture 212
maxilla, fracture 115, 115–16
McMurray's test 171
medical libraries, use of 19–28
medulla oblongata 279–80
medullary nails 220–1, 224
Ménière's disease 101–3
  physiotherapy 103
meniscectomy 194
meniscus of knee, damage 171,
  192–4
menstrual cycle, variations 70
mental symptoms with cerebral
  lesions 292
metacarpals, fracture 238–41
metatarsals, fracture 250–1
midbrain 279–80
mid-thigh amputation 135–6
mobilisation, early 50
Monteggia's fracture 232–3, 235
multiple injuries 206–9

muscle atrophy and imbalance 46,
  54–6
  physiotherapy 56
muscles, contusions 184–5
  injuries 183–6
  rupture 185
  strain 183–4
myelography 330
myomectomy 74

nasal sinusitis 104–5
  physiotherapy 105
nasogastric tube 37
naso-pharyngeal suction 49
National Library of Medicine
  Classification 22–3
nephrectomy 41–2
nerve conductivity tests in facial
  palsy 96
nerve entrapment syndrome 70–1
nose, fracture 115, 116
nucleus pulposus 197, 339–41
nystagmus 285, 292

obesity 83, 85
occipital lobe 276
oedema in stump, control 143–8
oophorectomy 74
ovarian cystectomy 74
ovary, biopsy (wedge section) 74

painful arc syndrome 166–7
papilloedema 291
paralytic ileus 40
parietal lobe 276
parkinsonian syndrome 279, 314–
  17
  physiotherapy 316–17
patella, fracture 244–5, 247
  tap 171–2
pedicle flaps 111
pelvic exenteration 74
pelvic floor 67–8
  exercises 76–7
  restoration of function 83–8
  tilting 76
  weak muscles 78
pelvic inflammatory disease
  (P.I.D.) 69

Pelvic inflammatory disease – *cont.*
  treated by short wave diathermy
    91–2
pelvis, fractures 252–5
perineometer 85
periodicals 23–5
peritendonitis of tendo-calcaneus
    188–9
Pfannenstiel incision 72–3
  coughing following 76
phalanges of hand, fracture 238–9
physiotherapy, for or after:
  abdominal surgery 37
  adrenalectomy 38
  amputation, lower limb 138–57
    upper limb 157–8
  anterior cervical decompression
    and fusion 348–50
  athletic and sports injuries 202–5
  block dissection of cervical lymph
    glands 93–4
  breast surgery 38–40
  cerebellar tumours 311–12
  cerebello-pontine angle tumours
    314
  cleft lip and palate 117
  colonic and rectal surgery 40
  common carotid artery ligation
    305–6
  compound fractures 129
  cordotomy 353–4
  cranial surgery 296
  crush injuries of hand 118
  deep vein thrombosis 51, 75–6
  facial fractures 116–17
  facial palsy 96–8
  flap treatment of pressure sores
    125
  fractures 222–6, 228–55
  general surgery 31–4
  genito-urinary surgery 41–3
  gynaecological disease 75–7,
    83–92
  hemilaminectomy 347–8
  hemiplegia 308–9
  hernia repair 43–4
  hypophysectomy 98–9
  intervertebral disc lesions 200,
    342

intracranial aneurysms 304
intracranial tumours 310,
    311–12, 314
inversion injury of ankle 190–1
laminectomy 200–1, 348
laryngectomy 101
ligament injuries 190, 191, 192
lumbar disc herniation 343–5
lumbar stenosis 351
lymphoedema 39, 126–7
malignant melanoma 126
Ménière's disease 103
meniscectomy 194
meniscus damage 193–4
muscle atrophy and imbalance 56
muscle injuries 184, 184–5
nasal sinusitis 105
parkinsonian syndrome 316–17
pelvic inflammatory disease 69,
    91
peritendonitis 189
pollicisation 125
pre- and postoperative states
    48–50
pressure sores 53–4
spinal cord surgery 336–9
synovectomy 122
synovitis 177
  endon injuries and repairs 120,
    187, 188
trauma 256–70
upper abdominal surgery 30
wound infection 52
plaster casts 217–18
plastic surgery 108–32
plating of fracture 220
Pneumatic Post-Amputation
    Mobility Aid (PPAM AID)
    148, 157
pneumonia, aspiration 47–8
  postoperative 47
pollicisation 124–5
pons 279–80
port wine stains 130
posterior rhizotomy 352–3
postoperative pneumonia 47
postoperative pulmonary collapse 47
postoperative treatment in cranial
    surgery 298–9

Pott's disease 335–6
presacral neurectomy 75
pressure sores 52–4
  flap treatment 125
    physiotherapy 125
  physiotherapy 53–4
  postoperative 46
  prevention 53
  treatment 125
procallus 214
prostatectomy 42
prosthesis, immediate postoperative
    fitting 155–6
  after lower limb amputation
    149–52
  after upper limb amputation 158
provocative exercise 194
pulse and blood pressure in cerebral
    lesions 292
pylon 148, 149–54, 157

radio-isotope scanning 290
radius fractures:
  head 232–3
  lower end 238–41
  neck 232–3
  shaft 234–7
rectocele 80
references, distinguishing 25–6
  for publication 27–8
rehabilitation, advanced, following
    trauma 256–70
  debatable points 262–4
  do's and don'ts 265–70
  treatment required 259–60
rehabilitation centres 260–2
respiratory complications of surgery
    45, 46–50, 300–1
respiratory rate in cerebral lesions
    292
rheumatoid arthritis 121–2
rhinoplasty 129
ribs, fracture 206–8
rotator cuff injury 166–7, 167,
    181–2
Ryle's tube 37

salpingectomy 74
salpingo-oophorectomy 74

scaphoid, fracture 238–41
scapula, fracture, 230–1
scar revision 131–2
secretions, removal 49–50
Shirodkar suture 71
short wave diathermy, for
    gynaecological conditions 77,
    88–91
  contra-planar 89–90
  cross-fire 89
  for nasal sinusitis 105
shoulder
  acute inflammation 164
  examination 162–8
  fractures 230–1
  frozen 167–8
  history 162
  joint line palpation 164
  movement 165–6
  shrugging exercises 93–4
skin 108–9
  flaps and pedicles 110–13
  grafts 109–10
  ulcers 128
slings 217
Smith-Petersen pin 219, 224
Smith's fracture 238–41
soft tissues, injuries 161–201
spastic tetraparesis 347
speech disorders with cerebral
    lesions 293
spinal cord 321–2
  compression 322–35
  hemisection 324–5
  neoplasms 332–5
  surgery 321–55
    physiotherapy 336–9
spine, fractures of 254–5
  infections of 335–9
spinothalamic cordotomy 353–4
  physiotherapy 353–4
split skin grafts 110
springing of joint 165, 171
sprung back 192
stab wounds 209
Steinmann's pin 223
stereotaxy 315
sternoclavicular lesions 165
strapping 217

strength-duration curves in facial palsy 96
stress incontinence, operations 75
stump, above- and through-knee bandaging 145-6
  below-knee bandaging 146-7
  control of oedema 143-4
  strengthening 140
  upper limb 157-8
subacromial (subdeltoid) bursitis 164, 181
suction after cranial surgery 301
Sudek's atrophy 240-1
supraspinatus tendonitis 164
surgical drains 36
surgical incisions 35-6
surgical procedures 34-6
surgical tubes 37
swan neck deformity 122
Symes amputation 138
syndactyly 124
synovectomies, prophylactic 121-2
synovitis 176-8
  physiotherapy 178

team concept 29-30
temporal lobe 276, 293
tendo-calcaneus, rupture 187-8
  peritendonitis 188-9
tendon repairs 118-20
  rupture 186-8
tenosynovitis 179-80
thalamotomy 318-19
Thomas's splints 218, 223
Thompson operation 126
thyroidectomy 106-7
tibia fractures:
  malleolus 248-50
  plateau 244-6
  shaft 248-50
tibial collateral ligament damage 170
tracheostomy in cranial surgery 301-2
transposition flaps 111
trismus 116, 117

trunk, strengthening and mobilising after amputation 143
tuberculosis of spine 335-6

ulcers of skin 128
ulna fractures:
  olecranon 232-7
  shaft 232-7
ulna styloidectomy 124
ultrasound therapy 52, 184-5, 189, 190, 191
unaffected leg, strengthening and mobilising after amputation 140-1
universal decimal classification 22
upper abdominal surgery, physiotherapy 30
urethrocele 80
uterus 62-4
  prolapse 81

vagina, laxity 81
  discomfort treated by short wave diathermy 91
vaginal pressure gauge 85
venous thrombosis following surgery 45, 50-1
ventricular system of brain 285, 299
ventriculography 289
ventrosuspension 74
vertebrae, fractures 254-5
  neoplasms 334-5
vertigo 103, 293
vital capacity (V.C.), reducuon following surgery 47
vomiting, with cerebral lesions 292
vulvectomy 72

Wolfe grafts 110
wound infections 45, 51-2
woven bone 215
wrist and hand fractures 238-41

Z-plasty 131-2
zygoma, fracture 115, 116